Manual of
Clinical Paramedic
Procedures

PETE GREGORY AND IAN MURSELL

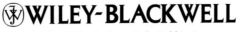

WILEY-BLACKWELL

A John Wiley & Sons, Ltd., Publication

This edition first published 2010
© 2010 by Pete Gregory and Ian Mursell

Blackwell Publishing was acquired by John Wiley & Sons in February 2007. Blackwell's publishing programme has been merged with Wiley's global Scientific, Technical, and Medical business to form Wiley-Blackwell.

Registered office
John Wiley & Sons Ltd, The Atrium, Southern Gate, Chichester, West Sussex, PO19 8SQ, United Kingdom

Editorial offices
9600 Garsington Road, Oxford, OX4 2DQ, United Kingdom
2121 State Avenue, Ames, Iowa 50014-8300, USA

For details of our global editorial offices, for customer services and for information about how to apply for permission to reuse the copyright material in this book please see our website at www.wiley.com/wiley-blackwell.

Library of Congress Cataloging-in-Publication Data

Gregory, Pete, BSc.
  Manual of clinical paramedic procedures / Pete Gregory and Ian Mursell.
    p. ; cm.
  Includes bibliographical references and index.
  ISBN 978-1-4051-6355-2 (pbk. : alk. paper)   1. Emergency medicine-Handbooks, manuals, etc.   2. Emergency medical technicians-Handbooks, manuals, etc.   I. Mursell, Ian.   II. Title.
  [DNLM: 1. Emergency Treatment-methods-Handbooks.   2. Emergency Medical Technicians-Handbooks. WB 39 G823m 2009]
  RC86.8.G743 2009
  616.02'5-dc22

                                                                                        2009005456

A catalogue record for this book is available from the British Library.

Set in 9 on 12 pt Interstate light by Toppan Best-set Premedia Limited
Printed and bound in Singapore by Fabulous Printers Pte Ltd

1   2010

Contents

Contents

Foreword

The *Manual of Clinical Paramedic Procedures* is unique in its extensive use of references to support the practical guidance that it offers. Evidence-based medicine is a core principle of practice in the modern UK National Health Service and in many other health providers throughout the world. Its application in pre-hospital care is, however, still under-developed, but this text goes a long way towards addressing this deficiency.

Both authors are experienced paramedics and educators, and draw on a considerable body of expertise to meet the needs of their readers. The appropriate audience for this book includes student paramedics, who will find this a rich source of material to support their studies, but also the broadest range of practitioners in pre-hospital care, resuscitation, and emergency medicine, including registered paramedics, doctors, nurses, resuscitation officers, and medical students.

Each chapter starts with a definition of the topic to be addressed. Where appropriate, the relevant anatomy and physiology are briefly but helpfully reviewed, followed by a detailed description of each clinical procedure. The use of copious colour pictures adds significantly to the utility of the clear, concise, and eminently readable text. Scenarios are used to establish the context of each chapter in true-to-life clinical settings, and break-out boxes prompt the reader to apply the principles described as they read through the material. Step-wise descriptions of each procedure are supported by detailed rationales for each sub-process and provide an important insight into the concepts behind each technique. Key points boxes emphasise particularly critical issues and summarise chapter contents, and each chapter ends with an extensive reference and further reading list. The use of this wide range of methods for presenting information means that this book will suit most readers, regardless of their preferred learning style, will aid retention, and prevent boredom.

I am naturally a lazy reader when studying, preferring to disappear into a good science fiction novel rather than a textbook. Yet I can enthusiastically recommend the *Manual of Clinical Paramedic Procedures* as the book that I wish had been available to me when I was studying to become a paramedic, and the one which I wish I had written myself! It should take pride of place on the bookshelf of any student or experienced practitioner of pre-hospital care – but should be re-read at regular intervals to support the highest standards of clinical practice that we all aspire to.

Malcolm Woollard, PA02584, MPH, MBA, MA(ED), DipIMC (RCSED), PGCE, RN, MCPara, NFESC, FASI, FHEA, FACAP

Professor in Pre-hospital and Emergency Care and Director, Pre-hospital,
Emergency & Cardiovascular Care Applied Research Group, Coventry University
Chair, College of Paramedics
Honorary Consultant Paramedic, West Midlands & South East Coast Ambulance
Service NHS Trusts
Professor in Pre-hospital Care, Charles Sturt University, NSW, Australia
Adjunct Senior Research Fellow, Monash University, Victoria , Australia

Introduction

Clinical skills are fundamental in the day-to-day work of prehospital care providers, yet it is difficult to find a text book that not only demonstrates a step-by-step approach to clinical skills, but also provides evidence to support the approaches being advocated. At a time where pre-hospital providers are becoming ever more high-profile and public expectations are increasing, it is essential that Paramedics, Emergency Medical Technicians (EMT), and those working in the voluntary services adopt practices that are supported by the evidence. There is currently a dearth of high-quality research in prehospital care to either support or refute many of the activities carried out by prehospital providers but there is often good evidence from other disciplines that can be extrapolated to fill the void.

The Manual of Clinical Paramedic Procedures serves to review the available literature surrounding the application of key skills in prehospital care, challenges some current practices, and offers recommendations based upon the findings. The clear diagrams, pictures and supporting evidence will provide a sound reference text for those at the beginning of their health care careers through to those who are already established as competent practitioners. It will also serve the many proactive members of the voluntary ambulance organisations looking to enhance the service that they provide to their communities.

For the qualified Paramedic, the manual provides the evidence to underpin their practice and offers a ready source of information that will prove invaluable when mentoring paramedic students. It will also add to the Paramedic's portfolio of continuing professional development by challenging current thinking and allowing the Paramedic to reflect upon how the evidence has influenced changes in their practice. Many of the clinical skills discussed within the book also fall within the remit of non-paramedic prehospital practitioners so there is plenty of value for the EMT, first responder and members of a voluntary care organisation. For the Paramedic student, the book is invaluable for learning clinical skills and has the advantage over other texts in that it clearly cites its references, which can easily be integrated into academic essays and reflections.

The application of clinical skills in emergency care is rarely straightforward, especially in the hostile prehospital environment. It is hoped that by using this manual as a basis for performing clinical skills, the practitioner will be better placed to make decisions and will have the underpinning knowledge to perform the skills safely and to greatest patient benefit.

Chapter 1

Airway management

Content

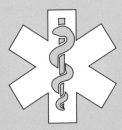

In emergency care, airway management is an essential first step as a means of achieving both oxygenation and ventilation. Failure to manage and maintain the airway can lead to neurological dysfunction and even death within minutes.[1] This chapter discusses the concept of a stepwise approach to airway management and provides the rationale for the airway interventions currently available to the paramedic.

Definition of airway management

Airway management may be defined as the provision of a free and clear passageway for airflow. Obstruction of the airway may be partial or complete and may occur at any level from the nose to the trachea. In the unconscious patient, the most common site of airway obstruction is at the level of the pharynx[2] and this obstruction has usually been attributed to posterior displacement of the tongue caused by reduced muscle tone. However, the cause of airway obstruction is often the soft palate and the epiglottis rather than the tongue.[3,4] Obstruction may also be caused by vomit or blood, swelling of the airway (e.g. anaphylaxis), a foreign body, or laryngeal spasm.

Concept of a stepwise approach

Airway management techniques range from basic manual manoeuvres to the more complex techniques of tracheal intubation and cricothyroidotomy. Each technique comes with its own inherent risks and it is essential that the paramedic is aware of the problems and limitations of each technique. It is advocated that a stepwise approach that leads from the least invasive to the most invasive technique be adopted.[1] The paramedic may choose to miss out certain steps based upon the needs of the patient, but a risk-benefit analysis should be undertaken to ensure that the most appropriate airway management technique is employed. It should be noted that measurement of airway adjuncts only provides a starting point for deciding on the appropriate size; it is essential to assess the effectiveness of any airway manoeuvre once undertaken.

Scenario

You are called to attend a 37-year-old female patient in cardiopulmonary arrest. On arrival you find that the patient is in the third trimester of pregnancy lying supine on the floor. What anatomical and physiological changes occur during pregnancy that may affect your airway management strategy? How would you manage the patient's airway?

Basic anatomy of the airway

See Figure 1.1.

Safe airway management requires sound knowledge of the relevant anatomy. This section provides an overview of the nose, pharynx, larynx, trachea and main bronchi; the practitioner is advised to refer to an appropriate anatomy text book for a deeper description of the airway.

Nose

The nose can be divided into external and internal portions. The external portion provides a supporting structure of bone and cartilage for the overlying muscle and skin; it is lined with a mucous membrane. The bony framework of the external nose is formed by the frontal bone, nasal bones and maxillae.

The internal portion lies inferior to the nasal bone and superior to the mouth and contains both muscle and a mucous membrane. It is worth remembering that the internal nares extend in an anterior-posterior direction, especially when inserting a nasopharyngeal airway.

Mouth

The mouth is not strictly a part of the airway, but as many airway management interventions involve the mouth, it is worth reviewing basic anatomy. The mouth is formed by the cheeks, hard and soft palates, and the tongue.[5] The lips surround the opening to the mouth and each lip is attached to its respective gum by the labial frenulum. The vestibule is the space between the cheeks or lips, and the teeth. The roof is formed by the hard and soft palates, whilst the tongue dominates the floor. The anterior portion of the tongue is free but connected to the underlying epithelium

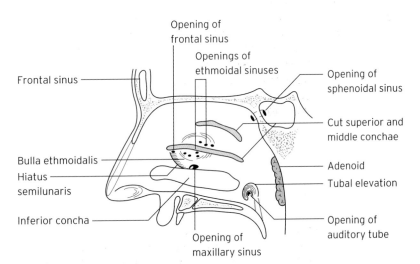

Figure 1.1 Lateral wall of nasal cavity. Reproduced from Faiz, O. and Moffat, D. *Anatomy at a Glance*, 2nd edn, copyright 2006, with permission of Blackwell Publishing.

by the lingual frenulum. The border between the mouth and the oropharynx extends from the dangling uvula to the base of the tongue.[6]

Pharynx

The pharynx is divided into three anatomical sections; the nasopharynx (extending from the internal nares to the posterior edge of the soft palate), the oropharynx (extending to the base of the tongue at the level of the hyoid bone) and the laryngopharynx (extending to the opening of the oesophagus).

Larynx

See Figures 1.2 and 1.3.

This is a very important structure in terms of airway management and it is essential to know the anatomy in depth. Basic anatomy is outlined here but it is recommended that revision should be undertaken with an appropriate anatomy text (see reference 5).

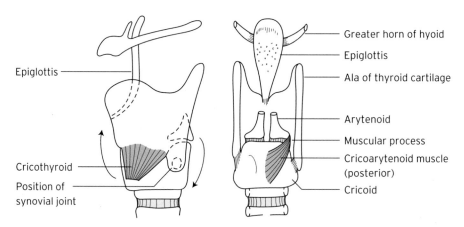

Figure 1.2 Cartilages of the larynx. Reproduced from Faiz, O. and Moffat, D. *Anatomy at a Glance*, 2nd edn, copyright 2006, with permission of Blackwell Publishing.

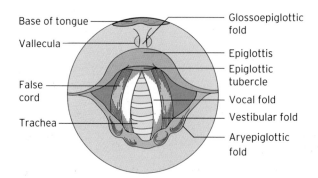

Figure 1.3 Larynx as viewed through a laryngoscope. Reproduced from Faiz, O. and Moffat, D. *Anatomy at a Glance*, 2nd edn, copyright 2006, with permission of Blackwell Publishing.

The larynx consists of nine cartilages; three paired and three single, as described below.

The epiglottis projects above the glottis and protects the larynx during swallowing. The thyroid cartilage forms most of the anterior and lateral surfaces of the larynx and tends to be more prominent in men. The cricoid cartilage is the ring-shaped cartilage that connects the larynx to the trachea. The three paired cartilages are found within the interior structure of the larynx and are the arytenoids, corniculate and cuneiform cartilages.

Trachea

See Figure 1.4.

The trachea is approximately 11–12 cm long and 2.5 cm in diameter. It is held open by 'C' shape cartilage, which is open posteriorly to allow for extension of the oesophagus during swallowing. The trachea bifurcates into the left and right main bronchi around the level of the 5th thoracic vertebra. The right main bronchus is

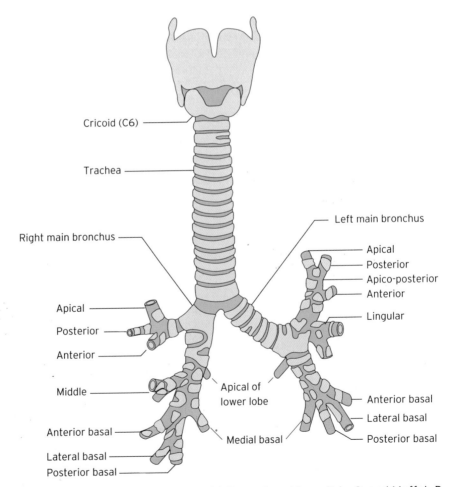

Figure 1.4 Trachea and main bronchi. Reproduced from Faiz, O. and Moffat, D., *Anatomy at a Glance* 2nd edn, copyright 2006, with permission of Blackwell Publishing.

larger in diameter than the left and extends at a steeper angle - an endotracheal tube that has been inserted too far is most likely to locate itself in the right side, as are foreign body obstructions.

Basic airway management manoeuvres

Head tilt and chin lift

This manoeuvre has been the mainstay of basic airway management for nearly 50 years with few changes advocated since the early 1960s. The rescuer's hand is placed on the patient's forehead and the head gently tilted back; the fingertips of the other hand are placed under the point of the patient's chin, which is gently lifted to stretch the anterior neck structures (Figure 1.5).

Jaw thrust

The jaw thrust is recommended where there is a risk of cervical spine injury but it may be used electively on any patient. Where there is no risk of spinal injury, the manoeuvre may be applied on its own or in conjunction with a head tilt manoeuvre.

The jaw thrust brings the mandible forwards and relieves obstruction by the soft palate and epiglottis. The practitioner places their index and other fingers behind the angle of the mandible and their thumbs on the mandible itself (Figure 1.6). The thumbs gently open the mouth whilst the fingers are used to apply pressure upwards and forwards. This movement causes the condyles of the mandible to sublux anteriorly in the temporomandibular joints. This displaces the mandible and tongue anteriorly, thereby clearing the airway.[7]

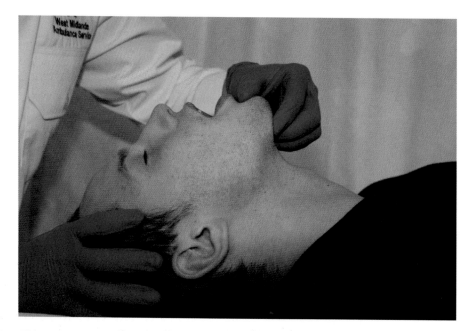

Figure 1.5 Head-tilt, chin-lift.

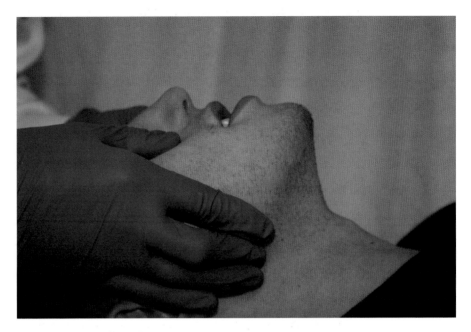

Figure 1.6 Jaw thrust.

THINK

Is there any circumstance where it would be permissible to perform a head tilt and chin lift manoeuvre in a patient with suspected cervical spine injury?

Basic airway adjuncts

Nasopharyngeal airway

See Figure 1.7.

The nasopharyngeal airway (NPA) is a simple airway adjunct that is used by a number of different healthcare disciplines. It has advantages over the oropharyngeal airway (OPA) in that it can be used in the presence of trismus, an intact gag reflex, or oral trauma.[8] Despite these advantages, the NPA is used less frequently than the OPA.[9,10]

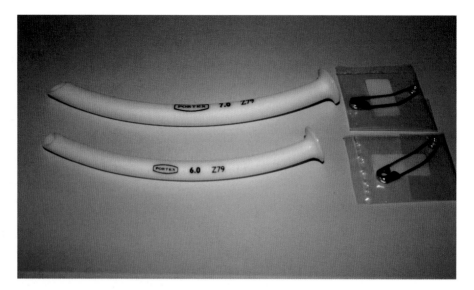

Figure 1.7 Nasopharyngeal airways.

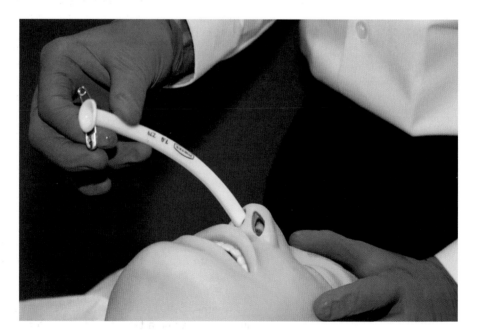

Figure 1.8 Bevel of NPA against the septum.

The NPA is designed to relieve soft tissue upper airway obstruction in a patient requiring airway support. The tube follows the natural curvature of the nasopharynx and extends to the posterior pharynx below the base of the tongue where it separates the soft palate from the pharynx. The distal end is bevelled to facilitate placing of the tube; the bevel should be placed against the nasal septum (Figure 1.8).

Sizing of an NPA

Traditional methods of sizing have tended to compare the NPA with the patients little finger or the size of their external nares; these methods are based on anecdote rather than evidence and are likely to be flawed. Both methods place emphasis on the diameter of the tube rather than the length despite an earlier study clearly showing that the length of the tube was more important than the diameter.[11] This study suggested that the tube should lie within 1cm of the epiglottis. If too short the airway would not separate the soft palate from the posterior wall of the pharynx and if too long would enter either the larynx and stimulate laryngeal reflexes, or enter the vallecula with the inherent risk of obstructing the airway.

One small study has shown that neither of the traditional methods for measuring the NPA correlated with the nasal anatomy of the subject, so are unreliable.[12] A clear correlation between patient height and their nares-epiglottis length has been demonstrated[11] so it is perhaps more sensible to base NPA size on the patient's height and sex. In the absence of a more accurate measurement, it is recommended that a size 6 (130mm length) be used for an average female and a size 7 (150mm length) for an average male.[8,12] Longer or shorter lengths may be considered for patients who are taller or shorter than average.

Once the initial choice has been made the NPA should be measured to ensure that only the correct length is inserted. A reasonable way of ascertaining this is to measure from the tip of the nose to the tragus of the ear. There is sufficient anatomical correlation for this to prove reliable although checks to ensure correct placement should be undertaken afterwards. When the length has been ascertained, the safety pin should be inserted into the proximal end of the NPA at the maximum point of insertion; this will prevent the NPA from being inserted too far into the pharynx and possibly into the oesophagus. For example, if a size 7 (150mm) had been selected and the measure from the tip of the nose to the tragus was 145mm, the pin should be placed 5mm distal to the flange of the NPA. The safety pin is not there to prevent loss of the NPA into the external nares. When inserting the safety pin, place to the side of the NPA to allow free passage for suction catheters if required.

Contraindications

A commonly taught contraindication to the use of an NPA is a potential or known basal skull fracture. Two published case reports of an NPA being inserted through a fractured cribriform plate into the cranial vault[13,14] may have been responsible for the development of this contraindication and it has been propagated by the Advanced Trauma Life Support Manual and courses. It is difficult to know whether these were isolated occurrences or whether further reports are less likely as it is no longer a novel complication, plus there may be a tendency to under report clinical errors.[15] The consensus appears to be that NPA placement may be necessary, even where relative contraindications exist, to avoid sub-standard airway management in patients with suspected or apparent base of skull fracture.

Complications

The most common complication is bleeding, which may cause serious airway obstruction if not managed. Blood tends to coagulate in the trachea and will form a solid occlusion to the passage of air. Patient positioning may help if bleeding does occur and suctioning will also be of benefit, although it is possible that suctioning may not be sufficient to maintain a clear airway.

If the bleeding is in the anterior portion of the nose, consider use of a tampon to stem the flow. If in the posterior portion of the nose, it may be necessary to insert a device such as a urinary catheter so that the balloon can be inflated to prevent aspiration of blood. Any practitioner who inserts an NPA must have a contingency plan for managing haemorrhage should it occur.

Necrosis of the anterior aspect of the nose may also occur if the diameter of the NPA is too large. If there is evidence of blanching around the external nares the NPA should be removed and a smaller one inserted. Necrosis will commence within about 20 minutes of the occlusion of blood supply and it is very difficult to cosmetically alter any damage.

Equipment required

- Range of nasopharyngeal airways
- Water-based lubricant
- Devices to arrest haemorrhage in both anterior and posterior portion of nose should it occur.

Technique for insertion

Procedure	Additional information/rationale
1. Select appropriate size, 7.0 as a starting point for an average adult male and 6.0 for an average adult female.	
2. Once the selection has been made, measure from the tip of the nose to the tragus of the ear. Insert safety pin to mark the maximum depth of insertion (this should be at the proximal end of the NPA).	If too short the airway would not separate the soft palate from the posterior wall of the pharynx; if too long may enter either the larynx or vallecula where the airway could become obstructed.
3. Where no risk of cervical spine injury exists, hyperextend the head and neck.	Stretches the anterior neck structures to relieve obstruction of the soft palate and epiglottis.
4. Lubricate the exterior of the tube with a water-soluble gel.	Minimises trauma during insertion.
5. If there is no obvious nasal deformity, it is recommended that the right nostril be used.[12]	The bevel of the NPA is designed to cause less trauma to the mucosa when inserted into the right nostril.
6. Where deformity exists, the most patent nostril should be selected.	

Procedure	Additional information/rationale
7. If inserting into the left nostril the bevel is placed alongside the septum and the airway rotated through 180° when it enters the nasopharynx.	To minimise trauma to the internal nares.
8. Insert the tube into the selected nostril and follow the nasal floor parallel to the mouth. It is imperative that the airway is not pushed in a cephalad direction.	This ensures correct location and reduces risk of cranial insertion where basal skull fracture exists.
9. Avoid pushing against any resistance. If resistance is felt, remove the airway, review technique and reinsert using the other nostril.	Pushing against resistance may cause bleeding and kinking of the NPA.
10. Verify appropriate position by listening for clear breath sounds and looking for chest rise and fall. Air may also be felt at the proximal end of the airway in the spontaneously breathing patient.	Ensures correct placement.
11. Check to make sure there is no blanching of the patient's nostrils. If there is, remove NPA and select a smaller diameter.	Prevents necrosis of the tissues.

Oropharyngeal airway

See Figure 1.9.

Oropharyngeal airways (OPA) are available in sizes suitable for neonate (00) to large adult (4). It is a curved plastic device designed to follow the curvature of the palate. It works to keep the tongue away from the posterior pharynx and to separate the soft palate from the pharyngeal wall. The OPA is designed to be used in unconscious patients requiring airway support and should only be inserted in those patients who have absent laryngeal and glossopharyngeal reflexes.[16] Use of an OPA in patients with these reflexes intact may cause vomiting or laryngospasm.

The oropharyngeal airway can become obstructed at three possible sites:[17] part of the tongue can occlude the end of the airway; the airway can lodge in the vallecula; and the airway can be obstructed by the epiglottis.

Sizing of an OPA

There is little evidence to support or contradict the traditional methods of sizing an OPA. Current teaching suggests that the length of the OPA should correspond with the vertical distance between the patient's incisors and the angle of the jaw (Figure 1.10).[16] This measurement is achieved by placing the flange of the OPA against the

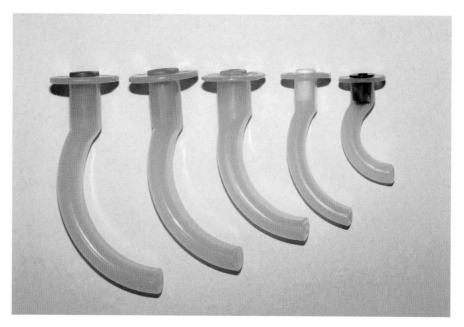

Figure 1.9 Oropharyngeal airways.

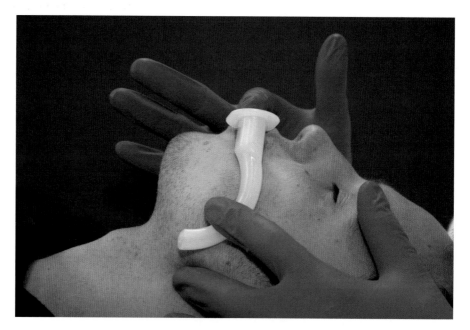

Figure 1.10 Measuring an OP airway.

patient's cheek, parallel to the front of the incisors and viewing the tip at the angle of the jaw.[18] If the airway is too long it may occlude the airway by locating within the vallecula and displacing the epiglottis; if too short it will not separate the soft palate or tongue from the posterior wall of the pharynx.

Contraindications

The OPA should not be used in any patient with an intact gag reflex.

Equipment required

Range of oropharyngeal airways.

Techniques for insertion

Procedure	Additional information/rationale
1. Select appropriate size.	If too short the airway would not separate the soft palate from the posterior wall of the pharynx; too long may displace the epiglottis.
2. Where no risk of cervical spine injury exists, hyperextend the head and neck. Grasp the patient's jaw and lift anteriorly.	Stretches the anterior neck structures to relieve obstruction of the soft palate and epiglottis.
3. Using other hand, hold the OPA at its proximal end and insert it into the patients mouth with the tip pointing towards the roof of the mouth.	Avoids unnecessary trauma to the delicate tissues in the mouth and inadvertent blocking of the airway by pushing the tongue back.
4. Once the tip reaches the level of the soft palate, gently rotate the airway 180° until it comes to rest over the tongue.	Brings the OPA into the alignment required for use.
5. The flattened, reinforced section of a correctly sized OPA should lie between the patient's teeth/dentures or gums. The lips should not be pulled over the flange of the OPA as this may cause damage to the labial frenulum.	Acts as a bite block.
6. Verify appropriate position by listening for clear breath sounds and looking for chest rise and fall.	Ensures correct placement.

See also Figures 1.11–1.14.

In small children the above technique should not be used due to the friable nature of the hard palate. Instead a tongue depressor should be employed and the OPA should be inserted 'right side up' with the tip pointing towards the tongue rather than the roof of the mouth.[19] This technique may also be utilised for adult patients where a tongue depressor is available.[18]

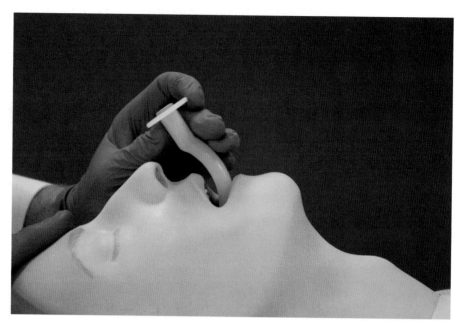

Figure 1.11 Insertion of an OPA.

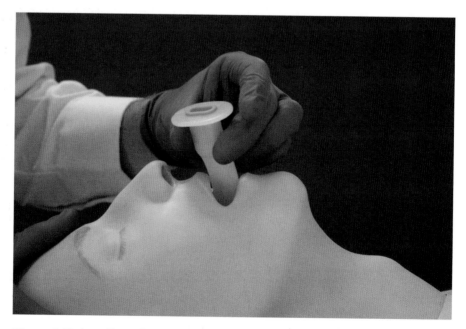

Figure 1.12 Insertion of an OPA.

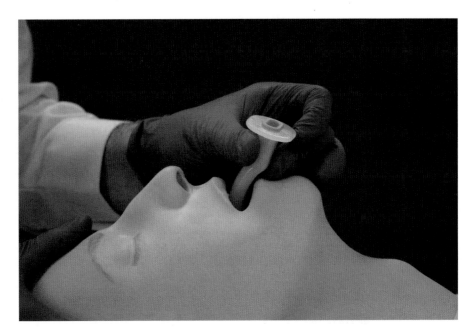

Figure 1.13 Insertion of an OPA.

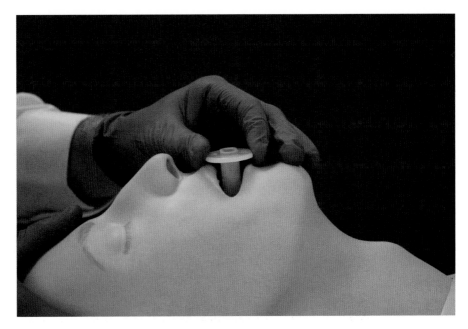

Figure 1.14 Insertion of an OPA.

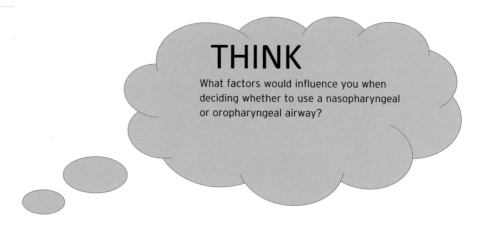

THINK

What factors would influence you when deciding whether to use a nasopharyngeal or oropharyngeal airway?

Advanced airway adjuncts and cricothyroidotomy

Laryngeal mask airway

See Figure 1.15.

The laryngeal mask airway (LMA) comprises a wide-bore tube with an elliptical inflatable cuff designed to seal around the laryngeal inlet.[16] The proximal end of the tube is fitted with a standard 15/22 mm connector. The LMA can be placed blind, requires less skill and is easier to insert than a tracheal tube.[20-26] The LMA provides for more efficient ventilation than with a bag-valve-mask (BVM) alone,[27] and when an LMA can be inserted without delay, it is recommended that bag-mask ventilation be avoided altogether.[16]

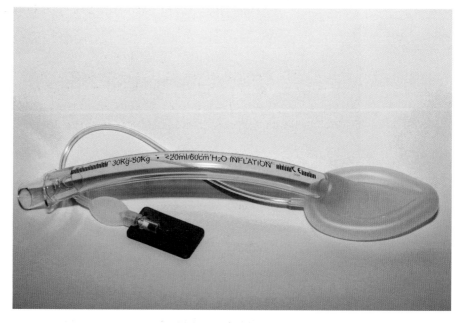

Figure 1.15 Laryngeal mask airway.

The LMA has been studied during cardiopulmonary resuscitation (CPR) but no studies have made a direct comparison with endotracheal intubation. The literature suggests that during CPR successful ventilation is achieved with an LMA in 72–98% of cases[28-34] and there is a reduction in the number of cases of regurgitation.[35] The perceived disadvantages of the LMA over endotracheal intubation surround the increased risk of aspiration and the inability to provide adequate ventilation for those with low lung or chest compliance.[16] There is currently no evidence demonstrating whether it is possible to perform continuous chest compressions with an LMA in situ; this may be one of the main benefits of endotracheal intubation.

A case series suggests that the LMA may have a use in the prehospital management of critically ill patients with inaccessible airways following trauma,[36] a contention supported by a manikin-based study comparing LMA with endotracheal intubation or Combitube in a simulation of restricted access to the patient's airway.[37] Times to ventilation with the LMA were much more rapid than with either of the other options but further research is required before a categorical recommendation can be made. Given the current level of evidence it is reasonable to suggest that where basic airway adjuncts do not provide the level of airway support required and endotracheal intubation is constrained by poor access to the patient's airway, the LMA should be considered as an alternative.

There are significant concerns regarding the intubation success of paramedics (mainly from literature in the USA [see later in this chapter]) and the LMA may be a reasonable alternative where endotracheal intubation has failed, or electively as part of a stepwise approach to airway management.

Sizing of a laryngeal mask airway

Sizing of the LMA is based upon the weight of the patient and this information can normally be found on the sterile packet and the LMA device itself. Table 1.1 gives typical ranges, but these values may change depending upon the brand of LMA used.

Contraindications

The LMA cannot be used in a patient with an intact gag reflex.

As the LMA is less effective at preventing aspiration, consideration needs to be given to alternative methods in patients at higher risk of regurgitation; for example, patients who are pregnant or who have a hiatus hernia.[38]

Table 1.1 Typical values for LMA

Size	Age/weight range	Maximum cuff inflation (mL air)
1	Neonates up to 5 kg	4
1.5	Children 5-10 kg	7
2	Children 10-20 kg	10
2.5	Children 20-30 kg	14
3	Children 30-50 kg	20
4	Small/normal adults	30
5	Normal/large adults	40

Equipment required

- LMA – range of sizes
- 50 mL syringe
- Tie
- Lubrication
- Stethoscope.

Procedure

Note: this describes the 'classic' technique; modified techniques exist for specific situations and LMA devices.

Procedure	Additional information/rationale
Check and prepare all equipment:	
1. Check the cuff by inflating it with 50% more air than is required.	
• Completely deflate the cuff, conforming it so that no folds appear near the tip; this may be achieved by pressing the device, cuff down, on a flat surface. Use the inside of the sterile LMA packet to minimise the risk of contamination.	Reduces the risk of inserting a device that will fail. To ensure that the cuff will inflate and seal correctly when in situ. Hygiene.
• Lubricate the base of the device with a water-soluble lubricant.	Minimise trauma during insertion.
2. The patient should be preoxygenated prior to insertion and ventilation should be interrupted for no more than 30 seconds to achieve correct placement. Before inserting the LMA, the patient's neck is flexed and the head extended ('sniffing position') by pushing the head from behind with the non-dominant hand.[39]	Preoxygenation replaces the primarily nitrogenous mixture of ambient air, which constitutes the patient's functional residual capacity, with oxygen, so increases the interval before desaturation in a patient who is hypoventilating or apnoeic.
3. Place the index finger of the dominant hand in the notch between the tube and the cuff	
4. Open the patient's mouth and slide the convex side of the airway against the roof of the patient's mouth.	Guides the LMA and avoids pushing the tongue backwards with the risk of airway obstruction.
5. Use your finger to push against the hard palate and advance past the tongue; once past the tongue, the LMA should advance easily. It is usually necessary to remove the dominant hand from the tube in order to facilitate final positioning of the LMA into the hypopharynx. Maintain a hold of the LMA with the sub-dominant hand whilst the dominant hand is withdrawn and then ease the LMA into its final position with the dominant hand.	

Procedure	Additional information/rationale
6. Inflate the cuff with the appropriate amount of air and, if properly positioned, the LMA should move out of the airway slightly (1-2 cm).	Inflation of the cuff forms a seal around the laryngeal inlet.
7. Following inflation, ventilate the patient and look for rise and fall of the chest. Auscultate the chest to confirm air entry.	Re-oxygenates the patient and ensures correct placement.
8. Secure the tube with an appropriate tie and consider using a rigid cervical collar to reduce flexion and extension of the head and neck.	The LMA was not designed to be used in patients who are being transported so careful attention must be paid to the airway during any patient manoeuvres.

Complications

Complications from LMA use can be categorised into mechanical, traumatic and pathophysiological.[40] Mechanical complications relate to the technical performance as an airway device and include failed insertion (0.3-4%), ineffective seal (<5%), and malposition (20-35%).[40] Traumatic complications relate to local tissue damage and include sore throat (10% with ranges between 0-70%), dysphagia (4-24%), and dysarthria (4-47%).[40] Pathophysiological complications relate to the LMA's effects on the body and include coughing (<2%), vomiting (0.02-5%) detectable regurgitation (0-80%), and clinical regurgitation (0.1%).[40]

There is little evidence available from prehospital studies so the figures presented above are derived largely from studies in the operating department. It has been stated that prehospital LMA success rates are lower than those seen in the hospital cardiac arrest or elective surgical patient but the data are old and may not reflect current trends.[41]

An incident of gastric rupture associated with paramedic use of the LMA during CPR has been reported although there appears to be only one published report of such an occurrence;[42] healthcare professionals should not discount the use of the LMA on the basis of one case report.

Endotracheal intubation

Endotracheal intubation (ETI) is considered to be the 'gold standard' of airway management[43] and involves the introduction of a cuff-sealed tube into the trachea. The cuffed tube seals the trachea up to peak pressures of approximately 50 mbar and prevents aspiration of solid or liquid foreign material.[44] Endotracheal intubation confers numerous advantages over the bag-valve-mask:[44]

- Secure ventilation with patient-adjusted airway pressures
- Optimum protection against aspiration
- Option of administering medication (e.g. epinephrine, lidocaine, atropine, naloxone)
- Bronchial suction.

The indications for prehospital ETI may be dependent upon the availability of sedatives or neuromuscular-blocking agents to facilitate endotracheal intubation; without pharmacological adjuncts, the practitioner may be unable to intubate unless the patient has a severely reduced level of consciousness.

There are numerous concerns surrounding out-of-hospital intubation by paramedics as studies evaluating either survival or neurological outcome following out-of-hospital ETI have failed to show any significant benefits.[45-59] It is acknowledged that there are weaknesses in many of these studies in that they were mainly retrospective analyses of trauma patients involving a single centre or countrywide trauma register. Studies tended to evaluate survival to discharge only rather than long-term follow-up, and often inferred neurological outcome based on discharge destination, e.g. to home, to rehabilitation centre; none used formal neurological scales to measure outcomes. Not all studies took into account the confounding factors that may have affected patient outcome, which is a major factor in retrospective studies, and some did not adjust outcomes for severity of injury or illness.

Although there are inherent weaknesses in the studies, it has to be recognised that multiple studies have arrived at similar conclusions.

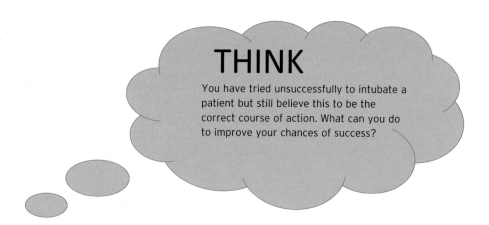

THINK

You have tried unsuccessfully to intubate a patient but still believe this to be the correct course of action. What can you do to improve your chances of success?

Equipment required

- Oxygen and ventilation equipment
- Laryngoscope handle and blades
- Endotracheal tube, bougie
- 10 mL syringe
- Water-soluble lubricant (see notes below)
- Magill forceps
- Tape, tie or commercial tube securing device
- Suction.

Preparation of equipment and discussion

- **Oxygen:** Ensure adequate supply of oxygen with which to ventilate the patient.

- **Endotracheal tube:** Select correct tube size. The size of the tube is printed on the sterile package as well as on the tube itself. Traditionally, the largest diameter was advocated to minimise resistance to airflow; 9 mm for an adult male, 8 mm for an adult female and 7 mm for an adolescent[60] (see Table 1.2 for paediatric sizes). Balance the desire for a large diameter with the risk of mucosal damage that may be caused by an oversized tube.[60]
  - Inflate the cuff with 10 mL of air and check there are no leaks.
  - Check to ensure that the connector is firmly attached to the proximal end of the tube.
  - There is debate as to whether tubes should be cut or uncut; cutting tubes to the appropriate length reduces the risk of right bronchial intubation and may reduce movement and rotation of the tube when connected to a ventilator.
- **Laryngoscope blades and handle:** It is best to have a selection of blades available as some patients may be easier to intubate with one rather than another. Check the integrity of the blade, and the brightness and tightness of the bulb. A straight[61] or McCoy blade[62] may improve the view at laryngoscopy; however, extra skill and training are required for these laryngoscopes to be effective. There is no evidence to suggest that it is appropriate to have either the straight or the McCoy blade available for paramedics.[63] A recent device, the Airtraq laryngoscope has proved successful in manikin trials,[64,65] and will be discussed later in this chapter.
- **Bougie:** Bougies are 60 cm long tracheal tube introducers with an external diameter of 5 mm to accommodate tracheal tubes >6 mm internal diameter. There is generally a 'coudé' tip, which comprises a 35 degree angle 2.5 cm from the distal end; this facilitates insertion of the bougie through the vocal cords when only the epiglottis (Grade III view) or tip of the arytenoids (Grade II view) can be visualised. The traditional technique has been for a 2nd operator to thread the tube over the bougie although there is sense in having the tube already positioned on the bougie in prehospital care given the emergency nature of the intubation.
  - A literature review recommended that the bougie should be available to paramedics as long ago as 2000[66] but it is likely that many paramedics do not have access to, or have not been trained in their use.[63] A shaped bougie has been shown to be better than a straight bougie,[67] and JRCALC are now advocating that a bougie be available for all prehospital intubation. Given that the practitioner should be aiming for a first time successful intubation, it is reasonable to assert that a bougie should be used for EVERY intubation rather than visualising first only to find a grade III view.
  - **Recommendation:** All ambulance paramedics should have access to and be trained in the use of bougies. Paramedics should routinely use a bougie for tracheal intubations to avoid delays created when a poor view is obtained through laryngoscopy.
- **Magill forceps:** Magill forceps are curved forceps that may be useful for removing obstructions under direct vision, or helping to guide the tip of the tube towards the trachea.
- **Lubricant:** Tubes for orotracheal intubation are usually lubricated prior to use as a matter of routine based on tradition. Searches have identified no literature to support the use of water-based lubricant to ease the passage of the tube and products such as KY Gel have been shown not to reduce the incidence of postoperative sore throat.[68] There has been a report of obstruction of a lubricated

tracheal tube with a flexible clear membrane said to be 'like a lump of glue'.[69] Analysis suggested that the most likely contaminant that caused the problem was a water-based lubricant.[70]

- It has been stated that lubricants may result in tube obstruction and interfere with inspection of the tube[70] and there appears to be nothing to be gained from lubricating oral tracheal tubes.[71]
- **Recommendation:** Routine lubrication of orotracheal tubes is to be discouraged until evidence shows that benefits outweigh the potential problems.

Table 1.2 Recommended tracheal tube sizes for children

Age	Diameter (mm)	Length (cm)
Birth	3	10
1 month	3	10
3 months	3.5	11
6 months	4	12
9 months	4	12
12 months	4.5	13
18 months	4.5	13
2 years	5	14
3 years	5	14
4 years	5	15
5 years	5.5	15
6 years	6	16
7 years	6	16
8 years	6.5	17
9 years	6.5	17
10 years	7	18
11 years	7	18

Reference: Joint Royal Colleges Ambulance Liaison Committee. *UK Ambulance Service Clinical Practice Guidelines*. London: JRCALC, 2006.

Confirming placement of the tube

There has been concern over the safety of endotracheal intubation by paramedics in the prehospital environment. At time of writing no studies have taken place in the UK to evaluate paramedic success rates although the College of Paramedics (CoP) Research and Audit Committee are looking to facilitate this study. Reports suggest that between 5.8% and 25% of endotracheal intubations carried out by paramedics are misplaced and unrecognised on arrival at the emergency department (ED).[72,73,74,75]

In a 2004 survey, 76% of UK ambulance services provided nothing more than a stethoscope to confirm tube placement.[63] A stethoscope on its own is unreliable to confirm correct placement as breath sounds have been shown to be present in 48% of oesophageal intubations.[76]

Additional measures for confirming tube placement

- **Oesophageal detector devices:** The oesophageal detector device (ODD) is a suction device fitted to an endotracheal tube (ETT) and depends on anatomical differences between the oesophagus and the trachea. When suction is applied with an oesophageal ETT placement, the oesophageal wall collapses and very little air can be suctioned. The person operating the device will notice a marked resistance. With correct ET tube placement, the rigidity of the tracheal cartilage prevents collapse so air can be suctioned and no resistance will be noticed.
  - Reports on the effectiveness of the ODD have varied. One report found that only 50% of oesophageal intubations were detected,[77] whilst two other studies found the ODD to have high sensitivity for oesophageal intubation but low specificity for tracheal intubation (meaning correctly placed tubes may have been removed)[78,79] A further study found the ODD to be more specific for tracheal intubation than end tidal CO_2 in the context of cardiac arrest although this study was undertaken in the ED rather than out of hospital.[80]
  - **Recommendation:** The ODD is useful as a further adjunct to confirm tube placement but it is neither sensitive enough nor specific enough to be used as the sole measure of correct placement.
- **Capnometry:** Capnometry measures the amount of CO_2 in a gas sample. Capnometers may use colorimetric or electronic technology. Colorimetric capnometers use a chemical reaction to detect the presence of CO_2 in exhaled gas. A filter containing metacresol purple is placed between the ETT and ventilation device and when CO_2 is greater than 2%, the filter turns yellow. This reaction is rapid and should occur with each breath.[38] Electronic capnometers detect and calculate the amount of CO_2 in each breath and provide real-time indication of the patient's CO_2 levels. It should be noted that capnometry is one of the minimum standards used by UK anaesthetists[81] and its use should be compulsory in pre-hospital care.
- **Condensation in the tube:** Teaching related to condensation in the tube is based on tradition rather than evidence. Only one study has been conducted to evaluate the value of misting in the tube and that was conducted on dogs so has limited applicability to humans. In this study, condensation appeared in 100% of tracheal intubations and 83% of oesophageal intubations.[82]
  - **Recommendation:** Evidence is limited but condensation in the tubing should not be relied upon as an indicator of tracheal tube placement.

Key Point

No single method of assessing tube placement is infallible so practitioners should use more than one methodology. Combined use of visualisation, ODD, capnography, auscultation, and patient condition should conspire to improve the recognition rate for misplaced intubations.

How many attempts?

- A large multi-centre prospective study looked at the number of attempts required by paramedics, out-of-hospital nurses and physicians to accomplish out-of-hospital ETI.[83] Cumulative success for the first three attempts was 69.9%, 84.9% and 89.9% respectively with an overall success rate of 91.8%. When considering the number of attempts, the practitioner needs to assess the time taken to undertake ETI. Rapid sequence induction has been shown to add 10.7 minutes to on scene times whilst standard ETI added a mean of 5.2 minutes.[84]
  - **Recommendation:** It would be reasonable to suggest a maximum of three attempts at ETI as the overall success rate does not increase with subsequent attempts but the increased time to secure an airway, the delay on scene and the emergency nature of the intubation suggest that fewer attempts should be made. Where an intubation fails, consider if another member of the team is better placed to successfully perform the task. It may be better to limit the number of intubation attempts on any patient to a maximum of two to minimise the risks to the patient.

Airway positioning and manipulation

- **Head position:** The 'sniffing' position has been widely accepted as the correct position for alignment of the airway.[85,86] In cases of Cormack and Lehane grade III view under direct laryngoscopy, elevation of the patient's head beyond the sniffing position and external laryngeal pressure may improve the view.[87] The utility of the 'sniffing' position for intubation outside the hospital environment has not been established.[88]
- **Cricoid pressure v Bimanual laryngoscopy v BURP:** Initially described by Sellick in 1961,[89] cricoid pressure is used during laryngoscopy to prevent regurgitation of stomach contents into the lungs by compressing the oesophagus. The value of this manoeuvre has been questioned in a study that found that the oesophagus was lateral to the larynx in >50% of study subjects and that cricoid pressure caused a small amount of airway compression in 81% of the subjects studied.[90] Cadaver studies have demonstrated the efficacy of cricoid pressure [91] and clinical studies showing that gastric insufflation with air during mask ventilation is reduced when cricoid pressure is applied.[92]

Studies have demonstrated that the quality of laryngeal view is likely to be worsened by cricoid pressure.[93,94]

Bimanual laryngoscopy – the manipulation of the larynx by the free hand of the intubationist – has been shown to improve the laryngeal view compared with cricoid pressure and backwards, upwards, right pressure (BURP) on the thyroid cartilage, or no manipulation.[95]

- **Recommendations:** The sniffing position is important in prehospital intubation but where a grade III view exists, the practitioner should consider asking an assistant to elevate the head beyond the sniffing position and applying external laryngeal pressure. Cricoid pressure should not be used to improve the view during laryngoscopy but may be useful when ventilating with a bag-valve-mask. Bimanual laryngoscopy should be taught and practitioners should use this technique in preference to cricoid pressure or BURP of the thyroid cartilage.

Preoxygenation

Preoxygenation replaces the primarily nitrogenous mixture of ambient air, which constitutes the patient's functional residual capacity, with oxygen, so increasing the interval before desaturation in a patient who is hypoventilating or apnoeic. The effectiveness of preoxygenation has been found to be limited in those with significant cardiopulmonary pathology such as congestive heart failure and respiratory failure complicated by excessive secretions,[96] and it is likely that patients who will be intubated in the prehospital environment will be physiologically compromised. Preoxygenation may be difficult to achieve but effort should be expended to ensure that the patient is well oxygenated before intubation attempts take place. There is no categorical evidence as to how much preoxygenation is required but it is likely to be more than the 4-8 vital capacity breaths used in elective preoxygenation.[97] It is suggested that SpO_2 levels should be 100% for two minutes prior to intubation and should not be allowed to fall below 96%[38] although SpO_2 readings will not be available in a cardiac arrest situation.

Procedure

Procedure	Additional information/rationale
1. Check, prepare and assemble equipment.	
• Ask colleague to preoxygenate patient whilst equipment is being prepared	Increases interval before desaturation during intubation attempt
• Remove the patient's upper and lower dentures, if present, immediately before laryngoscopy.	Provides greater aperture for inserting laryngoscope and tubes.
• Position patient in the 'sniffing' position.	Aligns the axes of the airway
2. Holding the laryngoscope in the left hand, insert blade in right hand side of mouth and displace tongue to the left. Move the blade towards the midline and advance until the distal end is located in the vallecula; lift the laryngoscope handle slightly upward and towards the feet without levering back on the teeth or gums. At this point check the position of the blade – it may need to be adjusted to visualise the cords.	A curved blade should be placed in the vallecula, a straight blade is normally used to lift the epiglottis directly.
3. Visualise the larynx and insert the ETT under direct vision. Consider use of bimanual laryngoscopy and/or repositioning of the patient's head if the view is sub-optimal.	
4. Use a bougie to aid tracheal placement.	
5. The black mark on the distal end of the tube should pass just beyond the vocal cords.	Reduces the risk of intubation of the right main bronchus and prevents inflation of the cuff between the vocal cords.

Procedure	Additional information/rationale
6. Inflate the cuff with just enough air to stop the leaking sound around the tube. In a correctly sized tube this should require only 4-6 mL[38]. Ventilate the patient using BVV or mechanical ventilator.	Forms a seal to prevent aspiration.
7. Check tube placement by listening across the stomach and then across the lungs for bilateral breath sounds. Use ODD, and capnometry as per local guidelines. When in doubt, remove the tube and re-ventilate.	Ensures correct placement of endotracheal tube.
8. Insert OP airway.	Acts as a bite block.
9. Secure tube with commercially produced device, tape or bandage.	Helps to maintain correct tube positioning during patient movement.
10. Consider applying cervical collar.	Minimises tube movement during transportation of the patient.
11. Recheck tube placement periodically, especially after patient movement.	Ensure that the tube is still correctly located.

Airtraq®

The Airtraq is an anatomically shaped laryngoscope with two separate channels: An enclosed channel that contains a high definition optical system, and a guiding channel that holds the endotracheal tube (ETT) and guides it through the vocal cords. It is a single-use device that can be used with any standard endotracheal tube. Recent studies have shown that the device improves the view, reduces time for tracheal tube placement, and appears to be easier for less experienced intubationists to acquire the skills of intubation.[98-100] At time of writing the device is not available for use by UK paramedics, but it is felt that this is such an important breakthrough that its inclusion is warranted.

Procedure

Procedure	Additional information/rationale
Preparation	
1. Check, prepare and assemble equipment.	
2. Ask colleague to preoxygenate patient whilst equipment is being prepared.	Increases interval before desaturation during intubation attempt.
3. Remove the patient's upper and lower dentures, if present, immediately before laryngoscopy.	Provides greater aperture for inserting Airtraq and tubes.

Procedure	Additional information/rationale
4. Use of the 'sniffing the morning air' position is less important with the Airtraq but the patient's head should not be hyperextended on the neck.	
5. Select the ETT size and the corresponding Airtraq.	
6. Turn the light ON. Wait until the light stops blinking if the patient is breathing spontaneously.	When the light stops blinking, the lens is heated to prevent misting. This is only necessary in a breathing patient.
7. Lubricate the ETT and place it into the Airtraq's guiding channel.	Facilitates easy passage of tube through Airtraq device.

Airtraq placement

1. Insert the Airtraq into the midline of the patient's mouth.	
2. Slide the Airtraq through the oropharynx and larynx, keeping it in the midline.	
3. Look through the eyepiece to view the airway and to identify structures.	
4. Place the tip of the Airtraq at the vallecula. Gently lift up the Airtraq to expose the vocal cords.	
5. Alternatively the tip can be placed under the epiglottis (Miller style).	

ETT insertion

1. Align the centre of the visual field by gently moving the tip of the Airtraq.	
2. Advance the ETT by gently pushing it down the guiding channel until you see the ETT passing through the vocal cords.	
3. If the ETT won't advance, slowly repeat the BACK & UP manoeuvre until vocal cords are centred in the view field: BACK: Rotate the Airtraq back, taking it away from the glottis. UP: Gently pull the Airtraq Up.	Should help to align the tip of the ETT with the opening of the glottis.

Procedure	Additional information/rationale
Verification, Airtraq removal and disposal	
1. Verify ETT placement and insertion length as previously described. Inflate the ETT cuff, connect the ETT to the breathing circuit and verify placement and seal.	
2. Separate the ETT from the Airtraq by pulling it laterally and then rotate the Airtraq backwards. Make sure to hold the ETT.	
3. Insert OP airway.	Acts as a bite block.
4. Secure tube with commercially produced device, tape or bandage.	Helps to maintain correct tube positioning during patient movement.
5. Consider applying cervical collar.	Minimises tube movement during transportation of the patient.
6. Recheck tube placement periodically, especially after patient movement.	Ensure that the tube is still correctly located.

Needle cricothyroidotomy

Needle cricothyroidotomy is a technique used as a temporary life-saving procedure when it is determined that the airway and ventilation cannot be maintained in any other way[101]. It represents the final step in the Difficult Airway Society's guidelines for managing the 'can't intubate, can't ventilate' emergency.[102] Needle cricothyroid-otomy involves the insertion of a 14/16 gauge cannula into the trachea via the crico-thyroid membrane with ventilation achieved via a low-pressure oxygen set-up or, less commonly, jet ventilator. Needle cricothyroidotomy is inferior to the surgical procedure due to the limited airflow afforded by the narrow lumen but has been shown to be the technique of choice in the prehospital and emergency depart-ment.[103-108] The use of a low-pressure oxygen delivery system is ineffective and all ambulance services should be provided with high-pressure jet ventilation systems.[101] Needle cricothyroidotomy should be considered as an emergency procedure to be used for no longer than 15-45 minutes until a more definitive airway can be secured.[109]

Indications for use

Can't intubate; can't ventilate emergencies.

Complications

* The technique provides high flow of oxygen to the lungs but does not allow for proper ventilation. CO_2 levels will rise quickly so transportation should be expedited rapidly in order to secure a definitive airway.

- Bleeding may occur at the wound site although this is rare.
- Subcutaneous emphysema through incorrect catheter placement and excessive air leakage around the insertion site.
- Risk of barotrauma or pneumothorax when using jet ventilation – this can be minimised by opening the release valve only long enough to ensure adequate rise of the chest.

Equipment required

- 14/16 gauge catheter-over-needle cannula with 10 mL syringe attached
- Alcohol swab
- Oxygen tubing with 3-way tap
- Oxygen cylinder and flow-meter
- Tape.

Procedure

Procedure	Additional information/rationale
1. Check, prepare and assemble equipment.	Remove the blood reservoir from the rear of the cannula and attach the 10 mL syringe.
2. Maintain attempts at oxygenating the patient and clearing obstruction whilst preparing equipment.	May prevent the need for the procedure if the airway can be cleared by other means.
3. Identify the cricothyroid membrane in the midline between the thyroid cartilage and cricoid cartilage.	Locates the correct point of insertion.
4. Swab the site and then insert tip of cannula through the membrane angled at 45° towards the feet; aspirate on the syringe as the needle is inserted.	Tracheal entry can be confirmed when air freely enters the syringe.
5. Railroad the cannula over the needle into the trachea and secure with tape.	
6. Connect one end of oxygen tubing to the catheter and the other end to the jet ventilator.	This can be achieved by connecting the oxygen supply via a Y-connector – give 15 L/min for an adult.
7. Open the release valve on the jet ventilator and adjust the pressure to provide adequate chest rise.	
8. Auscultate over both apices and lung bases, and over the epigastrium.	To confirm placement.

Chapter Key Points

1. Airway management is a key feature of prehospital care.
2. It is essential to understand the anatomy of the airway in order to perform airway management knowledgably.
3. Airway management techniques should be used in a step-wise approach.
4. The practitioner needs to be able to justify airway management decisions.
5. Each airway technique has its own inherent problems; the practitioner should be aware of the problems and limitations associated with each technique and have tools to remedy them.

References and Further reading

1 Gregory P, Ward A. *Sander's Paramedic Textbook*. London: Elsevier, 2009.
2 Baskett TF. Arthur Guedel and the oropharyngeal airway. *Resuscitation* 2004;63:3–5.
3 Boidin MP. Airway patency in the unconscious patient. *Br J Anaesth* 1985;57:306–310.
4 Nandi PR, Charlesworth CH, Taylor SJ, Nunn JF, Dore CJ. Effect of general anaesthesia on the pharynx. *Br J Anaesth* 1991;66:157–162.
5 Tortora GJ, Derrikson B. *Principles of Anatomy and Physiology*, 11th edn. New York: Wiley, 2006.
6 Martini FH, Bartholemew EF. *Essentials of Anatomy and Physiology*, 4th edn. San Francisco: Pearson, 2007.
7 Tong JL, Ashworth DR, Smith JE. Cardiovascular responses following laryngoscope assisted, fibreoptic orotracheal intubation. *Anaesthesia* 2005;60:754–758.
8 Roberts K, Whalley H, Bleetman A. The nasopharyngeal airway: dispelling myths and establishing the facts. *Emerg Med J* 2005;22:394–396.
9 Roberts K, Allison KP, Porter KM. A review of emergency equipment carried and procedures performed by UK front line paramedics. *Resuscitation* 2003; 58(2):153–158.
10 Allison K, Porter K. Nasopharyngeal airways: an under-utilised pre-hospital resource. *Pre-Hosp Immediate Care* 2000;4(4):192–193.
11 Stoneham MD. The nasopharyngeal airway. *Anaesthesia* 1993;48:575–580.
12 Roberts K, Porter K. How do you size a nasopharyngeal airway. *Resuscitation* 2003;56:19–23.
13 Muzzi DA, Losasso TJ, Cucchiara RF. Complication from a nasopharyngeal airway in a patient with a basilar skull fracture. *Anesthesiology* 1991;74:366–368.
14 Schade K, Borzotta A, Michaels A. Intracranial malposition of nasopharyngeal airway. *J Trauma* 2000;49:967–968.
15 Ellis DY, Lambert C, Shirley P. Letters – Intracranial placement of nasopharyngeal airways: is it all that rare? *Emerg Med J* 2006;23:661.
16 Nolan JP, Deakin CD, Soar J, Böttiger BW, Smith G. European Resuscitation Council Guidelines for Resuscitation 2005 Section 4. Adult advanced life support. *Resuscitation* 2005;67S1, S39–S86.
17 Marsh AM, Nunn JF, Taylor SJ, Charlesworth CH. Airway obstruction associated with the use of the Guedel airway. *Br J Anaesth* 1991;67:517–523.
18 Bledsoe BE, Porter RS, Cherry RA. *Essentials of Paramedic Care*. New York: Prentice Hall, 2005.

19 Jevon P. *Paediatric Advanced Life Support*. London: Butterworth-Heinemann, 2003.

20 Davies PR, Tighe SQ, Greenslade GL, Evans GH. Laryngeal mask airway and tracheal tube insertion by unskilled personnel. *Lancet* 1990;336:977-979.

21 Flaishon R, Sotman A, Ben-Abraham R, Rudick V, Varssano D, Weinbroum AA. Antichemical protective gear prolongs time to successful airway management: a randomized, crossover study in humans. *Anesthesiology* 2004;100:260-296.

22 Ho BY, Skinner HJ, Mahajan RP. Gastro-oesophageal reflux during day case gynaecological laparoscopy under positive pressure ventilation: laryngeal mask vs. tracheal intubation. *Anaesthesia* 1998;53:921-924.

23 Reinhart DJ, Simmons G. Comparison of placement of the laryngeal mask airway with endotracheal tube by paramedics and respiratory therapists. *Ann Emerg Med* 1994;24: 260-263.

24 Rewari W, Kaul HL. Regurgitation and aspiration during gynaecological laparoscopy: comparison between laryngeal mask airway and tracheal intubation. *J Anaesth Clin Pharmacol* 1999;15:67-70.

25 Pennant JH, Walker MB. Comparison of the endotracheal tube and laryngeal mask in airway management by paramedical personnel. *Anesth Analg* 1992;74:531-534.

26 Maltby JR, Beriault MT, Watson NC, Liepert DJ, Fick GH. LMA-Classic and LMA-ProSeal are effective alternatives to endotracheal intubation for gynecologic laparoscopy. *Can J Anaesth* 2003;50:71-77.

27 Alexander R, Hodgson P, Lomax D, Bullen C. A comparison of the laryngeal mask airway and Guedel airway, bag and face mask for manual ventilation following formal training. *Anaesthesia* 1993;48:231-234.

28 Rumball CJ, MacDonald D, The PTL. Combitube, laryngeal mask, and oral airway: a randomized prehospital comparative study of ventilatory device effectiveness and cost effectiveness in 470 cases of cardiorespiratory arrest. *Prehosp Emerg Care* 1997;1:1-10.

29 Verghese C, Prior-Willeard PF, Baskett PJ. Immediate management of the airway during cardiopulmonary resuscitation in a hospital without a resident anaesthesiologist. *Eur J Emerg Med* 1994;1:123-125.

30 Tanigawa K, Shigematsu A. Choice of airway devices for 12,020 cases of nontraumatic cardiac arrest in Japan. *Prehosp Emerg Care* 1998;2:96-100.

31 The use of the laryngeal mask airway by nurses during cardiopulmonary resuscitation: results of a multicentre trial. *Anaesthesia* 1994;49:3-7.

32 Grantham H, Phillips G, Gilligan JE. The laryngeal mask in prehospital emergency care. *Emerg Med* 1994;6:193-197.

33 Kokkinis K. The use of the laryngeal mask airway in CPR. *Resuscitation* 1994;27:9-12.

34 Leach A, Alexander CA, Stone B. The laryngeal mask in cardiopulmonary resuscitation in a district general hospital: a preliminary communication. *Resuscitation* 1993;25:245-248.

35 Stone BJ, Chantler PJ, Baskett PJ. The incidence of regurgitation during cardiopulmonary resuscitation: a comparison between the bag valve mask and laryngeal mask airway. *Resuscitation* 1998;38:3-6.

36 Hulme J, Perkins GD. Critically injured patients, inaccessible airways, and laryngeal mask airways *Emerg Med J* 2005;22:742-744.

37 Hoyle JD Jr, Jones JS, Deibel M, Lock DT, Reischman D. Comparative study of airway management techniques with restricted access to patient airway. *Prehosp Emerg Care* 2007;11(3):330-336.

38 Margolis GS. *Airway Management: Paramedic*. Boston: Jones and Bartlett, 2004.

39 Asai T, Morris S. The laryngeal mask airway: its features, effects and role. *Can J Anaesth* 1994;41(10):930-960.

40 Brimacombe JR. Problems with the laryngeal mask airway: prevention and management. *Int Anesth Clin* 1998;36:139-154.

41 Grantham H, Phillips G, Gilligan JE. The laryngeal mask in pre-hospital emergency care. *Emerg Med* 1994;28:97-102.

42 Haslam N, Campbell GC, Duggan JE. Gastric rupture associated with use of the laryngeal mask airway during cardiopulmonary resuscitation. *BMJ* 2004;329;1225-1226.

43 Baskett PJF, Bossaert L, Carli P *et al*. Guidelines for the advanced management of the airway and ventilation during resuscitation. *Resuscitation* 1996;31:201-230.

44 Dörges V. Airway management in emergency situations. *Best Pract Res Clin Anaesthesiol* 2005;19(4):699-715.

45 Bulger EM, Copass MK, Sabath DR *et al*. The use of neuromuscular blocking agents to facilitate prehospital intubation does not impair outcome after traumatic brain injury. *J Trauma* 2005;58:718-723.

46 Davis DP, Hoyt DB, Ochs M *et al*. The effect of paramedic rapid sequence intubation on outcome in patients with severe traumatic brain injury. *J Trauma* 2003;54:444-453.

47 Davis DP, Peay J, Sise MJ *et al*. The impact of prehospital endotracheal intubation on outcome in moderate to severe traumatic brain injury. *J Trauma* 2005;58:933-939.

48 Gausche M, Lewis RJ, Stratton SJ *et al*. Effect of out-of-hospital pediatric endotracheal intubation on survival and neurological outcome a controlled clinical trial. *JAMA* 2000;283:783-790.

49 Lockey D, Davies G, Coats T. Survival of trauma patients who have prehospital tracheal intubation without anaesthesia or muscle relaxants observational study [abstract]. *BMJ* 2001;323:141.

50 Murray JA, Demetriades D, Berne TV *et al*. Prehospital intubation in patients with severe head injury. *J Trauma* 2000;49:1065-1070.

51 Sloane C, Vilke GM, Chan TC *et al*. Rapid sequence intubation in the field versus hospital in trauma patients. *J Emerg Med* 2000;19:259-264.

52 Stockinger ZT, McSwain NE Jr. Prehospital endotracheal intubation for trauma does not improve survival over bag-valve-mask ventilation. *J Trauma* 2004;56:531-536.

53 Wang HE, Peitzman AB, Cassidy LD *et al*. Out-of-hospital endotracheal intubation and outcome after traumatic brain injury. *Ann Emerg Med* 2004;44:439-450.

54 Winchell RJ, Hoyt DB. Endotracheal intubation in the field improves survival in patients with severe head injury Trauma Research and Education Foundation of San Diego. *Arch Surg* 1997;132:592-597.

55 Bochicchio GV, Ilahi O, Joshi M *et al*. Endotracheal intubation in the field does not improve outcome in trauma patients who present without an acutely lethal traumatic brain injury. *J Trauma* 2003;54:307-311.

56 Christensen EF, Hoyer CC. Prehospital tracheal intubation in severely injured patients a Danish observational study. *BMJ* 2003;327:533-534.

57 Cooper A, DiScala C, Foltin G *et al*. Prehospital endotracheal intubation for severe head injury in children a reappraisal. *Semin Pediatr Surg* 2001;10:3-6.

58 DiRusso SM, Sullivan T, Risucci D *et al*. Intubation of pediatric trauma patients in the field predictor of negative outcome despite risk stratification. *J Trauma* 2005;59: 84-90.

59 Suominen P, Baillie C, Kivioja A *et al*. Intubation and survival in severe paediatric blunt head injury. *Eur J Emerg Med* 2000;7:3-7.

60 Dolenska S, Dala P, Taylor A. *Essentials of Airway Management*. London: Greenwich Medical Media, 2004.

61 Henderson JJ. The use of paraglossal straight blade laryngoscopy in difficult tracheal intubation. *Anaesthesia* 1997;52:552-560.

62 Chisholm DG, Calder I. Experience with the McCoy laryngoscope in difficult laryngoscopy. *Anaesthesia* 1997;52:906-908.

63 Ridgway S, Hodzovic I, Woollard M, Latto IP. Prehospital airway management in Ambulance Services in the United Kingdom. *Anaesthesia* 2004;59 (11):1091-1094.

64 Woollard M, Lighton D, Mannion W. Airtraq vs standard laryngoscopy by student paramedics and experienced prehospital laryngoscopists managing a model of difficult intubation. *Anaesthesia* 2008;63:26-31.

65 Woollard M, Mannion W, Lighton D. Use of the Airtraq laryngoscope in a model of difficult intubation by prehospital providers not previously trained in laryngoscopy. *Anaesthesia* 2007;62:1061-1065.

66 Pitt K, Woollard M. Should paramedics bougie on down? *Pre-hosp Imm Care* 2000;49: 68-70.

67 Hodzovic I, Wilkes AR, Latto IP. To shape or not to shape – simulated bougie-assisted difficult intubation in a manikin. *Anaesthesia* 2003;58:791-797.

68 Stock MC, Downs JB. Lubrication of tracheal tubes to prevent sore throat from intubation. *Anesthesiology* 1982;57:418-420.

69 Tackley R. Transparent obstruction of RAE tube. *Anaesthesia* 2001;56(3):279-280.

70 Badrakumar A, Ball DR, Jefferson PD. Why KY? *Anaesthesia* 2001;56(8):799-820.

71 Sprague NE, Moffett SP. Oral tracheal tubes. Is lubrication necessary? *Today's Anaesthetist* 1989;4:140-142.

72 Jones JH, Murphy MP, Dickson RL, Somerville GG, Brizendine EJ. Emergency physician-verified out-of-hospital intubation: miss rates by paramedics. *Acad Emerg Med* 2004;11:707-709.

73 Jemmett ME, Kendal KM, Fourre MW, Burton JH. Unrecognized misplacement of endotracheal tubes in a mixed urban to rural emergency medical services setting. *Acad Emerg Med* 2003;10:961-965.

74 Wirtz DD, Ortiz C, Newman DH, Zhitomirsky I. Unrecognized misplacement of endotracheal tubes by ground prehospital providers. *Prehosp Emerg Care* 2007;11:213-218.

75 Katz SH, Falk JL. Misplaced endotracheal tubes by paramedics in an urban emergency medical services system. *Ann Emerg Med* 2001;37:62-64.

76 Caplan RA, Posner KL, Ward RJ, Cheney FW. Adverse respiratory events in anaesthesiology. A closed claims analysis. *Anesthesiology* 1990;72:828-833.

77 Pelucio M, Halligan L, Dhindsa H. Out-of-hospital experience with the syringe esophageal detector device. *Acad Emerg Med* 1997;4:563-568.

78 Takeda T, Tanigawa K, Tanaka H, Hayashi Y, Goto E, Tanaka K. The assessment of three methods to verify tracheal tube placement in the emergency setting. *Resuscitation* 2003;56(2):153-157.

79 Tanigawa K, Takeda T, Goto E, Tanaka K. Accuracy and reliability of the self-inflating bulb to verify tracheal intubation in out-of-hospital cardiac arrest patients. *Anesthesiology* 2000;93:1432-1436.

80 Bozeman WP, Hexter D, Liang HK, Kelen GD. Esophageal detector device versus detection of end-tidal carbon dioxide level in emergency intubation. *Ann Emerg Med* 1996;27:595-599.

81 Association of Anaesthetists of Great Britain and Ireland. *Recommendations for Standards of Monitoring During Anaesthesia and Recovery*. London: AAGBI, 2000.

82 Kelly JJ, Eynon CA, Kaplan JL, de Garavilla L, Dalsey WC. Use of tube condensation as an indicator of endotracheal tube placement. *Ann Emerg Med* 1998;31:575-578.

83 Wang HE, Yealy DM. How many attempts are required to accomplish out-of-hospital endotracheal intubation? *Acad Emerg Med* 2006;13:372-377.

84 Cudnik MT, Newgard CD, Wang H *et al.* Endotracheal intubation increases out-of-hospital time in trauma patients. *Prehosp Emerg Care* 2007;11:224-229.

85 Magill IW. Technique in endotracheal anaesthesia. *BMJ* 1930;2:817-819.

86 Benumof J. *Conventional (Laryngoscopic) Orotracheal and Nasotracheal Intubation (Single-Lumen Tube)*. St Louis, MO: Mosby, 1996.

87 Schmitt HJ, Mang H. Head and neck elevation beyond the sniffing position improves laryngeal view in cases of difficult direct laryngoscopy. *J Clin Anesthes* 2002;14:335-338.

88 Walz JM, Zayaruzny M, Heard SO. Airway management in critical illness. *Chest* 2007;131:608-620.

89 Sellick BA. Cricoid pressure to control regurgitation of stomach contents during induction of anaesthesia. *Lancet* 1961;2:404-406.

90 Smith KJ, Dobranowski J, Yip G *et al.* Cricoid pressure displaces the esophagus: an observational study using magnetic resonance imaging. *Anesthesiology* 2003;99: 60-64.

91 Salem M, Joseph N, Heyman H *et al.* Cricoid compression is effective in obliterating the esophageal lumen in the presence of a nasogastric tube. *Anesthesiology* 1985;63:443-446.

92 Lawes EG, Campbell I, Mercer D. Inflation pressure, gastric insufflation and rapid sequence induction. *Br J Anaesth* 1987;59:315-318.

93 Noguchi T, Koga K, Shiga Y *et al.* The gum elastic bougie eases tracheal intubation while applying cricoid pressure compared to a stylet. *Can J Anaesth* 2003;50:712-717.

94 Haslam N, Parker L, Duggan JE. Effect of cricoid pressure on the view at laryngoscopy. *Anaesthesia* 2005;60:41-47.

95 Levitan RM, Kinkle WC, Levin WJ *et al.* Laryngeal view during laryngoscopy: a randomized trial comparing cricoid pressure, backward-upward-rightward pressure, and bimanual laryngoscopy. *Ann Emerg Med* 2006;47:548-555.

96 Mort TC. The value of preoxygenation in the critically ill patients requiring emergency intubation. *Crit Care Med* 2005;33:2672-2675.

97 Mort TC. Complications of emergency tracheal intubation: immediate airway-related consequences: Part II. *J Intensive Care Med* 2007;22:208-215.

98 Maharaj CH, Costello JF, Higgins BD, Harte BH, Laffey JG. Learning and performance of tracheal intubation by novice personnel: a comparison of the Airtraq® and Macintosh laryngoscope. *Anaesthesia* 2006;61(7):671-677.

99 Maharaj CH, Ni Chonghaile M, Higgins B, Harte B, Laffey J. Tracheal intubation by inexperienced medical residents using the Airtraq and Macintosh laryngoscopes – a manikin study *Am J Emerg Med* 2006;24(7):769-774.

100 Mahara CH, Costello JF, McDonnell JG, Harte BH, Laffey JG. The Airtraq® as a rescue airway device following failed direct laryngoscopy: a case series. *Anaesthesia* 2007; 62(6):598-601.

101 Scrase I, Woollard M. Needle vs surgical cricothyroidotomy: a short cut to effective ventilation. *Anaesthesia* 2006;61:962-974.

102 Henderson JJ, Popat MT, Latto IP, Pearce AC. Difficult Airway Society. Difficult Airway Society guidelines for management of the unanticipated difficult intubation. *Anaesthesia* 2004;59:675-694.

103 Roberts K, Allison KP, Porter KM. A review of emergency equipment carried and procedures performed by UK front line paramedics. *Resuscitation* 2003;58:153-158.

104 Ridgway S, Hodzovic I, Woollard M, Latto IP. Prehospital airway management in Ambulance Services in the United Kingdom. *Anaesthesia* 2004;59:1091-1094.

105 Ryder IG, Paoloni CC, Harle CC. Emergency transtracheal ventilation: assessment of breathing systems chosen by anaesthetists. *Anaesthesia* 1996;51:764-768.

106 Porter K, Allison KP, Greaves I. Variations in equipment on UK front line ambulances. *Pre-Hospital Immediate Care* 2000;4:126-131.

107 Ratnayake B, Langford RM. A survey of emergency airway management in the United Kingdom. *Anaesthesia* 1996;51:908-911.

108 Wong DT, Lai K, Chung FF, Ho RY. Cannot intubate cannot ventilate and difficult intubation strategies: Results of a Canadian national survey. *Anesthes Analges* 2005;100:1439-1446.

109 TinUnalli JE, Kelen GD, Stapczynskl JS. Surgical airway management. In: *Emergency Medicine: A Comprehensive Study Guide*, 6th edn. New York, NY: McGraw-Hill, 2004, pp. 119-124.

Chapter 2
Assisted ventilation

Content

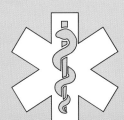

Assisted ventilation is one of the core skills of the prehospital practitioner. There has been a tendency to view assisted ventilation as a simple skill for ambulance practitioners yet it can be difficult to ventilate a patient correctly in the prehospital environment. This chapter discusses the indications for assisted ventilation and the equipment and techniques that can be used in the field.

Definition of assisted ventilation

Assisted ventilation is where the practitioner offers ventilatory support to a patient whose alveolar ventilation is inadequate to maintain normal partial pressures of oxygen and carbon dioxide. This can be achieved by using either mechanical or manually generated positive pressure and may be a lifesaving treatment. In prehospital care the pressure may be generated using expired air ventilation (mouth-to-mouth/nose), a mechanical ventilator such as the Pneupac® paraPAC, or a bag-valve-mask (BVM) (Figures 2.1 and 2.2). Either may be used with a mask or endotracheal tube/laryngeal mask airway.

Normal inspiration occurs when the diaphragm (primary muscle of inspiration) contracts, causing an increase in the size of the thoracic cavity. As a result, intrathoracic pressure falls to below that of atmospheric pressure and air is drawn into the lungs. Assisted ventilation creates a positive pressure that pushes air into the lungs. Failure to provide adequate ventilation for an indicated patient will lead to hypoxia, retention of CO_2, development of acidosis and cardio-respiratory arrest.

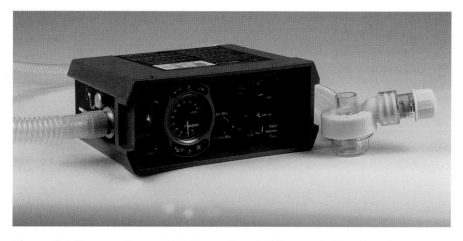

Figure 2.1 Pneupac® paraPAC. Reproduced with permission of Smiths Medical International.

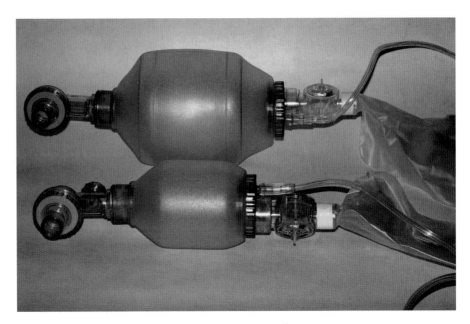

Figure 2.2 Silicone bags.

Scenario

You are called to attend an elderly male patient who is known to suffer from COPD. On arrival you are confronted with a centrally cyanosed obese male patient with poor respiratory effort – you assess his respiratory rate to be 5 breaths per minute. The patient opens his eyes to voice but is unable to speak due to inadequate ventilation. You notice he has a full moustache and beard.

- Make a list of the problems you may encounter when attempting to support the ventilation of this patient and identify some techniques you may be able to use to overcome them.
- Would you use a bag-valve-ventilator or mechanical ventilator? Provide a rationale for your answer.

Indications for assisted ventilation

Inadequate ventilation is the overriding indication for assisted ventilation. In cases of apnoea, the indication is unequivocal but, for patients with depressed ventilation, the requirement may be less obvious. Artificial ventilation should be provided as soon as possible in any patient in whom spontaneous ventilation is inadequate or absent.[1]

Patients with a life-threatening respiratory emergency will present in either respiratory failure or respiratory distress.[2] Those with respiratory distress are still able to compensate for the effects of their illness, and urgent treatment may prevent their further deterioration. These patients present with signs and symptoms indicative of increased work of breathing but may show few signs of the systemic effects of hypoxia or hypercapnia. Patients with respiratory failure tend not to show evidence of increased work of breathing as exhaustion overrides their ability to compensate. These patients will normally exhibit signs of the systemic effects of hypoxia and hypercapnia, and immediate treatment will be required to prevent cardiac arrest. Box 2.1[2] shows the key findings associated with increased work of breathing and weak respiratory effort; these are indicative of a patient with a life-threatening respiratory condition. For these patients, it is suggested that assisted ventilation should be undertaken if the respiratory rate is <10 or >29/min (adult), titrated to SpO_2.[2] However, some patients presenting with respiratory rates between 10 and 29/min will still benefit from assisted ventilation; it is a clinical judgement for the paramedic to make based upon ALL physical observations not just the respiratory rate.

Increased work of breathing

- Stridor associated with other key findings
- Use of accessory muscles
- Adopting orthopnic position (sat upright)
- Tracheal tug
- Intercostal recession
- Expiratory wheeze associated with other key findings
- Cessation of expiratory wheeze without improvement in condition
- Inability to speak in whole sentences
- Respiratory rate <10 or >29

Weak respiratory effort

- Decreased, asymmetrical, or absent breath sounds
- Oxygen saturation <92% on air or <95% on high concentration oxygen
- PEFR <33% of normal
- Hypercapnia (measured with end tidal CO_2 monitor where available)
- Tachycardia (≥120) or bradycardia (late and ominous finding)
- Arrhythmias
- Pallor and/or cyanosis (particularly central cyanosis)
- Cool clammy skin
- Falling blood pressure (late and ominous finding)
- Changed mental status – confusion, feeling of impending doom, combativeness
- Falling level of consciousness
- Exhaustion (+/–muscular chest pain)

Box 2.1 Key findings indicating increased work of breathing or weak respiratory effort[2]

Fatigue induced by a prolonged, severe asthma attack, head injury induced hypoventilation, and drug induced respiratory depression (e.g. opiates) are typical causes of inadequate ventilation requiring assisted ventilation. Apnoea is an absolute indication for assisted ventilation irrespective of the cause.

The literature and complications associated with assisted ventilation

The most common initial form of ventilatory assistance in the emergency clinical setting is usually accomplished using bag-valve-ventilation (BVV) techniques. The BVV mask was developed in 1955 by Henning Ruben in Denmark and has been the most common method of ventilating a patient in respiratory or cardiac arrest since that time.[3] Performing ventilation with a bag-valve-mask device is regarded as a relatively simple task that all healthcare personnel should be able to perform with little training. Ventilation utilising this technique is accepted worldwide and considered to be the standard of care in a variety of clinical settings.[4,5]

Even though the technique is considered to be safe and effective and has been used in the emergency setting for many years, it has some potentially fatal complications. Among them are decreased oxygenation, lung aspiration due to gastric dilatation, or even gastric rupture.[6] The main complications should be recognised early but it is questionable as to whether problems are always rectified. Gastric over-distention, aspiration of gastric contents, and barotrauma can lead to the premature death of a patient.[7] By utilising too much pressure whilst ventilating, the rescuer may overcome the lower oesophageal sphincter pressure and produce aspiration.[8]

In a patient with an unprotected airway, the distribution of inspiratory gas volume between lungs and stomach during bag-valve-mask ventilation depends on several variables. These variables include: upper airway pressure, inspiratory flow rate, airway resistance and compliance, and lower oesophageal sphincter pressure.[9] The lower oesophageal sphincter pressure is normally 20 to 25 cm H_2O in a healthy adult, but is significantly reduced in patients with cardiac arrest.[10] Bag-valve-mask (BVM) ventilation is often applied with a high flow rate over a short inflation time, which inevitably produces a high peak airway pressure. If the peak airway pressure exceeds the lower oesophageal sphincter pressure during ventilation, the stomach is inflated. Thus, it is essential to keep the peak airway pressure to a minimum during ventilation of a non-intubated patient.

Several strategies are available to reduce peak inspiratory flow rates, and therefore, peak airway pressure. These include the use of a paediatric bag-valve-mask instead of an adult one, use of cricoid pressure, or a mechanical ventilator.[11,12] Studies looking at the efficacy and safety of mechanical ventilators suggest that pulmonary barotrauma may result from excessive peak inspiratory flow rates, so a recommendation has been made that lower peak inspiratory flow rates should be used.[13] There have been few studies investigating the effectiveness of mechanical ventilators although one study does suggest significant benefits of a mechanical ventilator over BVV. The study found that when compared with the resuscitation ventilator, the bag-valve-mask resulted in significantly higher peak airway pressure and significantly lower oxygen saturation.[14] This study suggests that the mechanical ventilator may be a suitable alternative to BVM even in the non-intubated patient.

A further option is offered by the SMART BAG®, which has a pressure-responsive flow-limiting valve. If properly squeezed, there are no differences in performance between this valve and a standard valve. The piston provides both a tactile and visual feedback to the provider when excessive pressure is applied and prevents excessively high peak airway pressure. In simulated scenarios, this bag provided ventilation performance that was more consistent with current guidelines and delivered similar tidal volumes when compared with ventilation with a traditional bag-valve-mask resuscitator.[15] However, in the patient with low compliant lungs it is possible that this bag will not allow for adequate ventilation.

The ventilation rate is also very important as hyperventilation of a patient during cardiac arrest is linked with adverse haemodynamic effects and decreased cerebral perfusion, which translate into increased mortality.[16] Several studies have documented high respiratory rates during pre-hospital resuscitation,[17,18] despite the recommended rate of 10 breaths per minute.[1]

THINK

Can you remember the last time you ventilated a patient with a BVM? Did you ventilate once every 6 seconds as per the guidelines? How can you improve your performance?

There are many potential reasons for the apparent failings in assisted ventilation, including stress, fatigue, the inability to convert training into real world situations, failings in training manikins, and an erroneous belief that in cardiac arrest the patient can never receive too much oxygen. The use of a correctly set-up mechanical ventilator may overcome many of these issues although the question of bag or machine remains unanswered.

When using a mask rather than a tube, the seal between face and mask is the key component to minimising the risk of leakage and hypoventilation (Figure 2.3). Traditionally, ambulance staff have been expected to perform this as a single-handed operator in the rear of a moving vehicle, but it is unlikely that this is an effective procedure due to movement, stress and the need to undertake other tasks. This is particularly true in the case of obese patients or those without teeth or with abundant facial hair. In addition, practitioners with smaller hands may not be able to squeeze the bag sufficiently to ventilate the patient.[19] When using a ventilator with a mask it is best practice for one person to hold the mask in place whilst maintaining the patient's airway and the second person squeezes the bag, paying particular attention not to overinflate[20] (Figure 2.4). This would require a second person to squeeze a

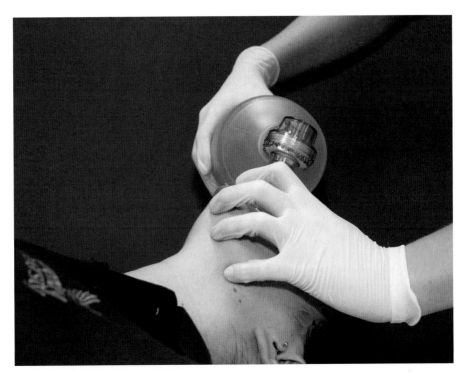

Figure 2.3 Making a seal (single-operator).

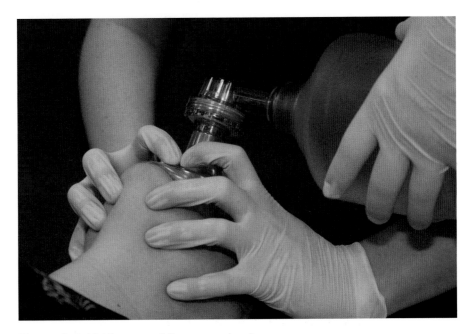

Figure 2.4 Making a seal (two-operators).

BVV device (not always available), so it may be necessary to connect the mask to a mechanical ventilator in order to achieve this.

In an intubated patient or a patient with an LMA in situ, use of a mechanical ventilator has been shown to allow paramedics to accomplish extra tasks, improve documentation and provide better patient care.[21] In addition, side effects are no different between the automatic transport ventilator and the bag valve ventilator.

Equipment and procedures for assisted ventilation

Bag-valve-ventilator

The bag-valve-ventilator comprises of a squeezable bag, oxygen reservoir and oxygen connection tubing, one way valve, and 15 mm/22 mm universal connector (Figure 2.2). When squeezed, the increase in pressure forces air forward to the patient's lungs via a one-way valve; when released, the bag self-inflates and draws air from the ambient atmosphere or oxygen reservoir if attached. The valve is designed to function during both spontaneous and manually controlled ventilation. A self-inflating bag can be connected to a face mask, tracheal tube, or alternative airway device.[1]

There are many types of face masks, varying in design, size, and construction materials. Transparent masks are preferred because they allow for inspection of lip colour, condensation, secretions, and vomitus.[22] The mask's size and shape must conform to the facial anatomy if a good seal is to be achieved, thus several different mask shapes and sizes should be available.

Suction should be available and normal airway management techniques should be utilised prior to attempting ventilation (see Chapter 1).

Procedure

Procedure	Additional information/rationale
Preparation	
1. Test the bag-valve device's capability for delivering positive-pressure ventilation before use.	To ensure that the device will function correctly. Seal the bag-valve device connector with the thumb and squeeze the bag with reasonable force. If it is difficult to compress the bag or if air is forced between the connector and thumb, positive pressure can be delivered.
2. Connect mask to patient delivery valve and oxygen tubing to oxygen supply.	
3. Turn on oxygen (normally 15 L/min for an adult) and allow reservoir to fill.	

Procedure	Additional information/rationale
One-hand technique[23]	
1. Place the thumb and index finger on the body of the mask while your other fingers pull the jaw forward and extend the head (see Figure 2.3).	Helps to maintain the airway and creates a seal with the mask. **Caveat:** Extreme caution is advised in patients with cervical spine injuries, in which flexion or extension of the neck is contraindicated. In this situation, the jaw-thrust manoeuvre without head extension is indicated.[25]
2. Place your middle and ring fingers on the ridge of the mandible and the fifth finger behind the angle of the mandible.[22,24]	Prevents obstruction of the airway created by pushing the tongue against the palate.[24]
3. Minimize the pressure applied to the submandibular soft tissues.	
4. Maintain an adequate seal whilst extending the patient's head, thrusting the jaw forward, and then squeeze the bag with the other hand.	
5. Ventilate the lungs at 10 breaths min with a tidal volume of no more than 10 ml/kg.[1] Deliver each breath over approximately 1 sec and give a volume that corresponds to normal chest movement.	This represents a compromise between giving an adequate volume, minimising the risk of gastric inflation, and allowing adequate time for chest compression during CPR.[1]
6. Assess adequacy of ventilation by inspecting and auscultating the chest and abdomen.	Rising and falling of the chest and breath sounds synchronous with the delivered tidal volume suggest adequate ventilation. Epigastric sounds and abdominal distension indicate gastric insufflation and poor ventilation
Two-hand technique[23]	
1. Hold the mask with two hands, with each hand positioned as described in the one-hand technique (see Figure 2.4).	
2. A second person should compress the bag-valve device in the same way as described above.	
3. Assess adequacy of ventilation using the same techniques as for one-hand technique.	

Mechanical ventilator

There are many different transport mechanical ventilators available but this section will discuss the Pneupac® paraPAC as it is the most commonly used in UK prehospital practice (Figure 2.5). The figure lays out the controls and the functions of each; this will be useful reference when viewing the procedures.

The Pneupac® paraPAC is suitable for transportation use by trained prehospital providers. It has dual controls that allow easy selection of tidal volume and frequency to match the patient's ventilatory requirements, and is suitable for ventilation during controlled or emergency transportation.

The paraPAC includes a CPR setting, CMV/Demand* (SMMV**), air mix, integrated pressure monitoring/alarm system and a separate tidal volume control, allowing for selection of optimum ventilation. The 'demand' system detects spontaneous breathing by an adult patient and inhibits the ventilator appropriately to the level of breathing. The tidal volume required to completely inhibit the ventilator is about 450 ml.

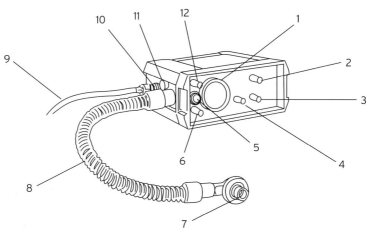

Figure 2.5 Controls and features of ParaPac 20D.
1.   Inflation pressure monitor
2.   Frequency Control
3.   Tidal Volume Control
4.   Air mix control
5.   Supply gas failure alarm
6.   Main pneumatic switch (Demand - CMV/Demand)
7.   Patient valve
8.   Patient hose
9.   Input hose
10. Inlet connection
11. Audible alarm
12. Relief pressure control

*CMV/Demand = Continuous mandatory ventilation.
**SMMV = Synchronised minimum mandatory ventilation.

Functional check and procedures[26]

- Functional check

1. Check the ventilator controls as follows:
   a. Main pneumatic switch   'Demand' (model 20D)
   b. '0'   (model 20)
   c. Frequency   12 b/min (detent position)
   d. Tidal volume   800 ml
   e. Air mix switch   'No air mix'
   f. Relief pressure   30 cmH$_2$O
2. Connect the probe on the input hose to an appropriate gas outlet.
3. If connected to a cylinder regulator, turn on cylinder valve slowly.
4. Check that the visual alarm for supply gas failure has changed from red to white.
5. Switch the main pneumatic switch to 'CMV/Demand (model 20D) or '1' (model 20). The ventilator should commence cycling. Occlude the output port on the patient valve and check that the manometer gives a reading of between 30 and 50 cmH$_2$O during each inspiratory phase. The audible alarm should sound. Check that the unit cycles every 5 seconds.
6. Switch over to air mix and repeat step 5; the change in the manometer reading should not exceed 5 cmH$_2$O.
7. Set the 'tidal volume' to its minimum setting, occlude the output port and check that at least 20 cm pressure is attained on the manometer. Gradually increase the flow setting and observe how the pressure rises. At the end of the green segment, the pressure should be attaining the nominal set value.
8. Reset the 'tidal volume' to its minimum setting and select 'no air mix'. Occlusion of the output port should now cause the manometer to rise sharply to between 30 and 50 cmH$_2$O and the alarm should sound.
9. Set the 'frequency' and 'tidal volume' controls to the extremes of their range. By listening to the gas flow, check that the ventilator is responding to the controls and that no irregularities of performance can be discerned.
10. Finally, set the controls as specified in step 1 so that the ventilator is left set for emergency use.

THINK

Why set the tidal volume at 800 ml when the average adult tidal volume is only around 500 ml?

Procedure	Additional information/rationale
Operation	
This equipment should only be used and operated by personnel trained and competent in its use.	For patient safety.
1. Connect supply hose to gas supply.	
2. Turn on gas supply slowly (if relevant).	
3. Check that the visual alarm for supply gas failure has changed from red to white.	Determines problem with gas supply or unit.
4. Turn the main pneumatic switch to 'CMV/Demand (model 20D) or '1' (model 20).	CMV ventilates the non-breathing patient, demand overrides.
5. Set ventilation parameters to suit patient.	Ensure correct volumes and rates are chosen for age of patient.
6. Briefly occlude the patient connection port of the patient valve with the thumb and check that the peak inflation pressure reading on the manometer is appropriate for the patient and that the audible alarm sounds.	Safety check prior to commencing ventilation.
7. Having ensured a clear airway, apply face mask to patient, or connect patient valve to ET tube/LMA.	
8. Check chest movement and Inflation Pressure Manometer is appropriate to ensure correct ventilation.	
9. Make adjustments as necessary.	

The patient's condition and chest movement, as well as the inflation pressure monitor should be kept under constant observation so that adverse ventilation conditions can be detected and corrected before the patient is put at risk. When ventilating with a mask, the peak inflation pressure should be kept below 20 cmH$_2$O to minimise the risk of gastric insufflation.

Chapter Key Points

1. Artificial ventilation should be provided as soon as possible in any patient in whom spontaneous ventilation is inadequate or absent.
2. The most common initial form of ventilatory assistance in the emergency clinical setting is usually accomplished using the bag-valve ventilation technique. Even though the technique is considered to be safe and effective and has been used in the emergency setting for many years, it has some potentially fatal complications.
3. A high flow rate over a short inflation time inevitably produces a high peak airway pressure in an unprotected airway. High peak airway pressure overcomes the pressure of the lower oesophageal sphincter and causes gastric inflation.
4. Use of a paediatric BVM, cricoid pressure, or mechanical ventilation may help to overcome the high pressures involved.
5. The ventilation rate is very important as hyperventilation of a patient during cardiac arrest is linked with adverse haemodynamic effects and decreased cerebral perfusion; the recommended rate is 10 breaths per minute.
6. When using a ventilator with a mask it is best practice for one person to hold the mask in place whilst maintaining the patient's airway and the second person squeezes the bag, paying particular attention not to overinflate.
7. In an intubated patient or a patient with an LMA in situ, use of a mechanical ventilator has been shown to allow paramedics to accomplish extra tasks, document better, and provide better patient care.

References and Further reading

Website with flash animation of issues surrounding BVV http://vam.anest.ufl.edu/checkout/check-sirb.html

1 Nolan JP, Deakin CD, Soar J, Böttiger BW, Smith G. European Resuscitation Council Guidelines for Resuscitation 2005 Section 4. Adult advanced life support. *Resuscitation* 2005;67(S1):S39–S86.
2 Woollard M, Greaves I. The ABC of community emergency care; 4 shortness of breath. *Emerg Med J* 2004; 21:341–350.
3 Ruben H. A new non-rebreathing valve. *Anesthesiology* 1995;16:643–645.
4 Noordergraaf GJ, van Dun PJ, Kramer BP, Schors MP, Hornman HP, de Jong W. Airway management by first responders when using a bag-valve device and two oxygen-driven resuscitators in 104 patients. *Eur J Anaesthesiol* 2004;21:361–366.
5 Dorges V, Knacke P, Gerlach K. Comparison of different airway management strategies to ventilate apneic, nonpreoxygenated patients. *Crit Care Med* 2003;31:800–804.
6 Smally AJ, Ross MJ, Huot CP. Gastric rupture following bag-valve-mask ventilation. *J Emerg Med* 2002;22:27–29.
7 Wenzel AH, Idris AH, Banner MJ *et al.* Respiratory system compliance decreases after cardiopulmonary resuscitation and stomach inflation impact of large and small tidal volumes on calculated peak airway pressure. *Resuscitation* 1998;38:113–118.

8 Zecha-Stallinger A, Wenzel V, Wagner-Berger HG, von Goedecke A, Lindner KH, Hormann C. A strategy to optimize the performance of the mouth-to-bag resuscitator using small tidal volumes effects on lung and gastric ventilation in a bench model of an unprotected airway. *Resuscitation* 2004;61:69-74.

9 Wenzel V, Idris AH. The current status of ventilation strategies during cardiopulmonary resuscitation. *Curr Opin Crit Care* 1997;3:206-213.

10 Rabey PG, Murphy PJ, Langton JA, Barker P, Rowbotham DJ. Effect of the laryngeal mask airway on lower oesophageal sphincter pressure in patients during general anaesthesia. *Br J Anaesth* 1993;70:380-381.

11 Wenzel V, Idris AH, Banner MJ, Kubilis PS, Williams JL. Influence of tidal volume on the distribution of gas between the lungs and stomach in the nonintubated patient receiving positive pressure ventilation. *Crit Care Med* 1998;26:364-368.

12 Stallinger A, Wenzel V, Wagner-Berger H *et al*. Effects of decreasing inspiratory flow rate during simulated basic life support ventilation of a cardiac arrest patient on lung and stomach tidal volumes. *Resuscitation* 2002;54:167-173.

13 Guidelines 2000 for cardiopulmonary resuscitation and emergency cardiovascular care. International consensus on science. *Circulation* 2000;102(Suppl):1-384.

14 von Goedecke A, Wenzel V, Hormann C *et al*. Effects of face mask ventilation in apneic patients with a resuscitation ventilator in comparison with a bag-valve-mask. *J Emerg Med* 2006;30:63-67.

15 Busko JM, Blackwell TH. Impact of a pressure-responsive flow-limiting valve on bag-valve-mask ventilation in an airway model. *Can J Emerg Med* 2006;8(3):158-163.

16 O'Neill JF, Deakin CD. Do we hyperventilate cardiac arrest patients? *Resuscitation* 2007;73:82-85.

17 Aufderheide TP, Sigurdsson G, Pirrallo RG *et al*. Hyperventilation-induced hypotension during cardiopulmonary resuscitation. *Circulation* 2004;109:1960-1965.

18 Aufderheide TP, Lurie KG. Death by hyperventilation: a common and life-threatening problem during cardiopulmonary resuscitation. *Crit Care Med* 2004;32:S345-351.

19 Thomas AN, Dang PT, Hyatt J, Trinh TN. A new technique for two-hand bag valve mask ventilation. *Br J Anaesthes* 1992;69:397-398.

20 Roberts I *et al*. Airway management training using an LMA: a comparison of two different training programmes. *Resuscitation* 1997;33(3):211-214.

21 Weiss SJ, Ernst AA, Jones R, Ong M, Filbrun T, Augustin C, Barnum M, Nick TG. Automatic transport ventilator versus bag valve in the EMS setting: a prospective, randomized trial. *South Med J* 2005;98(10):970-976.

22 Miller RD (Ed) *Miller's Anesthesia*, 6th edn. New York: Churchill Livingstone, 2005.

23 Ortega R, Mehio AK, Woo A, Hafez DH. Positive-pressure ventilation with a face mask and a bag-valve device. *N Engl J Med* 2007;357:e4.

24 Barash PG, Cullen BF, Soelting RK. *Clinical Anesthesia*, 5th edn. Philadelphia: Lippincott Willams & Wilkins, 2006.

25 Wilson WC, Grande CM, Hoyt DB. *Trauma: Emergency Resuscitation, Perioperative Anesthesia, Surgical Management*. New York: Informa Healthcare, 2007.

26 Smiths Medical. *paraPAC20 and 20D Ventilator User's Manual*. Issue 4. Luton: Smiths Medical, 2003.

Chapter 3

Cardiopulmonary resuscitation and basic life support

Content

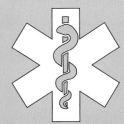

Sudden death as a result of cardiac arrest is a leading cause of ischaemic heart disease deaths in Europe.[1] Survival rates calculated from cardiac arrest to hospital discharge is estimated to be 10.7% in all types of cardiac arrest with cardiac arrest of ventricular fibrillation origin having the highest survival rate at 21.2%.[1] However these figures are a culmination of both in-hospital and out of hospital cardiac arrests; taken in isolation, out of hospital cardiac arrests have a survival rate of approximately 6.4%.[2] The provision of cardiopulmonary resuscitation is paramount in the management of all patients in cardiac arrest by potentially maintaining low level circulation to key organs.[1] This chapter discusses cardiopulmonary resuscitation across the age continuum, including the use of mechanical chest compression devices. In addition procedures allied to life support in the treatment of foreign body airway obstruction and the unconscious casualty will be reviewed.

Definitions

Cardiac arrest is defined as the sudden and complete loss of cardiac output due to asystole, ventricular fibrillation, ventricular tachycardia or loss of mechanical cardiac function.[3] The clinical diagnosis is based upon the patient being unconscious and pulseless (breathing can take some time to stop after cardiac arrest). Death is virtually inevitable unless effective treatment is given.

Cardiopulmonary resuscitation (CPR) or basic life support (BLS) consists of a series of manoeuvres that attempt to maintain a low level of circulation to perfuse the vital organs such as the heart and brain until more definitive treatment such as defibrillation or advanced life support can be given or there is a return of spontaneous circulation.[1,4] For the purposes of this chapter CPR and BLS are used interchangeably.

The chain of survival

The chain of survival (Figure 3.1) is a sequence of events that are necessary to maximise the chances of survival following a cardiac arrest. The chain is based upon the principle that a patient in cardiac arrest is most likely to survive if all of the links

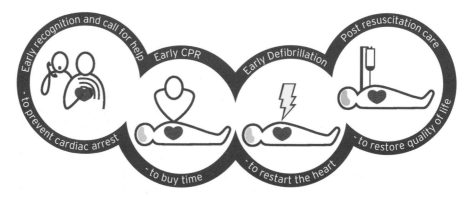

Figure 3.1 The chain of survival. Reproduced with kind permission of Laerdal Medical Ltd.

in the chain are present and timely. The focus of this chapter will be upon steps 1 and two of the chain. Further information regarding the following steps of the chain is provided in other chapters (e.g. defibrillation).

The importance of CPR

CPR is aimed at providing oxygen delivery to vital organs until more definitive treatment or spontaneous circulation can be restored and is therefore of great significance in the management of cardiac arrest. Several studies have supported the role of early CPR in cardiac arrest, with improved outcomes, including the role of bystander CPR in successful cardiac arrest outcome.[5-9] It is believed that successful outcomes from cardiac arrest are improved by CPR due to the creation of a 'bridge to successful defibrillation', whereby CPR prolongs the phase of ventricular fibrillation which has a higher successful resuscitation rate.[1,10] With such a wealth of evidence supporting the use of CPR in cardiac arrest and subsequent outcomes, a clear understanding of the process of CPR is imperative.

Lay rescuers versus healthcare providers

There is a distinct difference between the provision of CPR between the trained healthcare provider and the lay person. It is important to bear this in mind when attending a scene where bystander CPR is underway. This chapter will describe the process of CPR for the trained healthcare provider, however the main differences between the processes are highlighted below:

- Lay rescuers are not taught to assess for pulses or signs of life. The lay rescuer may commence CPR in an unresponsive patient with abnormal breathing.
- The lay rescuer may not perform rescue breathing or 'mouth-to-mouth' ventilation due to fears of contamination.[13]

The change to recent guidelines for the lay person not to assess for a pulse or absence of breathing is a result of studies into the ability of the lay person (and healthcare professionals) to undertake carotid pulse checks.[11] In addition confusion has been found over the presence of agonal breathing and an association as normal breathing.[12] Therefore it may be found that the lay person has undertaken CPR on a premise that differs from the trained healthcare provider.

Adult basic life support

This section contains the guidelines for single rescuer CPR. The recommendations of this are based upon the 2005 International Consensus Conference on Cardiopulmonary Resuscitation and Emergency Cardiovascular Care Science document[13] and European Resuscitation Council Guidelines,[1] with further supporting evidence included.

Figure 3.2 shows the adult CPR algorithm, whilst it is designed for the lay rescuer the principles remain the same for the trained healthcare provider. This chapter will outline the process of basic life support, for further information and guidance upon principles raised such as airway management and defibrillation please see the relevant chapters of this text.

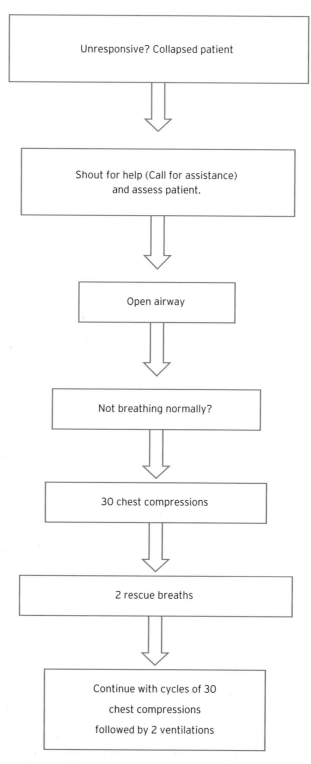

Figure 3.2 Adult basic life support algorithm. Reproduced with permission of Resuscitation Council UK.

The main principle of basic and advanced life support is the adherence to the ABC approach.

A   Airway

B   Breathing

C   Circulation

You should remain on each level until any major deficiencies are rectified. Source: Resuscitation Council UK.[1]

Sequence of BLS

1. Ensure personal/patient and bystander safety:
    *   This is of undoubted importance to all healthcare providers and lay persons.
2. Check the victim for a response:
    *   Gently shake the shoulders and ask loudly 'are you all right?'
    *   Consider any suggestion of cervical spine injury and provide support for the c-spine during shaking the shoulders as required. This can be achieved by holding the head still with one hand whilst shaking the patient's shoulders.
3. If the patient responds:
    *   Urgent medical assessment may be required.
    *   During this time consider oxygen therapy, clinical assessment and treatment.
4. If the patient does not respond:
    *   Consider requesting assistance.
    *   Turn the patient onto their back (considering c-spine injury).
    *   Open the airway, if no c-spine injury suspicion use the head tilt and chin lift technique. See airway management chapter for guidance.
    *   If there is suspicion of c-spine injury consider a jaw thrust or chin lift with assistance from others to manually stabilise the head and neck. If a life threatening airway obstruction persists, despite airway manoeuvres add a head tilt gently a small amount at a time. The lack of patency of an airway overrides the hypothetical risk of a cervical spine injury.
5. Keeping the airway open look, listen and feel for breathing for no more than 10 seconds:
    *   Look for chest movement.
    *   Listen for breath sounds.
    *   Feel for air upon your cheek.
    *   In the first few minutes after cardiac arrest a victim may be breathing (barely) or be taking infrequent noisy gasps, this shouldn't be confused for normal breathing.[1,13]
6. Check for the presence of a carotid pulse for no more than 10 seconds. This can be undertaken at the same time as checking for the presence of normal breathing for those who are experienced in clinical assessment. Inexperienced providers may check for a carotid pulse after checking for breathing:
    *   There may be other signs of life such as movement which may contradict the absence of a palpable pulse. Remember to view the patient as a whole.

7. If the victim is breathing normally and has a pulse:
    * Turn the patient into the recovery position. This is discussed later in the chapter.
    * Continue to monitor airway status, breathing and pulse.
    * Continue to perform a medical assessment and required interventions.
8. If there is a pulse but no breathing:
    * Ventilate the patient's lungs using a bag-valve-mask, pocket mask or mouth to mouth ventilations. This should be at a rate of 10 min^{-1}, the easiest way to determine this is to provide a breath when you would need a breath. Be careful not to hyperventilate or over-inflate.
    * To provide mouth-to-mouth ventilation:
        a. Ensure head tilt and chin lift.
        b. Pinch the soft part of the nose closed with the index finger and thumb of your hand on the forehead.
        c. Open the mouth a little, but maintain the chin upwards.
        d. Take a breath and place your lips around the mouth, making sure that you have a good seal.
        e. Blow steadily into the mouth over about 1–1.5 sec watching for chest rise.
        f. Maintaining head tilt and chin lift, take your mouth away from the victim and watch for the chest to fall as air comes out.
        g. Only those who are confident and competent in assessing for breathing and a pulse will be able to make this diagnosis. If in doubt treat as if the patient is in cardiac arrest.
9. If there is abnormal breathing, no pulse or signs of life:
    * Commence CPR.
    * Kneel beside the patient. Place the heel of one hand in the centre of the chest.
    * Place the heel of the other hand on top of the other hand.
    * Interlock the fingers and ensure that pressure is not applied over the ribs but over the sternum (Figure 3.3). Do not apply pressure over the upper abdomen or lower part of the sternum.
    * Position yourself vertically above the victim's chest with the arms straight.
    * Press the sternum down approximately 4–5 cm.
    * After each compression release the pressure off of the chest, without losing contact between the hands and the sternum.
    * Repeat at a rate of 100 min^{-1} for 30 compressions.
    * Compression and release should take equal amounts of time.
10. Follow with two rescue breaths:
    * After 30 compressions, re-open the airway and provide two ventilations using a bag-valve mask, pocket mask or mouth to mouth ventilation.
    * Use an inspiratory time of 1 second and provide enough volume to produce a chest rise as in normal breathing.
    * Allow for the chest to fall prior to the second ventilation.
    * If a ventilation fails repeat until successful up to a maximum of five attempts.
11. Recommence chest compressions as before. This cycle should continue until definitive care is reached or provided.
12. Reassess the patient only if changes occur such as signs of life. If not continue CPR.
13. If assistance is available consider changing rescuer every two minutes to avoid fatigue and subsequent reduction in quality of CPR.[1]

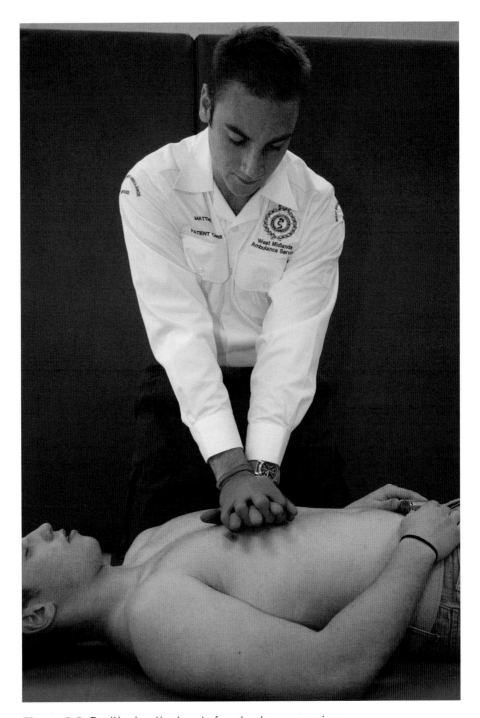

Figure 3.3 Positioning the hands for chest compressions.

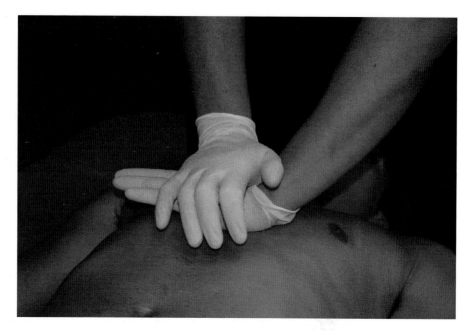

Figure 3.4 Overhead CPR.

14. In the case of lone rescuer or CPR in confined spaces, overhead CPR or straddle CPR may be used for resuscitation.[1] See Figure 3.4.
    - Note that the hands must be positioned so that the heel of the bottom hand is over the sternum as with the 'standard' chest compression position. This reduces pressure over the ribs and ensures compressions are delivered to the correct area with reduced likelihood of rib fracture.

Rescuer danger

The safety of the rescuer and victim are paramount during resuscitation. There have been a relative few incidences of rescuers suffering adverse effects from CPR, with isolated reports of infections such as tuberculosis and severe acute respiratory distress syndrome being transmitted via mouth-to-mouth ventilation.[1] There have been no reported incidences of HIV being transmitted during CPR. With the availability of filters, barrier devices and one way valves it is recommended that rescuers take appropriate precautions and risk assess each situation.

Initial rescue breaths

During the first few minutes following non-asphyxial cardiac arrest blood oxygen remains high and lack of oxygenation to the vital organs is limited more by the lack of cardiac output. It is therefore less important to provide initial rescue breaths than to provide chest compressions.[14] In addition it is recognised that rescuers are often unwilling to undertake mouth-to-mouth ventilation, therefore the emphasis has been placed upon effective chest compressions as opposed to ventilation.

Chest compressions

Chest compressions produce blood flow by increasing intrathoracic pressure and directly compressing the heart.[13] Chest compressions are able to produce systolic blood pressures of 60-80 mmHg, this enables a crucial amount of blood flow to the vital organs.[15] There is little evidence to support the specific placement of the hands during chest compressions, however the placement of the hands in the current position is aimed at being simplistic and reducing injury to underlying tissues.[16]

Chest compression depth is aimed at providing an adequate intra-thoracic pressure and compression of the heart to allow for the forcing of blood to the vital organs. The recommended depth for adult chest compression is 4-5 cm. The majority of evidence that supports the recommended compression depth is based upon animal studies due to the ethical nature of such research. It is believed that blood flow increases with compression force and depth during CPR, thus improving circulation.[17,18] However studies suggest that in both out of hospital cardiac arrest and in hospital cardiac arrest that compression depths are often inadequate.[19] It is suggested in a small scale animal study that a reduction in compression depth of 30% can significantly reduce coronary perfusion pressure and subsequent successful resuscitation.[20] However no large scale study has been undertaken to validate these results.

Compression rate is recommended at 100 min^{-1}; this rate is suggested as a speed for compressions not as a target for the number of compressions to be given per minute. This number will be reduced by a number of interruptions such as airway management and defibrillation. The rate of compressions is aimed at maintaining coronary perfusion pressure (CPP) and to allow for the heart to refill with blood following each ejection. Therefore rates that are too slow will allow CPP to fall thus reducing perfusion, whereas rates that are too high will cause reduced cardiac filling and subsequent falls in CPP.[13] Whilst there is little evidence to support the recommended rate mathematical models suggests that this rate would achieve best blood flow.[13]

Compression to ventilation ratio

Insufficient human studies have been undertaken to support a specific compression to ventilation ratio, however a small number of animal studies suggest that a ratio above 15:2 is required to optimise blood flow and oxygen delivery.[21] Interruptions to chest compressions should be minimised as stopping chest compressions causes the coronary flow to decrease substantially; on resuming chest compressions, several compressions are necessary before the coronary flow recovers to its previous level. Therefore a ratio of 30 compressions to 2 ventilations is now recommended. Studies utilising this new ratio suggest that CPR has been improved with increased chest compression numbers and reduced time where no CPR was being performed,[22] with a perceived benefit to patient outcome being identified.[23] However this is yet to be demonstrated in a large scale prospective study.

Compression only CPR

Both lay persons and healthcare professionals are often reluctant to perform mouth-to-mouth ventilation when no device is available to provide protection from contamination. Animal studies have demonstrated that compression only CPR may be as effective as standard CPR in the first few minutes following non-asphyxial cardiac arrest.[24] In adults chest compression only CPR has also been demonstrated to be more effective than no CPR on survival rates.[25] Recent human observational studies have supported this concept finding no significant differences in survival rates between standard CPR and compression only CPR by lay persons.[26,27] It has been suggested but yet to be empirically proven that compression only CPR may provide some level of passive airflow to ventilate patients when the airway is open and elastic recoil of the chest allows for air exchange.[28,29] Based upon current evidence it is recommended that compression only CPR should be undertaken as an alternative to no resuscitation.

> ### Key Point
>
> Basic life support and CPR follows a stepwise approach to patient assessment and management. It is important that any deficits at each level are rectified prior to moving onto the next step. If acting without equipment (i.e. in a non professional capacity) chest compression only CPR may suffice in the event that artificial ventilations are not possible.

Basic life support in pregnancy

Cardiac arrest seldom occurs late in pregnancy, however survival from such an event is exceptional.[30] There are a number of physiological changes that are peculiar to pregnancy that may affect life support and resuscitative measures, these include relative haemodilution (increased blood volume but relatively less red blood cells); increased gastric pressure due to the enlarged uterus and laryngeal oedema making airway management more difficult.[30,31] However in the third trimester the most important physiological change is the compression of the inferior vena cava by the gravid uterus (aortocaval compression). In a full term patient (without known obstetric abnormality) the vena cava may be completely occluded when in the supine position, this is believed to occur in up to 90% of cases and may result in a stroke volume of only 30% of the value expected in a non pregnant patient.[32] During cardiac arrest or when in the supine position the gravid uterus in a noticeably pregnant woman should be displaced to the left, either by manually displacing the uterus using two hands or by tilting the pelvis to the left by between 15° and 30° (a wedge or pillow/blankets may be used to achieve this),[32] Angles of greater than 30° will greatly inhibit adequate chest compressions and should therefore be avoided. It is recommended that a lateral tilt or manual displacement of the uterus is achieved or considered in any third trimester patient, this can be seen in Figure 3.5.

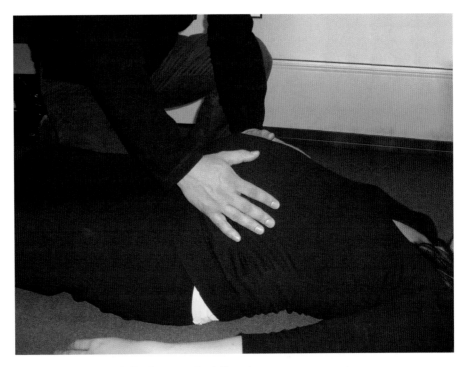

Figure 3.5 Manual displacement of the uterus.

Key Point

The gravid uterus may significantly reduce cardiac output during CPR, therefore displacement of the uterus is paramount in effective CPR.

Mechanical chest compression devices

Following concerns over a variety of factors within CPR, such as provider fatigue and the health and safety issues of performing CPR on a stretcher in a moving ambulance,[33] a series of mechanical devices have been designed to provide continuous chest compressions. An example of this is the LUCAS device (Lund University Cardiopulmonary Assist System) which is a gas driven CPR device which provides active compression/decompression (ACD) CPR.[34] ACD devices lift the anterior chest actively during decompression. Decreasing intra-thoracic pressure during the decompression phase increases venous return to the heart. This theoretically enables an increased cardiac output, coronary/cerebral perfusion pressures during the compression phase. In randomised animal studies, the use of ACD devices has been demonstrated to improves cardiac output and coronary perfusion pressure.[31,35] However throughout a series of studies no consensus has been reached to support

59

a definitive use of or rejection of such devices, suggesting that greater research is required to fully validate the introduction of such devices.[36]

The recovery position

There are several variations of the recovery position, however there is no single position that will suit all patients and no evidence to support a single recovery position. The recovery position is designed to ensure that the unconscious casualty has a clear unobstructed airway which allows for postural drainage of any secretions or vomit that may occur. The position should be stable and be as near to lateral as possible, with no pressure upon the chest to inhibit breathing.

The Resuscitation Council UK recommends the following sequence of actions to place a patient in the recovery postion[1]:

1. Remove any spectacles or loosen any tight clothing around the neck.
2. Kneel beside the victim and ensure that both of the legs are straight.
3. Place the arm nearest to you out at right angles with the elbow bent with the palm uppermost (Figure 3.6).
4. Bring the far arm across the chest and hold the back of the hand against the patient's cheek nearest to you.
5. With the your other hand grasp the far leg, just above the knee and pull it up, keeping the foot upon the ground (Figure 3.7).
6. Keeping the hand pressed against the cheek pull on the far leg to roll the patient towards you onto their side.
7. Adjust the upper leg to place the knee and hip at right angles, this will provide stability for the patient.

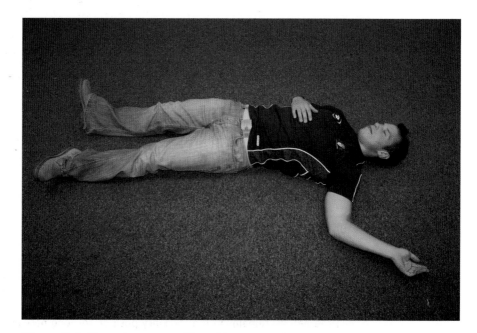

Figure 3.6 The recovery position: Step one.

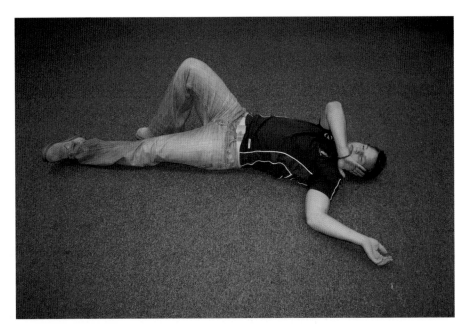

Figure 3.7 The recovery position: Steps two and three.

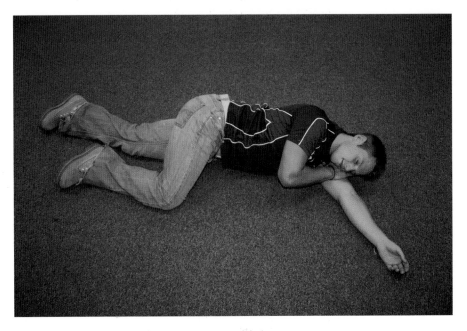

Figure 3.8 The completed recovery position.

8. Tilt the head back to ensure that the airway is open. If necessary adjust the hand under the cheek to keep the head tilted (Figure 3.8).
9. Ensure that the airway, breathing and circulation is re-checked frequently.
10. If the patient remains in the recovery position for long periods (>30 minutes) then consider alternating the sides to reduce pressure upon the lower arm.

Paediatric basic life support

Paediatric basic life support guidelines have been recently amended to include both the latest evidence and to allow for simplification to assist skill retention. The following guidance is recommended by the Resuscitation Council (UK)[1] and the European Resuscitation Council.[13]

Age definitions

New guidance upon paediatric resuscitation has allowed for a simplified defining of age groups in relation to basic life support protocols.

- An infant is a child under 1 year of age.
- A child is between 1 year and puberty. It is unnecessary and inappropriate to establish the onset of puberty formally. If you feel the patient is a child then the paediatric guidelines should be used.

Sequence of paediatric BLS

1. Ensure the safety of yourself, bystanders and the child.
2. Check the child's responsiveness:
   - Gently stimulate the child and ask loudly, 'Are you all right?'
   - Do not shake infants, or children with suspected cervical spine injuries as this may potentiate injury.
3. If the child responds by answering or moving:
   - Leave the child in the position in which you find him (provided no further danger).
   - Continue to monitor airway status, breathing and pulse.
   - Continue to perform a medical assessment and required interventions.
4. If the child does not respond:
   - Shout for help or call for assistance.
   - Turn the patient onto the back (considering c-spine injury).
   - Open the airway, if no c-spine injury suspicion use the head tilt and chin lift technique.
   - Do not push on the soft tissues under the chin as this may block the airway.
   - If you still have difficulty in opening the airway, use the jaw thrust method.
   - If there is a suspicion of cervical spine injury try to open the airway using chin lift or jaw thrust alone. If this is unsuccessful, add a head tilt a small amount at a time until the airway is open. The lack of patency of an airway overrides the hypothetical risk of a cervical spine injury.
5. Keeping the airway open, look, listen, and feel for normal breathing:
   - Putting your face close to the child's face and looking along the chest
   - Look for chest movements.
   - Listen at the child's nose and mouth for breath sounds.
   - Feel for air movement on your cheek.
   - Look, listen, and feel for no more than 10 sec before deciding that breathing is absent.

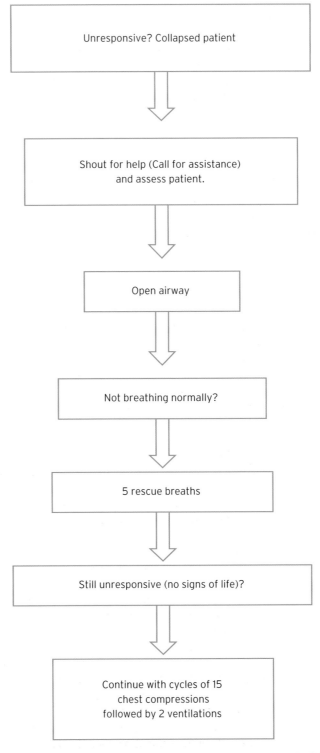

Figure 3.9 Paediatric basic life support algorithm. Reproduced with permission of Resuscitation Council UK.

6. If the child is breathing normally:
   - Turn the child onto his side into the recovery position (see adult recovery position above).
   - Monitor for continued breathing.
7. If the child is not breathing or is making agonal gasps (infrequent, irregular breaths):
   - Carefully remove any obvious airway obstruction.
   - Give 5 initial rescue breaths.
   - While performing the rescue breaths note any gag or cough response to your action.
   - Rescue breaths for a child over 1 year:
     a. Ensure head tilt and chin lift.
     b. Pinch the soft part of his nose closed with the index finger and thumb of your hand on his forehead.
     c. Open his mouth a little, but maintain the chin upwards.
     d. Take a breath and place your lips around his mouth, making sure that you have a good seal.
     e. Blow steadily into his mouth over about 1–1.5 sec watching for chest rise.
     f. Maintaining head tilt and chin lift, take your mouth away from the victim and watch for his chest to fall as air comes out.
     g. Take another breath and repeat this sequence 5 times. Identify effectiveness by seeing that the child's chest has risen and fallen in a similar fashion to the movement produced by a normal breath.
   - Rescue breaths for an infant:
     a. Ensure a neutral position of the head and apply chin lift.
     b. Take a breath and cover the mouth and nasal apertures of the infant with your mouth, making sure you have a good seal. If the nose and mouth cannot both be covered in the older infant, the rescuer may attempt to seal only the infant's nose or mouth with his mouth (if the nose is used, close the lips to prevent air escape).
     c. Blow steadily into the infant's mouth and nose over 1–1.5 sec sufficient to make the chest visibly rise.
     d. Maintain head tilt and chin lift, take your mouth away from the victim, and watch for his chest to fall as air comes out.
     e. Take another breath and repeat this sequence 5 times.
     f. If you have difficulty achieving an effective breath, the airway may be obstructed:
     g. Open the child's mouth and remove any visible obstruction. Do not perform a blind finger sweep as this may force an obstruction further into the airway.
     h. Ensure that there is adequate head tilt and chin lift but also that the neck is not overextended.
     i. If head tilt and chin lift has not opened the airway, try the jaw thrust method.
        Make up to 5 attempts to achieve effective breaths. If still unsuccessful, move on to chest compressions. **Please note:** This describes mouth to mouth ventilation for those trained to do so. If the equipment is available, the bag valve mask ventilation should be used. The airway management and ventilation chapters will demonstrate how this is achieved.

8. Check for signs of a circulation:
   - Take no more than 10 sec to look for signs of a circulation. These include any movement, coughing, or normal breathing (not agonal gasps - these are infrequent, irregular breaths).
   - Check the pulse (if you are trained and experienced) but ensure you take no more than 10 seconds to do this:
     a. In a child over 1 year - feel for the carotid pulse in the neck.
     b. In an infant - feel for the brachial pulse on the inner aspect of the upper arm.

9. If you are confident that you can detect signs of a circulation within 10 sec:
   - Continue rescue breathing, if necessary, until the child starts breathing effectively.
   - Turn the child onto his side (into the recovery position) if they remain unconscious.
   - Re-assess the child frequently.

10. If there are no signs of a circulation or no pulse, or a slow pulse (less than 60 min^{-1} with poor perfusion), or you are not sure:
    - Start chest compressions.
    - Combine rescue breathing and chest compressions.
    - For all children, compress the lower third of the sternum:
    - To avoid compressing the upper abdomen, locate the xiphisternum by finding the angle where the lowest ribs join in the middle. Compress the sternum one finger's breadth above this.
    - Compression should be sufficient to depress the sternum by approximately one-third of the depth of the chest.
    - Release the pressure, then repeat at a rate of about 100 min^{-1}.
    - After 15 compressions or 30 if a lone rescuer, tilt the head, lift the chin, and give two effective breaths.
    - Continue compressions and breaths in a ratio of 15:2.
    - Lone rescuers may use a ratio of 30:2, particularly if they are having difficulty with the transition between compression and ventilation.
    - Although the rate of compressions will be 100 min^{-1}, the actual number delivered will be less than 100 because of pauses to give breaths. The best method for compression varies slightly between infants and children.

11. Chest compression in infants:
    - The lone rescuer should compress the sternum with the tips of two fingers (Figure 3.10).
    - If there are two or more rescuers, use the encircling technique:
    - Place both thumbs flat, side by side, on the lower third of the sternum (as above), with the tips pointing towards the infant's head.
    - Spread the rest of both hands, with the fingers together, to encircle the lower part of the infant's rib cage with the tips of the fingers supporting the infant's back.
    - Press down on the lower sternum with your two thumbs to depress it approximately one-third of the depth of the infant's chest (See Figure 3.11).

12. Chest compression in children over 1 year:
    - Place the heel of one hand over the lower third of the sternum (as above).
    - Lift the fingers to ensure that pressure is not applied over the child's ribs.

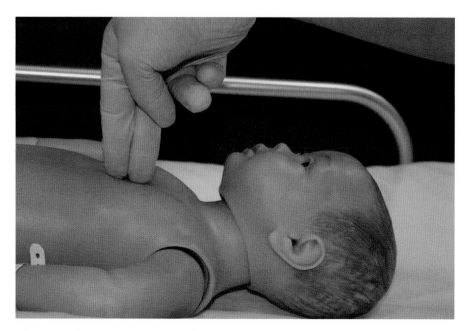

Figure 3.10 Two finger chest compressions.

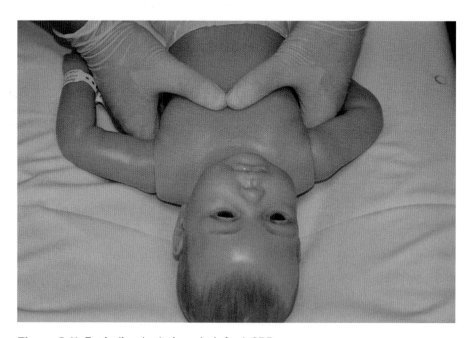

Figure 3.11 Encircling technique in infant CPR.

- Position yourself vertically above the victim's chest and, with your arm straight, compress the sternum to depress it by approximately one third of the depth of the chest.
- In larger children, or for small rescuers, this may be achieved most easily by using both hands with the fingers interlocked as with adult patients.

13. Continue resuscitation alternating between ventilations and chest compressions until:
    - the child shows signs of life (spontaneous respiration, pulse, movement) or further qualified help arrives.

14. If only one rescuer is present, undertake resuscitation for about 1min before going for assistance. To minimise interruptions in CPR, it may be possible to carry an infant or small child whilst summoning help.

Compression to ventilation ratio

Recent guidelines have sought to clarify the ratio of compressions to ventilation,[1,13] with a consensus that ratio should be based upon the number of rescuers. With 30:2 for lone rescuers to allow for simplicity. However in situations of two or more trained rescuers a ratio of 15:2 is recommended. This has been validated in both animal and mathematical studies, however for ethical reasons human studies are not applicable.[37-39]

Despite these recommendations there is little evidence to support the superiority of any ratio; however studies comparing 5:1 and 15:2 ratios suggest that a 5:1 ratio delivers too few chest compressions to be effective.[35,40]

Chest compression technique

The modified age definitions allow for a simplified approach to chest compressions. Previous guidance has been superseded in an effort to reduce compression of the upper abdomen as opposed to the chest.[41] Infant chest compression technique has remained the same however older children chest compressions have moved to a dynamic choice between one or two hands, with an emphasis upon providing adequate depth.[42]

> ### Key Point
>
> In paediatric life support 5 initial rescue breaths are provided due to the increased likelihood of a primary respiratory cause, this differs from adult guidance. A compression/ventilation rate of 30:2 is recommended for the lone rescuer, whereas 15:2 should be used in the event of 2 or more rescuers.

Newborn life support

During the birthing process the foetus experiences a potential period of hypoxia due to inadequate placental oxygen exchange. Although most babies are able to tolerate this experience, a few may require newborn life support post delivery.[1]

Newborn life support sequence

The following guidance is recommended by the Resuscitation Council (UK)[1] and the European Resuscitation Council[13] in the treatment of the newborn.

1. Keep the baby warm and assess:
   - Babies are born small and wet. They can experience rapid heat loss, especially if they remain wet and in a draught.
   - Whatever the problem, ensure the cord is securely clamped and then dry the baby, remove the wet towels, and cover the baby with dry towels.
   - For significantly preterm babies (30 weeks and below), there is now good evidence that placing the baby under a radiant heater and without drying the baby beforehand, immediately covering the head and body, apart from the face, with food-grade plastic wrapping, is the most effective way of keeping these very small babies warm during resuscitation or stabilisation at birth.
   - Drying the baby will provide significant stimulation and will allow time to assess colour, tone, breathing, and heart rate.
   - Reassess these observations regularly (particularly the heart rate) every 30 sec or so throughout the resuscitation process. The first sign of any improvement in the baby will be an increase in heart rate.
   - A healthy baby will be born blue but will have good tone, will cry within a few seconds of delivery, will have a good heart rate (the heart rate of a healthy newborn baby is about 120-150 beats min^{-1}), and will rapidly become pink during the first 90 seconds or so.
   - A less healthy baby will be blue at birth, will have less good tone, may have a slow heart rate (<100 beats min^{-1}), and may not establish adequate breathing by 90-120 seconds.
   - An ill baby will be born pale and floppy, not breathing and with a slow or very slow heart rate.
   - The heart rate of a baby is best judged by listening with a stethoscope. It can also be felt by gently palpating the umbilical cord but a slow rate at the cord is not always indicative of a truly slow heart rate - feeling for peripheral pulses is not helpful as the anatomy of the baby makes this difficult to achieve with confidence.
2. Before the baby can breathe effectively the airway must be open:
   - Place the baby on his back with the head in the neutral position, i.e. with the neck neither flexed nor extended. Most newborn babies will have a relatively prominent occiput, which will tend to flex the neck if the baby is placed on his back on a flat surface. This can be avoided by placing some support under the shoulders of the baby, but be careful not to overextend the neck.
   - If the baby is very floppy it may also be necessary to apply chin lift or jaw thrust.
3. If the baby is not breathing adequately by about 90 seconds give 5 inflation breaths. Until now the baby's lungs will have been filled with fluid. Aeration of the lungs in these circumstances is likely to require sustained application of pressures of about 30 cm of water for 23 sec - these are 'inflation breaths'.
   - If heart rate was below 100 beats min^{-1} initially then it should increase as oxygenated blood reaches the heart. If the heart rate does increase then it can be assumed that you have successfully aerated the lungs. If the heart

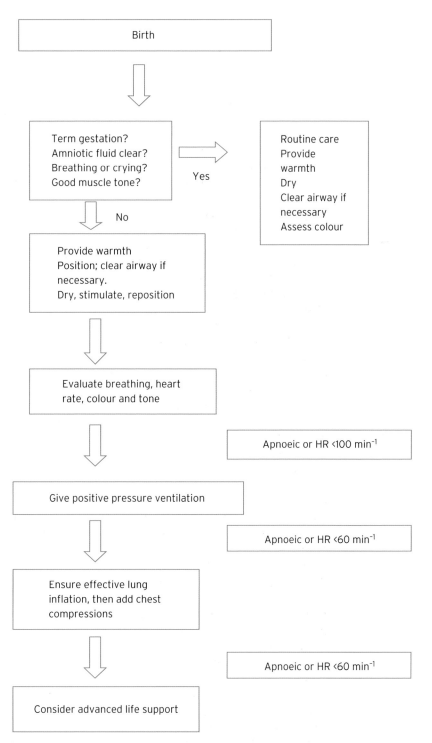

Figure 3.12 Newborn life support algorithm. Reproduced with permission of Resuscitation Council UK.

rate increases but the baby does not start breathing independently, then continue to provide regular breaths at a rate of about 30-40 min⁻¹ until the baby starts to breathe.

- If heart rate does not increase following inflation breaths, then either you have not aerated the lungs or the baby needs more than lung aeration alone. The most likely is failure to aerate the lungs effectively. If the heart rate does not increase, and the chest does not passively move with each inflation breath, then you have not aerated the lungs effectively.

4. If the heart rate remains slow (less than 60 min⁻¹) or absent following 5 inflation breaths, despite good passive chest movement in response to your inflation efforts, start chest compressions as indicated below:

5. Chest compressions should commence only when the lungs have been aerated successfully.

- In babies, the most efficient method of delivering chest compression is to grip the chest in both hands in such a way that the two thumbs can press on the lower third of the sternum, just below an imaginary line joining the nipples, with the fingers over the spine at the back.
- Compress the chest quickly and firmly, reducing the antero-posterior diameter of the chest by about one third.
- The ratio of compressions to inflations in newborn resuscitation is 3:1.
- Chest compressions move oxygenated blood from the lungs back to the heart. Allow enough time during the relaxation phase of each compression cycle for the heart to refill with blood. Ensure that the chest is inflating with each breath.

Key Point

In the newborn patient a slow pulse (below 60bpm) is an inadequate pulse rate for vital organ perfusion therefore CPR should be commenced at a compression/ventilation ratio of 3:1.

Foreign body airway obstruction (choking)

Definition

Choking is defined as the presence of a foreign body within the airway causing a partial or complete obstruction.[43] Foreign body airway obstruction (FBAO) is an uncommon but preventable cause of cardiac arrest,[44] with the key element of treatment being swift recognition followed by a set of simple steps.[1] Key signs and symptoms of the choking patient include:

- History – the patient may have been eating, or a child playing with a small toy.
- The victim may clutch their neck (universal choking sign).
- The victim may be coughing.

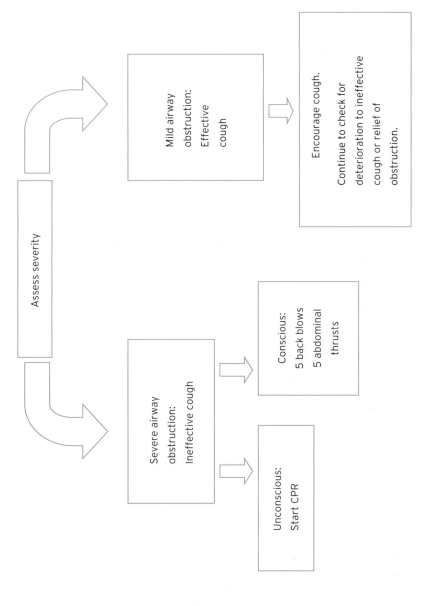

Figure 3.13 FBAO algorithm (adult). Reproduced with permission of Resuscitation Council UK.

- Inability to breathe or cough (severe airway obstruction).
- The victim may be unconscious.

Guidance for the treatment of the choking patient has been devised and standardised in the UK by the Resuscitation Council (UK)[1] and the European Resuscitation Council[13] utilising current best evidence and will therefore be recommended here.

Adult choking sequence

1. If the patient has a mild airway obstruction encourage them to cough. No other action is required.
2. If the patient shows signs of severe airway obstruction and is conscious:
   - Give up to five back blows.
   - Stand to the side of but slightly behind the patient.
   - Support the chest with one hand and lean the victim well forward, so that any obstructing objects that are removed comes out of the mouth rather than progresses down the airway.
   - Give up to five sharp blows between the shoulder blades with the heel of your other hand (Figure 3.14).
3. Check to see if each back blow has cleared the obstruction. If the obstruction is removed do not continue to give all five back blows.
4. If five back blows fail, continue to give up to five abdominal thrusts.
   - Stand behind the patient and put both hands around the upper part of the abdomen.
   - Lean the patient forward.

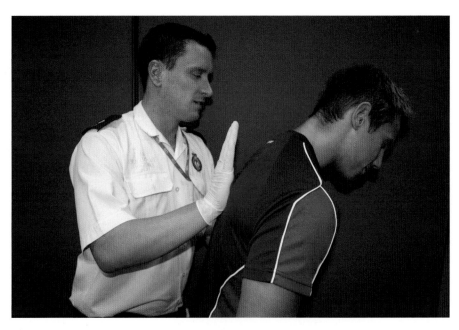

Figure 3.14 Deliver up to five sharp blows between the shoulder blades.

- Clench your fist and place it between the umbilicus and inferior to the xiphisternum.
- Grasp this hand with the other hand and pull sharply inwards and upwards (See Figure 3.15).
- Repeat up to five times.

5. If the obstruction is not relieved then continue to alternate five back blows with five abdominal thrusts.
6. If the patient becomes unconscious begin CPR as described earlier in this chapter. This should be undertaken even if the choking patient has a pulse, this is because chest compressions (thrusts) will reproduce pressure within the thoracic cage to potentially expel a FBAO.

A single method for relieving FBAO?

Clinical data for the relieving of FBAO is relatively sparse with mainly single case studies and retrospective data being used. However some of this data is influential in the care of the FBAO victim. Approximately 50% of all FBAO cases are not relieved by a single technique,[45] whereas the use of multiple techniques such as back blows, abdominal thrusts and chest thrusts significantly improves the likelihood of success.[46]

There is much debate as to what technique should be utilised to relieve FBAO, however no consensus has been reached. Cadaver and anaesthetised volunteer studies have demonstrated that chest thrusts can deliver a significantly higher airway pressure than abdominal thrusts, thus have the potential to be a more effective treatment for FBAO.[40,47] A similar study comparing abdominal thrust and back blows found that abdominal thrusts produced significantly higher airway pressures and where therefore more likely to dislodge a foreign body.[48] However there is no evidence of suitable quality to validate or dispute any of the suggested techniques or to change current practice.

Aftercare following a choking episode

There has been anecdotal evidence that suggests the use of FBAO relieving techniques, especially the abdominal thrust can result in underlying injury such as rib fracture, oesophageal rupture and gastric rupture among others.[40,49] Therefore it is always recommended that any victim of choking who has required abdominal thrusts should be reviewed by a doctor.[1,13]

Paediatric choking sequence

1. If the patient has a mild airway obstruction, encourage them to cough. No other action is required.

> ### Key Point
>
> If the patient is still able to cough effectively then supportive measures only are required. If the patient deteriorates then FBAO manoeuvres should be considered.

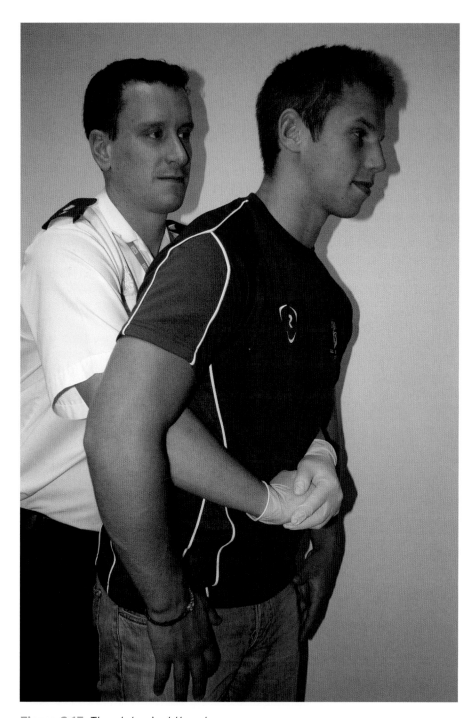

Figure 3.15 The abdominal thrust.

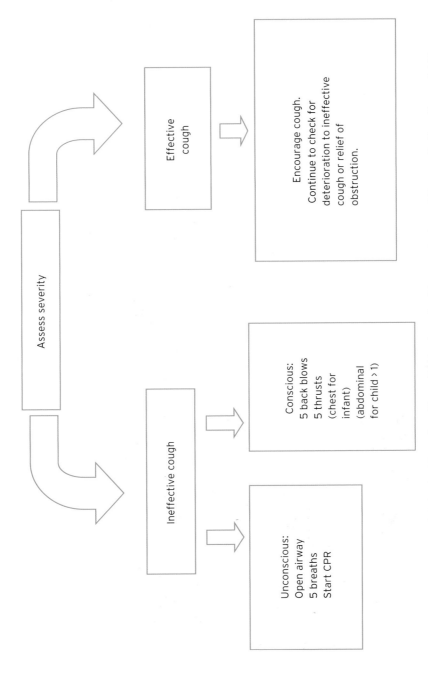

Figure 3.16 The paediatric choking algorithm. Reproduced with permission of Resuscitation Council UK.

2. If the patient shows signs of severe airway obstruction and is conscious:
   - Give up to five back blows as with the adult patient (see Figure 3.14 above).
3. If back blows do not relieve the FBAO then provide chest thrusts to infants or abdominal thrusts with children.
4. Back blows in an infant:
   - Support the infant in a head down position to allow for gravity to assist in removing the foreign body.
   - A seated or kneeling position may assist in this with the child across the lap.
   - Support the infants head by placing the thumb of one hand at the angle of the jaw and one or two fingers of the same hand at the same point on the other side of the jaw.
   - Deliver up to five sharp back blows with the heel of the other hand, aiming to relieve the obstruction with each blow.
5. In a child over 1 year this may be achieved with the same technique, or if a large child support the child in a forward position as with adults.
6. Chest thrusts are performed in the same way as with adults i.e. using a chest compression but sharper and at a slower rate.
7. Abdominal thrusts should only be performed in children over 1 year of age using the same technique as with adults. This is due to increased likelihood of underlying intra-abdominal injury in the younger child.
8. The cycle of back blows and abdominal thrusts or chest thrusts (in the child under 1) should continue until the obstruction is cleared.
9. In the unconscious child CPR should be commenced as with Paediatric Basic Life Support.

Chapter Key Points

1. Basic life support and foreign body airway obstruction is age specific. It is essential that you are comfortable with the processes involved in each age group so that you are less anxious and more prepared in the event of attending a paediatric or adult cardiac arrest or choking.
2. There is a clear step by step approach to resuscitation across the age continuum provided by the Resuscitation Council (UK) that is based upon current best evidence and provides standardised care.

References and Further reading

1 Resuscitation Council UK *Resuscitation Guidelines*. Resuscitation Council, UK, 2005.
2 Nichol G, Stiell I, Laupacis A, Pham B, Maio V, Wells G. A cumulative meta-analysis of the effectiveness of defibrillator-capable emergency medical services for victims of out-of-hospital cardiac arrest. *Ann Emerg Med* 1999;34:517–525.
3 Boon N, Colledge N, Walker B. (Eds) *Davidson's Principles and Practice of Medicine*, 20th edn. London: Churchill-Livingstone, 2006.
4 Deakin C, O'Neill J, Tabor T. Does compression only cardiopulmonary resuscitation generate adequate passive ventilation during cardiac arrest? *Resuscitation* 2007;75:53–59.

5 Becker L, Ostrander M, Barrett J, Kondos J. Outcome of CPR in a large metropolitan area – where are the survivors? *Ann Emerg Med* 1991;20(4):355-361.

6 Bang A, Biber B, Isaksson L, Lindqvist J, Herlitz J. Evaluation of dispatcher assisted cardio-pulmonary resuscitation. *Eur J Emerg Med* 1999;6(3):175-183.

7 Eisenberg M, Hallstrom A, Carter W, Cummins R, Bergner L, Pierce J. Emergency CPR instruction via telephone. *Am J Pub Health* 1985;75(1):47-50.

8 Engdahl J, Bang A, Lindqvist J, Herlitz J. Factors affecting short and long term prognosis among 1069 patients with out of hospital cardiac arrest and pulseless electrical activity. *Resuscitation* 2001;51(1):17-25.

9 Gallagher E, Lombardi G, Gennis P. Effectiveness of bystander cardiopulmonary resuscitation and survival following out of hospital cardiac arrest. *J Am Med Ass* 1995;274(24): 1922-1925.

10 Berg R, Sanders A, Kern K, Hilwig R, Heidenreich J, Porter M, Ewy G. Adverse hemodynamic effects of interrupting chest compressions for rescue breathing during cardiopulmonary resuscitation for ventricular fibrillation cardiac arrest. *Circulation* 2001;104:2465-2470.

11 Bahr J, Klingler H, Panzer W, Rode H, Kettler D. Skills of lay people in checking the carotid pulse. *Resuscitation* 1997;35:23-26.

12 Hauff S, Rea T, Culley L, Kerry F, Becker L, Eisenberg M. Factors impeding dispatcher assisted telephone cardiopulmonary resuscitation. *Ann Emerg Med* 2003;42:731-737.

13 International Consensus Conference on Cardiopulmonary Resuscitation and Emergency Cardiovascular Care Science: European Resuscitation Council. European Resuscitation Council Guidelines for Resuscitation. *Resuscitation* 2005;67S1:S7-S23.

14 Kern KB, Hilwig RW, Berg RA, Sanders AB, Ewy GA. Importance of continuous chest compressions during cardiopulmonary resuscitation: improved outcome during a simulated single lay-rescuer scenario. *Circulation* 2002;105:645-649.

15 Paradis NA, Martin GB, Goetting MG *et al.* Simultaneous aortic, jugular bulb, and right atrial pressures during cardiopulmonary resuscitation in humans. Insights into mechanisms. *Circulation* 1989;80:361-368.

16 Handley J. Teaching hand placement for chest compression – a simpler technique. *Resuscitation* 2002;53:29-36.

17 Ditchey R, Winkler J, Rhodes C. Relative lack of coronary blood flow during closed chest resuscitation in dogs. *Circulation* 1982;66:297-302.

18 Bellamy R, DeGuzman L, Pedersen D. Coronary blood flow during cardiopulmonary resuscitation in swine. *Circulation* 1984;69:174-180.

19 Tomlison A, Nyaether J, Kramer-Johansen J, Steen P, Dorph E. Compression force-depth relationship during out of hospital cardiopulmonary resuscitation. *Resuscitation* 2007;72: 364-370.

20 Ristagno G, Tang W, Jorgenson D, Russell J, Wang T, Sun S, Weil M. Effects of variable depth of chest compression on outcomes of CPR. *Circulation* 2006;114:1205-1206.

21 Sanders AB, Kern KB, Berg RA, Hilwig RW, Heidenrich J, Ewy GA. Survival and neurologic outcome after cardiopulmonary resuscitation with four different chest compression-ventilation ratios. *Ann Emerg Med* 2002;40:553-562.

22 Hostler D, Rittenberger J, Roth R, Callaway C. Increased chest compression to ventilation ratio improves delivery of CPR. *Resuscitation* 2007;74:446-452.

23 Olasveengen T, Wik L, Kramer-Johansen J, Sunde K, Pytte M, Steen P. Is CPR quality improving? A retrospective study of out of hospital cardiac arrest. *Circulation* 2007;116:384.

24 Kern KB, Hilwig RW, Berg RA, Sanders AB, Ewy GA. Importance of continuous chest compressions during cardiopulmonary resuscitation: improved outcome during a simulated single lay-rescuer scenario. *Circulation* 2002;105:645-649.

25 Becker LB, Berg RA, Pepe PE *et al.* A reappraisal of mouth to-mouth ventilation during bystander-initiated cardiopulmonary resuscitation. A statement for healthcare professionals from the Ventilation Working Group of the Basic Life Support and Pediatric Life Support Subcommittees, American Heart Association. *Resuscitation* 1997;35:189-201.

26 Bohm K, Rosenqvist M, Herlitz J, Hollenberg J, Svensson L. Survival is similar after standard treatment and chest compression only in out of hospital bystander cardiopulmonary resuscitation. *Circulation* 2007;116:2908-2912.

27 Iwami T, Kawamura T, Hiraide A *et al.* Effectiveness of bystander-initiated cardiac only resuscitation for patients with out of hospital cardiac arrest. *Circulation* 2007;116:2900-2907.

28 Berg RA, Kern KB, Hilwig RW, Ewy GA. Assisted ventilation during 'bystander' CPR in a swine acute myocardial infarction model does not improve outcome. *Circulation* 1997;96:4364-4371.

29 Deakin C, O'Neill J, Tabor T. Does compression only cardiopulmonary resuscitation generate adequate passive ventilation during cardiac arrest. *Resuscitation* 2007;75:53-59.

30 Morris S, Stacey M. ABC of resuscitation: resuscitation in pregnancy. *Br Med J* 2003;327:1277-1279.

31 Joint Royal Colleges Ambulance Liaison Committee. *UK Ambulance Service Clinical Practice Guidelines.* London: JRCALC, 2006.

32 Grady K, Howell C, Cox C. *Managing Obstetric Emergencies and Trauma: The MOET Course Manual*, 2nd edn. London: Royal College of Obstetricians and Gynaecologists, 2007.

33 Stapleton E. Comparing CPR during ambulance transport: Manual versus mechanical methods. *J Emerg Med Serv* 1991;16(9):63-72.

34 Steen S, Liao Q, Pierre L, Paskevisius A, Sjoberg T. Evaluation of LUCAS, a new device for automatic mechanical compression and active decompression resuscitation. *Resuscitation* 2002;55(3):285-299.

35 Rubertsson S, Karlsten R. Increased cortical cerebral blood flow with LUCAS; a new device for mechanical chest compressions compared to standard external compressions during experimental cardiopulmonary resuscitation. *Resuscitation* 2005;65:357-363.

36 Lafuente-Lafuente C, Melero-Bascones M. *Active chest compression – decompression for cardiopulmonary resuscitation.* Cochrane Database Systematic Review CD002751, 2004.

37 Berg RA, Hilwig RW, Kern KB, Babar I, Ewy GA. Simulated mouth-to-mouth ventilation and chest compressions (bystander cardiopulmonary resuscitation) improves outcome in a swine model of prehospital pediatric asphyxial cardiac arrest. *Crit Care Med* 1999;27:1893-1899.

38 Dorph E, Wik L, Steen PA. Effectiveness of ventilation compression ratios 1:5 and 2:15 in simulated single rescuer paediatric resuscitation. *Resuscitation* 2002;54:259-264.

39 Turner I, Turner S, Armstrong V. Does the compression to ventilation ratio affect the quality of CPR: a simulation study. *Resuscitation* 2002;52:55-62.

40 Whyte SD, Wyllie JP. Paediatric basic life support: a practical assessment. *Resuscitation* 1999;41:153-217.

41 Clements F, McGowan J. Finger position for chest compressions in cardiac arrest in infants. *Resuscitation* 2000;44:43-46.

42 Stevenson AG, McGowan J, Evans AL, Graham CA. CPR for children: one hand or two? *Resuscitation* 2005;64:205-208.

43 Ho P, Tung P, Law S, Wong J. Review of the Heimlich Manoeuvre. *Ann Coll Surg* 1999;3:7-10.

44 Langhelle A, Sunde K, Wik L, Steen P. Airway pressure with chest compressions versus Heimlich manoeuvre in recently dead adults with complete airway obstruction. *Resuscitation* 2000;44:105-108.

45 Redding JS. The choking controversy: critique of evidence on the Heimlich maneuver. *Crit Care Med* 1979;7:475-479.

46 International Liaison Committee on Resuscitation. Part 2. Adult Basic Life Support. 2005 International Consensus on Cardiopulmonary Resuscitation and Emergency Cardiovascular Care Science with Treatment Recommendations. *Resuscitation* 2005;67:187-200.

47 Ruben H, McNaughton FI. The treatment of food-choking. *Practitioner* 1978;221:725-729.

48 Day R, Crelin E, DuBois A. Choking: The Heimlich abdominal thrust vs back blows: An approach to measurement of inertial and aerodynamic forces. *Pediatrics* 1982;70(1):113-119.

49 Croom D. Rupture of stomach after attempted Heimlich manoeuvre. *J Am Med Ass* 1983;250:2602-2603.

Chapter 4

Defibrillation

Content

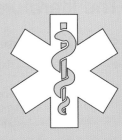

Out-of-hospital cardiac arrest is a public health problem that results in survival to hospital discharge rates of between 6% and 7%.[1] Ventricular fibrillation is the most common initial rhythm in out-of-hospital cardiac arrest[2] and has a significantly higher survival rate than patients presenting in non-shockable cardiac arrest rhythms. In some exemplary systems, survival to hospital discharge approaches 30%.[3] Early defibrillation is the key to successful resuscitation of these patients. External cardiac pacing is not commonly used in ambulance services but may have value in the management of symptomatic bradycardia that does not respond to pharmacological intervention.

Definition of defibrillation

Defibrillation is the only effective therapy for cardiac arrest caused by ventricular fibrillation and can be defined as an attempt to depolarise a critical mass of the myocardium in order to restore the synchronicity of the heart's electrical conduction system.[4] The overarching aim is to achieve the highest efficacy with the lowest possible energy and current, allowing for depolarisation of the myocardial cells with minimal or no myocardial damage.[5]

There are numerous factors that may impact on the effectiveness of defibrillation:

Scenario

You are a first responder called to attend a 55-year-old female patient in cardiac arrest following a short period of 'crushing' central chest pain. The patient has a previous history of ischaemic heart disease and has recently been discharged from hospital with unstable angina. You are the first on scene and the responding ambulance crew is not expected for another 5 minutes. The only other person at the location is the patient's mother who is 79 years of age.

1. What are your priorities with this patient given that you are the only health care professional on scene?
2. Given the history it is highly likely that this patient is in a shockable rhythm, when will you connect the defibrillator and what will you stop doing in order to achieve this?

The literature behind defibrillation

Strategies before defibrillation

Precordial thump

There is little high quality evidence to support the use of a precordial thump although 3 old case series suggest that VF or pulseless VT was converted to a perfusing rhythm by a precordial thump.[6,7,8] It has been suggested that an effective precordial thump may be delivered by the closed fist from between 5 and 40 cm.[9] There are suggestions that a precordial thump may lead to rhythm deterioration but it is not possible to judge the likelihood of this occurring. Current recommendations suggest that a single precordial thump may be considered after a monitored cardiac arrest if a defibrillator is not immediately available.[9]

CPR before defibrillation

In two studies, 1½–3 minutes of CPR by paramedics or EMS physicians before attempted defibrillation improved return of spontaneous circulation (ROSC) and survival rates for adults with out-of-hospital VF or VT when the response interval and time to defibrillation was ≥4 to 5 minutes.[10,11] A more recent trial contradicted these results and found no improvement in ROSC in adults with out-of-hospital VF or VT, in which 1 ½ minutes of paramedic CPR was delivered before defibrillation.[12] In animal studies of VF lasting 5 minutes, CPR (often with administration of epinephrine) before defibrillation improved haemodynamics and survival rates.[9]

Recommendation

In the case of out-of-hospital cardiac arrest attended, but unwitnessed, by healthcare professionals equipped with manual defibrillators, 2 minutes of CPR should be given prior to defibrillation (approximately 5 cycles of 30:2).[13]

Transthoracic impedance

Energy selection and transthoracic impedance are the two main determinants of intracardiac current flow during defibrillation. Transthoracic impedance (TTI) is the resistance to current flow created by body size and structure. Factors that determine TTI include energy selected, electrode size, paddle–skin coupling material, number and time interval of previous shocks, phase of ventilation, distance between electrodes (size of the chest), and paddle electrode pressure.[9]

Pad/paddle positioning and size

See Figure 4.1.

No human studies have evaluated the effect of pad/paddle position on defibrillation success or survival rates; most studies evaluated cardioversion or used secondary endpoints such as TTI.[9] A review of the science in 2005 suggests that placement of paddles or electrode pads on the superior-anterior right chest and the inferior-lateral left chest were effective, whilst alternative positions such as apex-posterior and anteroposterior positions were also reported to be effective.[9] Where paddles are being used it is suggested that the apical paddle should be placed longitudinally to maximise contact with the chest;[14] it is not clear if this is applicable to adhesive pads. Care should be taken to avoid placing pads or paddles directly on breast tissue as this has been shown to increase TTI.[15]

One human study[16] and one animal study[17] documented higher success rates with larger 12.8 cm paddles compared with 8 cm paddles. A number of studies have reported reduced TTI with larger paddles[15,18-23] and one animal study has shown significant myocardial damage when using small (4.3 cm electrodes) when compared with 8 cm or 12.8 cm pads.[24]

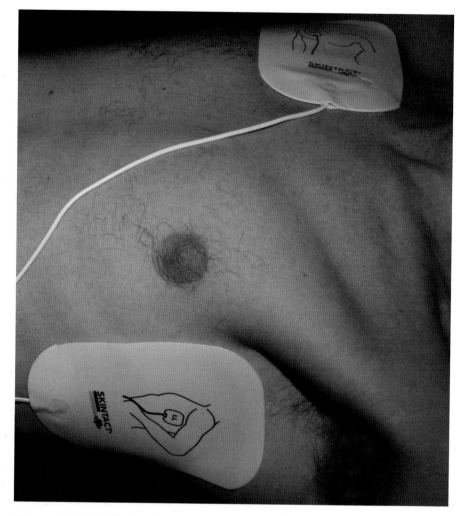

Figure 4.1 Defibrillation electrode position.

Recommendations[9]

- Pads should be placed on the superior-anterior right chest and inferior lateral left chest where possible.
- In large-breasted women it is reasonable to place the left electrode pad/paddle lateral to or beneath the breast, where paddles are used; the apical paddle should be placed longitudinally.
- Defibrillation success may be improved with 12.3 cm pads rather than 8 cm pads, small pads should be avoided to reduce the risk of myocardial injury.
- Where paddles are being used, the apical paddle should be placed longitudinally.

Adhesive pads or paddles?

Several studies reported in the 2005 International Consensus on Cardiopulmonary Resuscitation suggest that levels of TTI are similar with both paddles and pads. It has been suggested that TTI is reduced where an optimum 8 kg of pressure is applied to paddles but there are several safety and practical advantages to the use of pads, particularly in the prehospital environment.[9]

Ventilation status

During the inspiratory cycle the patient's lungs are filling with air, which increases TTI. Delivering shocks at the end of expiration when the lungs are deflated will reduce TTI and increase the chances of successful defibrillation.[4]

Recommendations

- Adhesive pads are safe and effective and suitable as an alternative to paddles.
- Defibrillation should coincide with the peak of expiration to minimise TTI.

Defibrillation waveform

Biphasic v monophasic defibrillation

Defibrillation waveforms are complex interventions; it is not important to understand the waveforms used by these defibrillators but it is important that the most effective devices are used. Monophasic waveforms vary in the speed at which the waveform returns to the zero voltage point - gradually (damped sinusoidal) or instantaneously (truncated exponential) - and deliver a current that proceeds in a single direction.[25] All new defibrillators produce a biphasic waveform, which means that the current flows initially in a positive direction and then, after a predetermined time reverses to a negative direction. The modern generation of biphasic defibrillators are calibrated to alter the waveform delivered to the patient based on TTI (that is, impedance compensated biphasic waveforms (ICB)). These devices aim to deliver a shock 'dose' that is proportional to each patient.[26]

This waveform has been shown to be more effective than the monophasic waveform defibrillators,[27] and is successful with fewer shocks.[28] Biphasic defibrillators are smaller and lighter than monophasic defibrillators and use lower energy levels so require less battery power.

Recommendation

- Biphasic waveform shocks are safe and effective for termination of VF when compared with monophasic waveform shocks.[9]

Energy levels for defibrillation

A metanalysis identified insufficient evidence for or against a specific energy level for either first or subsequent shocks when using a defibrillator.[9] It is reasonable to use energy levels of 150-200 joules with BTE waveform biphasic defibrillators, and 120 joules with the rectilinear biphasic waveform. An initial shock of 360 joules is considered reasonable when using a monophasic waveform defibrillator.[9]

Automated external defibrillation

Automated external defibrillators (AED) are sophisticated, computerised devices that deliver defibrillatory shocks to those in cardiac arrest caused by VF or ventricular tachycardia (VT).[29] AEDs use voice and visual prompts to guide the practitioner in the delivery of defibrillatory shocks and have become more sophisticated and safer over recent years. For AEDs to perform reliable ECG signal analysis and make a shock/no-shock decision, CPR must be discontinued due to the artefacts introduced by chest compressions and ventilations;[30] this introduces periods where there is no blood flow from compressions. One study identified that patients were not perfused for approximately 50% of the time when an AED was used in out-of-hospital cardiac arrest.[31] Animal studies have shown these delays to be linked to a worse outcome in cases of prolonged VF.[32]

A number of studies indicate that the use of AEDs by trained lay and professional responders has significantly improved the outcome for those who suffer an out-of-hospital VF cardiac arrest where an effective response plan is in place.[33-37] The evidence for the use of AEDs by trained responders (e.g. police and fire) is less clear with some studies indicating improved survival whilst others show no improvement.[9]

Recommendations

Use of AEDs by trained lay and professional responders is recommended to increase survival rates in patients with cardiac arrest. Use of AEDs in public settings (airports, casinos, sports facilities, etc) where witnessed cardiac arrest is likely to occur can be useful if an effective response plan is in place.[9] In order to minimise the time where there is no blood flow due to interruptions in compressions, professional ambulance staff should be trained in and have the use of manual defibrillators.

Procedure for defibrillation

Procedure	Additional information/ rationale
1. Perform CPR until defibrillator/monitor is attached.	Maximises perfusion whilst awaiting equipment.
2. Prepare patient's chest. Check for: • Patches (e.g. GTN) remove if found. • Jewellery or piercings in the pathway of defibrillation; remove if found. • Moisture: dry wet chests. • Pacemaker sites: avoid defibrillating over pacemaker sites. • Underwired bras: remove if found.	Maximises contact between pads and chest and reduces TTI.

Procedure	Additional information/ rationale
2. It may be necessary to shave chest hair for pad positioning but this should not delay defibrillation if no razor is available.	
3. Place the right (sternal) electrode to the right of the sternum, below the clavicle, and the apical paddle vertically in the mid-axillary line, approximately level with the V6 ECG electrode position or the female breast.	Ensures that the current passes through a critical mass of the myocardium.
4. Assess rhythm.	To identify shockable or non-shockable rhythm.
5. Select appropriate energy for defibrillator.	
6. Use strong verbal commands: 'VF/VT seen' 'Charging at 150 joules' (energy stated here is an example only).	Ensure safety during defibrillation
7. Confirm that nobody is in direct or indirect contact with the patient. Consider commands such as: 'Top, middle, bottom clear' whilst checking those specific areas of the patient.	
8. Ensure that oxygen is off and intravenous lines are down.	
9. State: 'stand clear'.	
10. Perform a final quick visual check to ensure that everyone is clear.	
11. Deliver shock.	
12. Immediately recommence CPR irrespective of the presenting rhythm.	

Definition of transcutaneous cardiac pacing (TCP)

External (transcutaneous) pacing is a temporary method of pacing a patient's heart during an emergency. Pulses of electrical current are delivered through the patient's chest to stimulate the cardiac muscle to contract. It restores electrical stimulation to the myocardium in an emergency setting and can be initiated quickly by any healthcare professional who has undertaken the necessary training.[38]

Terminology used in transcutaneous cardiac pacing

- **Capture:** The presence of a QRS complex after a pacing spike (electrical capture). If the patient has a palpable pulse consistent with the heart rate on the monitor then mechanical capture has also been achieved.
- **Demand pacing:** The provision of a pacing stimulus only when the patient's heart rate falls below a predetermined limit.
- **Fist (percussion) pacing:** The use of serial rhythmic blows with the closed fist over the left lower edge of the sternum to pace the heart. This will only be used in the emergency setting in P-wave asystole and profound bradycardia resulting in clinical cardiac arrest.[39]
- **Fixed-rate pacing:** The provision of a pacing stimulus irrespective of the patient's intrinsic heart rate.
- **Threshold:** The minimum energy required to maintain consistent capture.

Indications for use of transcutaneous cardiac pacing

The European Resuscitation Council Guidelines for resuscitation 2005 advocate TCP in bradycardia where there is no response to atropine, if atropine is unlikely to be effective or if the patient is severely symptomatic, particularly if there is high-degree block (Möbitz Type II or third-degree block).[40] The Joint Royal Colleges Ambulance Liaison Committee (JRCALC) also advocates the use of TCP where available.[41]

THINK

How does atropine work?
Can you explain how the different heart blocks manifest themselves on the ECG and relate them to the electrophysiology of the heart?

The literature behind transcutaneous cardiac pacing

There are few studies evaluating the use of transcutaneous pacing in the prehospital environment and all are over 15 years old. The conclusion of a systematic review of the literature suggests that there is no evidence to support the use of TCP in bradyasystolic cardiac arrest, and inadequate evidence to determine the efficacy of prehospital TCP in the treatment of symptomatic bradycardia.[42] However, temporary pacing has become the standard method for providing immediate treatment of severe bradycardias and certain tachycardias for the past 20 years.[43]

A pilot study has been undertaken to assess the feasibility of undertaking a randomised controlled trial (RCT) to evaluate the safety and effectiveness of prehospital TCP;[44] its results may help provide further evidence to support or refute the use of prehospital TCP.

Equipment

- Defibrillator/ECG monitor with TCP function.
- Pacing pads.
- Scissors.
- Analgesia may also be required.

Skin preparation

Prepare the patient by removing excess hair; this will help to improve contact between the electrodes and the patient's skin. It is recommended that scissors are used for this rather than a razor as any nicks in the skin can cause burns and excessive discomfort.[45,46] Consider cleaning the patient's skin with alcohol to remove salt residue from sweat as this has been linked to increased discomfort and a reduction in the effectiveness of pacing.[47]

Pad positioning

The positioning of the electrodes will depend upon whether the electrodes used are multi-function electrodes (MFE) capable of defibrillation and pacing, or pacing only electrodes.

Pacing only electrodes

An anterior/posterior (AP) position is recommended for use so that defibrillation pads can be applied rapidly in the event that defibrillation becomes necessary. The anterior electrode is placed on the left anterior chest (i.e. left of the sternum) centred over the position for lead V3. The posterior electrode should be placed to the left of the thoracic vertebrae, opposite the anterior electrode position.[45]

Multi-function electrodes

These electrodes are capable of defibrillation and monitoring as well as pacing. They must be placed in a position where defibrillation and chest compressions can be performed if required. Either an AP position or a right pectoral and apical position may be chosen. The AP position is preferred but should not be used if the patient is in cardiac arrest as compressions should not be interrupted to allow placement of the posterior electrode.[39]

Procedure for TCP

Procedure	Additional information/ rationale
1. Explain the procedure to the patient, gain consent and co-operation.	Legal requirement.
2. Attach ECG electrodes to the patient and connect to the ECG monitor.	
3. Prepare the patient's chest.	Reduces discomfort and improves effectiveness of pacing.
4. Remove excess hair (preferably trim with scissors) and consider cleaning chest with alcohol.	Improves electrode contact whilst reducing discomfort.
5. Following the instructions on the package, apply the MFE or pacing electrodes and connect to the pacing machine.	
6. Select the appropriate pacing mode – demand pacing is normally selected in the emergency setting.	
7. Set an appropriate rate; normally 60-90 beats/minute.[45] Start the output at the lowest setting and gradually increase until electrical capture is gained.	If the bradycardia was extreme, it is recommended that the initial pacing rate be lowered.[39]
8. The output needs to be higher than the threshold so it is recommended that output is increased by about 2mA.[45]	Allows capture to be maintained once threshold has been reached.
9. Monitor the patient's heart rate and rhythm to assess ventricular response to pacing; assess the haemodynamic response by palpating central pulses and taking blood pressure.[38]	Ensures mechanical as well as electrical capture and assesses the patient's physiological response to the procedure.
10. Administer analgesia as required and per guidelines.	To minimise pain.
11. Monitor and adjust output if capture is lost.	

Chapter Key Points

1. Defibrillation is the only effective therapy for cardiac arrest caused by ventricular fibrillation and can be defined as an attempt to depolarise a critical mass of the myocardium in order to restore the synchronicity of the heart's electrical conduction system.
2. A 1½ to 3-minute period of CPR may be considered before attempting defibrillation in adults with out-of-hospital VF or pulseless VT when the EMS response (call to arrival) interval is >4 to 5 minutes
3. Adhesive pads are safe and effective and suitable as an alternative to paddles.
4. Defibrillation should coincide with the peak of expiration to minimise TTI.
5. External (transcutaneous) pacing is a temporary method of pacing a patient's heart during an emergency.
6. The European Resuscitation Council Guidelines for resuscitation 2005 advocate TCP in bradycardia where there is no response to atropine, if atropine is unlikely to be effective or if the patient is severely symptomatic, particularly if there is high-degree block (Möbitz Type II second- or third-degree block).

References and Further reading

1 Nichol G, Stiell IG, Laupacis A, Pham B, De Maio VJ, Wells GA. A cumulative meta-analysis of the effectiveness of defibrillator-capable emergency medical services for victims of out-of-hospital cardiac arrest. *Ann Emerg Med* 1999;34:517-525.
2 Kuisma M, Repo J, Alaspää A. The incidence of out-of-hospital ventricular fibrillation in Helsinki, Finland, from 1994 to 1999. *Lancet* 2001;358(9280):473-474.
3 Cobb LA, Fahrenbruch CE, Walsh TR *et al.*, Influence of cardiopulmonary resuscitation prior to defibrillation in patients with out-of-hospital ventricular fibrillation. *JAMA* 1999;281:1182-1188.
4 Graham-Garcia J, Heath J, Andrews J. Defibrillation and biphasic shocks: Implications for perianesthesia nursing. *J Perianesthes Nurs* 2005;20(1):23-34.
5 Weisfeldt ML, Kerber RE, McGoldrick RP *et al.* American Heart Association Report on the Public Access Defibrillation Conference, December 8-10, 1994. Automatic External Defibrillation Task Force. *Circulation* 1995;92:2740-2747.
6 Befeler B. Mechanical stimulation of the heart: its therapeutic value in tachyarrhythmias. *Chest* 1978;73:832-838.
7 Volkmann HK, Klumbies A, Kühnert H, Paliege R, Dannberg G, Siegert K. Terminierung von Kammertachykardien durch mechanische Herzstimulation mit Präkordialschlägen [Terminating ventricular tachycardias by mechanical heart stimulation with precordial thumps]. *Z Kardiol* 1990;79:717-724.
8 Caldwell G, Millar G, Quinn E. Simple mechanical methods for cardioversion: defence of the precordial thump and cough version. *BMJ* 1985;291:627-630.
9 International Consensus on Cardiopulmonary Resuscitation. Part 3, Defibrillation. *Circulation* 2005;112:III-17-III-24.
10 Cobb LA, Fahrenbruch CE, Walsh TR, Copass MK, Olsufka M, Breskin M, Hallstrom AP. Influence of cardiopulmonary resuscitation prior to defibrillation in patients with out-of-hospital ventricular fibrillation. *JAMA* 1999;281:1182-1188.

11 Wik L, Hansen TB, Fylling F, Steen T, Vaagenes P, Auestad BH, Steen PA. Delaying defibrillation to give basic cardiopulmonary resuscitation to patients with out-of-hospital ventricular fibrillation: a randomized trial. *JAMA* 2003;289:1389-1395.

12 Jacobs IG, Finn JC, Oxer HF, Jelinek GA. CPR before defibrillation in out-of-hospital cardiac arrest: a randomized trial. *Emerg Med Australas* 2005;17:39-45.

13 Resuscitation Council (UK). *Adult Advanced Life Support.* Resuscitation Guidelines 2005 available online at www.resus.org.uk

14 Deakin CD, Sado DM, Petley GW, Clewlow F. Is the orientation of the apical defibrillation paddle of importance during manual external defibrillation? *Resuscitation* 2003;56:15-18.

15 Pagan-Carlo LA, Spencer KT, Robertson CE, Dengler A, Birkett C, Kerber RE. Transthoracic defibrillation: importance of avoiding electrode placement directly on the female breast. *J Am Coll Cardiol* 1996;27:449-452.

16 Dalzell GW, Cunningham SR, Anderson J, Adgey AA. Electrode pad size, transthoracic impedance and success of external ventricular defibrillation. *Am J Cardiol* 1989;64:741-744.

17 Thomas ED, Ewy GA, Dahl CF, Ewy MD. Effectiveness of direct current defibrillation: role of paddle electrode size. *Am Heart J* 1977;93:463-467.

18 Kerber RE, Grayzel J, Hoyt R, Marcus M, Kennedy J. Transthoracic resistance in human defibrillation: influence of body weight, chest size, serial shocks, paddle size and paddle contact pressure. *Circulation* 1981;63:676-682.

19 Dalzell GW, Cunningham SR, Anderson J, Adgey AA. Electrode pad size, transthoracic impedance and success of external ventricular defibrillation. *Am J Cardiol* 1989;64:741-744.

20 Samson RA, Atkins DL, Kerber RE. Optimal size of self-adhesive preapplied electrode pads in pediatric defibrillation. *Am J Cardiol* 1995;75:544-545.

21 Atkins DL, Sirna S, Kieso R, Charbonnier F, Kerber RE. Pediatric defibrillation: importance of paddle size in determining transthoracic impedance. *Pediatrics* 1988;82:914-918.

22 Atkins DL, Kerber RE. Pediatric defibrillation: current flow is improved by using 'adult' electrode paddles. *Pediatrics* 1994;94:90-93.

23 Killingsworth CR, Melnick SB, Chapman FW, Walker RG, Smith WM, Ideker RE, Walcott GP. Defibrillation threshold and cardiac responses using an external biphasic defibrillator with pediatric and adult adhesive patches in pediatric-sized piglets. *Resuscitation* 2002;55: 177-185.

24 Dahl CF, Ewy GA, Warner ED, Thomas ED. Myocardial necrosis from direct current counter-shock: effect of paddle electrode size and time interval between discharges. *Circulation* 1974;50:956-961.

25 Cummins RO, Hazinski MF, Kerber RE *et al.* Low-Energy Biphasic Waveform Defibrillation: Evidence-Based Review Applied to Emergency Cardiovascular Care Guidelines : A Statement for Healthcare Professionals From the American Heart Association Committee on Emergency Cardiovascular Care and the Subcommittees on Basic Life Support, Advanced Cardiac Life Support, and Pediatric Resuscitation. *Circulation* 1998;97:1654-1667.

26 Adgey AAJ, Spence MS, Walsh SJ. Theory and practice of defibrillation: (2) defibrillation for ventricular fibrillation. *Heart* 2005;91:118-125.

27 International Liaison Committee on Resuscitation. Part 3: Defibrillation. *Circulation* 2005;67:203-211.

28 Page RL, Kerber RE, Russell JK, Trouton T, Waktare J, Gallik D *et al.* for the BiCard Investigators. Biphasic versus monophasic shock waveform for conversion of atrial fibrillation. *J Am Coll Cardiol* 2002;39:1956-1963.

29 Handley AJ, Koster R, Monsieurs K, Perkins GD, Davies S, Bossaert L. European Resuscitation Council Guidelines for Resuscitation 2005 Section 2. Adult basic life support and use of automated external defibrillators. *Resuscitation* 2005;67S1:S7-S23.

30 Eilevstjønn J, Kramer-Johansen J, Eftestøl T, Stavland M, Myklebust H, Steen PA. Reducing no flow times during automated external defibrillation. *Resuscitation* 2005;67:95-101.

31 International Liaison Committee on Resuscitation. Part 3: Defibrillation. *Resuscitation* 2005;67:203-211.

32 Berg RA, Hilwig RW, Kern KB, Sanders AB, Xavier LC, Ewy GA. Automated external defibril-lation versus manual defibrillation for prolonged ventricular fibrillation: lethal delays of chest compressions before and after countershocks. *Ann Emerg Med* 2003;42:458-467.

33 The Public Access Defibrillation Trial Investigators. Public-access defibrillation and survival after out-of-hospital cardiac arrest. *N Engl J Med* 2004;351:637-646.

34 Valenzuela TD, Roe DJ, Nichol G, Clark LL, Spaite DW, Hardman RG. Outcomes of rapid defibrillation by security officers after cardiac arrest in casinos. *N Engl J Med* 2000;343:1206-1209.

35 Caffrey SL, Willoughby PJ, Pepe PE, Becker LB. Public use of automated external defibril-lators. *N Engl J Med* 2002;347:1242-1247.

36 O'Rourke MF, Donaldson E, Geddes JS. An airline cardiac arrest program. *Circulation* 1997;96:2849-2853.

37 Page RL, Joglar JA, Kowal RC, Zagrodzky JD, Nelson LL, Ramaswamy K, Barbera SJ, Hamdan MH, McKenas DK. Use of automated external defibrillators by a US airline. *N Engl J Med* 2000;343:1210-1216.

38 Gibson T. A practical guide to external cardiac pacing. *Nurs Stand* 2008;22(20):45-48.

39 Resuscitation Council UK. *Advanced Life Support*, 5th edn. London: Resuscitation Council UK, 2006.

40 Nolan JP, Deakin CD, Soar J, Böttiger BW, Smith G. European Resuscitation Council Guide-lines for Resuscitation 2005 Section 4. Adult advanced life support. *Resuscitation* 2005;67S1:S39-S86.

41 Fisher JD, Brown SN, Cooke MW (Eds) *UK Ambulance Service Clinical Practice Guidelines 2006*. Norwich: IHCD, 2006.

42 Sherbino J, Verbeek PR, MacDonald RD, Sawadsky BV, McDonald AC, Morrison LJ. Prehos-pital transcutaneous cardiac pacing for symptomatic bradycardia or bradyasystolic cardiac arrest: A systematic review. *Resuscitation* 2006;70:193-200.

43 Abate E, Kusumoto FM, Goldschlager NF. *Cardiac Pacing for the Clinician*. United States, Springer, 2007.

44 Morrison LJ, Long J, Vermeulen M, Schwartz B, Sawadsky B, Frank J, Cameron B, Burgess R, Shield J, Bagley P, Mauszl V, Brewer JE, Dorian P. A randomized controlled feasibility trial comparing safety and effectiveness of prehospital pacing versus conventional treat-ment: 'PrePACE'. *Resuscitation* 2008;76:341-349.

45 Craig K. How to provide transcutaneous pacing. *Nursing* 2005;35(10):52-53.

46 Jevon P. Cardiac Monitoring, Part 3. *Nursing Times* 2007;103(3):26-27.

47 Ellenbogen KA, Wood MA. *Cardiac Pacing and ICDs*. Oxford: Blackwell Publishing, 2005.

Chapter 5

Cardiovascular observations and examination techniques

Content

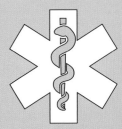

Assessment of vital signs is a very important aspect of health care and assessment as these can rapidly reflect basic health status or manifestations of physiological and psychological reactions of stress or disease processes. Vital signs or observations include areas such as pulse rate, respiratory rate, blood pressure and temperature, in addition, in advancing healthcare investigations such as blood glucose measurements, peak expiratory flow and oxygen saturations are common clinical observations that are measured.

In understanding disease processes and homeostatic mechanisms the body's physiological responses can be assessed through the accurate measurement of such vital signs. Therefore the ability to undertake and perform correct observation techniques is essential in patient monitoring. This chapter will guide the practitioner through the process of performing vital sign measurements and provide a theoretical underpinning for each skill using best evidence.

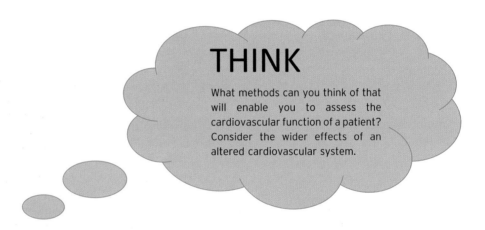

THINK

What methods can you think of that will enable you to assess the cardiovascular function of a patient? Consider the wider effects of an altered cardiovascular system.

The assessment of pulses

A pulse is the alternating expansion and recoil of arteries during each cardiac cycle; it is felt as the pressure wave passes through the arterial tree.[1] A pulse can be palpated in any artery that lies close to the surface of the body by compressing the artery against firm tissue such as bone; this provides a simple method of counting heart rate. Due to accessibility the radial pulse is the most routinely used, the radial artery surfaces prominently at the wrist. However there are a variety of sites that can be utilised and may be clinically important; these include:

- The carotid artery
- The subclavian artery
- The brachial artery
- The aorta
- The ulna artery
- The femoral artery
- The popliteal artery
- The dorsalis pedis artery.

The locations of and flow of these can be found in the majority of anatomy and physiology textbooks or on-line.

Indications for measuring a pulse

A pulse is taken for a variety of reasons, both clinically and psychologically, these include:

* To gather information on the patients cardiovascular status
* To gain a baseline measurement for future review and monitoring
* To provide reassurance and gain a bond with patients who may be anxious.

The pulse is palpated to assess for the following:

* Rate
* Rhythm
* Amplitude.

Pulse rate

Normal pulse rates vary across client groups with factors such as age (see Table 5.1) and health status affecting rate. The pulse may also vary due to posture, for example a healthy adult male may have a pulse of 66 beats per minute when laying down, however this may rise to 70 when sitting up and rise again to 80 upon standing. This may rise further during times of distress or vigorous exercise; rates of between 140-180 are not unusual at these times.[1]

A normal adult resting pulse rate is between 60-100 bpm,[2] with rates below 60 bpm termed as bradycardic and greater than 100 bpm tachycardic. These definitions are however arbitrary and should be taken in context of the clinical situation. There are numerous causes of both fast and slow pulse rates, examples of these can be seen in Table 5.2.

The pulse rate is a major factor in cardiac output, cardiac output is the volume of blood ejected by each ventricle per minute. This is a factor of stroke volume which is the volume pumped by each contraction of the ventricle and the heart rate. The relationship between these is shown in the following equation:

$$\text{Cardiac output} = \text{heart rate} \times \text{stroke volume}$$

The pulse rate of a healthy individual tends to be relatively constant, however in disease states or injury the stroke volume can be reduced, this is especially prominent in damage to cardiac muscle and reduced blood volume states.[2] In these cases cardiac output can only be maintained by increases in heart rate.

Table 5.1 Normal pulse rates per minute across the age continuum

Age (years)	<1	2-5	5-12	>12
Pulse range	110-160	95-140	80-120	60-100

Table 5.2 Causes of bradycardia and tachycardia, adapted from Douglas G, Nicol F, Robertson C. (2005) *Macleod's Clinical Examination*. London: Elsevier.[2]

Fast heart rate (tachycardia)	Slow heart rate (bradycardia)
Exercise	Sleep
Pain	Athletic training
Excitement/anxiety	Hypothyroidism
Fever	Medication (beta blockers, digoxin)
Medication (sympathomimetics, vasodilators)	Complete and second degree heart block
Hyperthyroidism	Sick sinus syndrome
Cardiac arrhythmia (atrial fibrillation, atrial flutter, supraventricular tachycardia, ventricular tachycardia)	Carotid sinus sensitivity

Pulse rhythm

The rhythm of a pulse is regular in health, due to the co-ordination of the cardiac muscle fibres. The heart has an independent, co-ordinated conduction system that is a function of gap junctions and the hearts intrinsic cardiac conduction system.[1,3] Gap junctions in cardiac muscle cells form interconnections between adjacent cells allowing for the passing of charged ions and therefore nervous impulses from cell to cell. The intrinsic cardiac conduction system consists of a group of non-contractile cardiac cells specialised in initiating and distributing impulses throughout the heart, so that it depolarises and contracts in an orderly manner.[1]

It is important to identify any irregularity of the pulse rhythm, considering whether this is a permanent change or an intermittent problem. A normal pulse may be altered by extra systoles, ectopic beats or cardiac arrhythmia. Common causes of an irregular pulse can be seen Box 5.1.

Often the pulse wave produced by an extra systole is difficult to palpate at the wrist as it is too weak, therefore this may produce a pulse deficit where the pulse felt at the wrist differs from the heart rate at the apex of the heart.[2] Ventricular ectopic beats (extra beats originating from within the ventricles) are followed by a compensatory diastolic pause to allow for increased ventricular filling, thus a delayed beat is noted following the extra systole.

The presence arrhythmias such as atrial fibrillation or second degree heart block cause an irregularity in pulse rhythm due to loss of co-ordination of the electrical conduction system this may be through rapid electrical discharge or delayed discharge. Pulse rhythms can be classed either regular or irregular, however variations exist as seen in Table 5.3.

Sinus arrhythmia
Atrial extrasystoles
Ventricular extrasystoles
Atrial fibrillation
Second degree heart block

Box 5.1 Common causes of an irregular pulse[2]

Table 5.3 Heart rate rhythm abnormalities[4]

Regular	Self explanatory. It should be noted that heart rate can accelerate with inspiration and decrease with expiration in the normal adult. This is due to reduced tone of the vagus nerve (which slows the heart) during inspiration[6]. This is often referred to as sinus arrhythmia.
Irregularly irregular	This is a completely random pattern of pulsation. This is normally associated with atrial fibrillation where irregular impulses reach the ventricles causing irregular pulsation with no discernable pattern.
Regularly irregular	It is possible to have an irregular beat that occurs in a regular pattern. This is commonly seen in second degree heart blocks and pulsus bigeminus.
Regular with ectopics	A normal heart rate may be interrupted by a beat that is out of sequence making the pulse feel irregularly irregular. This requires electrocardiography to confirm.

Pulse volume/character

Also referred to as amplitude, the strength of a pulse is a reflection of force of ejection of blood from the ventricles and the elasticity of the arterial wall. The flexibility of an elastic artery in a healthy young adult feels different from a hardened arteriosclerotic vessel. A large volume pulse may be felt during times of high cardiac output such as exercise, stress, heat and pregnancy. It may also occur with fever, thyrotoxicosis, anaemia, peripheral arteriovenous shunts and Paget's disease.[2] It may also be caused by aortic regurgitation, a condition which results in back flow of blood through the aortic valve. A low volume pulse is a sign of reduced stroke volume secondary to cardiovascular disease or peripheral vascular disease. A weak or thready pulse is most commonly seen in the hypovolaemic patient.[3,5]

The term character has a similar yet distinct meaning, with volume you are looking for the strength of a pulse, however with character the strength is assessed alongside how quickly or slowly this is achieved.[6] This is best assessed at the carotid artery as the source is nearer to the heart and less subject to damping and distortion from the arterial tree. This is not an easy skill to acquire and requires experience therefore further reading is suggested (see References).

Pulse symmetry

Symmetry of the major arteries can provide useful information, however this is not routinely required. The undertaking of these tests is usually as a result of clinical suspicion of conditions such as acute aortic dissection or obstruction of the arterial tree.[7] Pulses should be bilaterally equal and felt simultaneously, any delay or reduction of volume could indicate an abnormal pathology. Any delay between the radial artery and femoral artery on the same side may also indicate an underlying condition.

Technique for pulse taking

The technique for pulse taking applies to all pulses with only the location altering. A step by step guide to the process of pulse taking can be seen below.

The procedure for pulse taking

Procedure	Rationale
1. Explain and discuss the procedure to the patient.	This is vital for both consent and relaxing the patient to get a more accurate reading.
2. Place the first, second and third finger along the artery and press gently.	The thumb should not be used as it has a strong pulse which may be mistaken for the patient's pulse (although in stronger pulses such as the brachial or the carotid it may be used as there is less likelihood of confusion). Pressing hard will occlude the artery making it difficult to palpate the pressure wave in the artery.
3. The pulse should be counted for 15 seconds (minimum) and multiplied by 4 to provide the number of beats per minute.[7] If the beat is irregular or is either too rapid or too slow then a 60 second count may be more appropriate.[8,9] Make note of the strength and character of the pulse.	An irregular, slow or fast pulse may be poorly estimated using a short counting period, therefore a longer period will allow for a more accurate estimation of pulse rate.
4. Counting should start from 1 as opposed to 0.	This method has been proven more accurate in recording heart rate.[8]
5. Record the pulse rate on the patient record.	This allows for trends to be recognised over time.
6. Now palpate the opposite artery in the same manner. *This should not be undertaken with the carotid artery.*	If either pulse feels diminished in volume confirm the difference by simultaneously palpating the arteries. This may indicate conditions such as coarctation, blockage of any artery or aneurysm. You should not palpate both carotid arteries simultaneously as this will reduce cerebral blood flow.
7. In carotid artery palpation the patient should lie on a bed or couch.	Palpation of the artery may cause a reflex bradycardia; this may cause a reduction in blood pressure and subsequent syncope.

Locating the artery

There are four key arteries for pulse taking; the radial artery; the brachial artery; the femoral artery and the carotid artery. However, any artery may be of clinical significance, for example dorsalis pedis artery in the foot in extremity trauma, which is often used in assessing peripheral blood flow beyond the site of a leg injury.

The radial artery

The radial artery is most commonly palpated proximal to the wrist on the radial (thumb) side of the palmar aspect (inner) of the forearm. In some patients you may be able to see the pulsation of the artery; therefore it is often worth visually inspecting the area prior to locating the pulse.

The brachial artery

The brachial pulse is located medially to the bicep tendon in the crease of the elbow. In the anatomical position this will be on the medial aspect of the arm.

The femoral artery

This is palpated at the midway point between the upper extremity of the pubis and the anterior portion of the iliac spine.

The carotid artery

The carotid artery is located between the larynx and the anterior border of the sternocleidomastoid muscle. Gently pressing between these structures should allow for palpation of the artery.

The dorsalis pedis artery

This is often referred to as the pedal pulse and is located over the dorsum of the foot. This is felt by compressing over the tarsal bones of the mid-foot.

Key Point

It is important not only to assess for the presence of a pulse but to consider the rate, volume and rhythm as these factors may indicate altered physiology and disease processes.

Capillary refill time measurement

Capillary refill time (CRT) is defined as the time taken for blood that has been removed from the tissues by the application of pressure to return to the tissues.[10] Traditionally CRT has been taught as a tool for rapid cardiovascular assessment and an indication of the adequacy of tissue perfusion (often after traumatic injury). Normal CRT is proposed to be less than two seconds, with any time longer than this deemed as prolonged or abnormal, however there is considerable debate as to the accuracy of such a parameter.[11]

What can influence CRT?

In three studies that sought to verify the accuracy of a parameter for 'normal' CRT, results of up to 6 seconds were found.[12] Findings suggest that CRT is age, sex and environment dependant, with adult males and children having significantly shorter CRT than women and the elderly. It has also been noted that ambient and body temperature can significantly alter CRT with reduced temperatures increasing CRT.[12,13] There is also a potential influence upon CRT with the use of vasoactive medications such as inotropes in the critically ill.

Where do I measure?

Traditionally CRT is measured on the pulp of a digit,[11] however the sternum and forehead are also areas of common usage. In the assessment of tissue perfusion below the site of an injury then naturally the site must be distal to the injury for the assessment to be of use. There is little definitive evidence to suggest one area for measurement is superior to another; however the use of differing areas for measurement, such as the foot may be linked to an increase CRT in cooler ambient temperatures.[13]

Is this accurate?

In a series of studies into the predictive value of CRT as an indicator of severity of illness or hypovolaemic status there appears little confidence in CRT use, with little validity found. Holcomb et al.[14] and Schriger and Baraff[15] found that CRT had little specificity and sensitivity in recognising hypovolaemia in trauma field studies and lab based studies respectively. A further study by Klupp and Keenan,[16] suggests that CRT is a poor predictor of peripheral vascular supply and therefore limited in its application.

Whilst there is little evidence to support the use of CRT as a measure of haemodynamic status, it is perceived as a quick and easy test that can be undertaken in any condition[17] and is therefore likely to remain as a part of clinical practice in the near future. It must however be considered as a part of a holistic assessment process and not in isolation.

Technique for measuring capillary refill time

There is no evidence to support a specific process for the measurement of CRT, therefore guidance is based upon current opinion and practice.

Capillary refill time measurement procedure

Procedure	Rationale
1. Explain the procedure to the patient and gain informed consent.	This is vital in all episodes of patient care to ensure conformity to professional duty of care and legal implications of consent.
2. If using the pulp of the finger raise the hand to the level of the heart.	This will ensure assessment of arteriolar capillary and venous stasis refill.[11]
3. Apply pressure to the digit for five seconds to compress blood from the tissues. The pressure should be enough to produce blanching.	There is little evidence to support a specific time for this, however shorter times may not remove blood from the tissues and subsequently falsely reduce CRT. A single study in neonatal patients suggests that there is no significant difference between 3s–7s.[18] However in the absence of strong evidence a suggested time of at least 5 seconds is recommended.
4. Release the pressure and time how long it takes for the colour of the digit to return to the same colour as the surrounding tissues.	This is the capillary refill time.
5. Document the findings.	This is essential to monitor trends over time.
6. Remember to consider ambient temperature, patient temperature and other findings.	This will allow for more appropriate application of the findings.

Blood pressure measurement

Blood pressure is defined as the force per unit area exerted on a vessel wall by the contained blood.[1] Within the context of prehospital care blood pressure refers to systemic arterial blood pressure. The nearer a blood vessel is to the heart the higher the blood pressure. It is this pressure gradient that maintains blood movement throughout the body.[1] Blood pressure is highest during the systolic phase of the cardiac cycle following contraction of the ventricle and lowest during the diastolic phase when the ventricles relax and refill. Blood pressure is usually expressed in term of millimetres of mercury (mmHg); this is the force exerted by a column of mercury of a height stated in millimetres. It is recorded as a systolic value over a diastolic value, for example 135/76 mmHg. The gap between the systolic pressure and the diastolic pressure is known as the pulse pressure.[1]

Blood pressure is a function of two main factors: (i) how much the elastic arteries near to the heart can be stretched and (ii) the volume of blood forced into them at any one time.[1]

Indications for monitoring blood pressure

Blood pressure is monitored for a variety of reasons including:

1. To record a baseline for future measurements
2. To record changes in response to treatments or condition
3. To monitor haemodynamic status.

What Influences blood pressure?

Influences upon blood pressure are wide and varied. Blood pressure can be affected by weight, age, diet, time of day, pain, pregnancy, anxiety and further wide ranging medical conditions.[19,20] The circumstances of the measurement itself may also be a factor in blood pressure readings with rises in systolic blood pressure of over 20 mmHg being attributed to anxiety and a perceived 'white coat effect'.[21] White coat hypertension is a condition in which a normotensive subject becomes hypertensive during blood pressure measurement, but then becomes normotensive again outside of the medical environment.

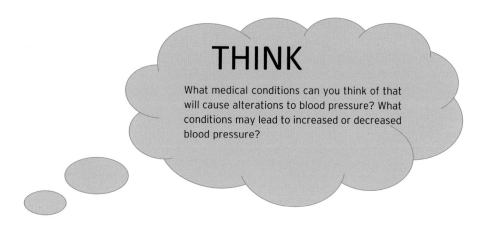

THINK

What medical conditions can you think of that will cause alterations to blood pressure? What conditions may lead to increased or decreased blood pressure?

Normal blood pressure

Normotension is a difficult notion as blood pressure can vary in individuals and can fluctuate due to a variety of factors. General consensus suggests that systolic readings of around 120 mmHg and diastolic readings around 80 mmHg are considered 'normal'.[22] However these may vary between 140/90 mmHg to 100/60 mmHg.[3] Any blood pressure reading must be taken in context as a blood pressure of 100/60 mmHg in a patient who has a normal blood pressure of 180/110 mmHg may well be hypotensive.

Hypertension

Hypertension is an elevation of the blood pressure that may be acute or chronic. In an adult this is generally considered to be any values above 140/90 mmHg and defined as 'the level of blood pressure at which there is evidence that blood pressure reduction does more good than harm'.[23] With variations in blood pressure measurement and the fluctuating nature of blood pressure, diagnoses of high blood pressure are not made upon single measurement but upon a series of measures. Hypertension is a significant risk factor for cardiovascular diseases such as myocardial infarction and stroke, therefore early diagnosis and treatment are key.

Hypotension

Hypotension or low blood pressure is generally defined as a systolic reading below 100 mmHg.[1] It may simply be a variation in blood pressure, however in the acutely ill patient it may be an indication of hypovolaemia, sepsis or cardiogenic shock.[24] Orthostatic or postural hypotension is a fall in systolic blood pressure of at least 20 mmHg or 10 mmHg in diastolic blood pressure within three minutes of quiet standing.[25] This may be asymptomatic or cause the patient to feel light-headed and in older patients this is linked with falls and poor mobility.[26]

Mean arterial pressure

Mean arterial blood pressure is the average pressure required to move blood through the circulatory system. The mean arterial pressure may be calculated mathematically or electronically. Mathematically it is calculated as below:

$$\text{Mean arterial pressure} = \frac{1}{3}\,\text{Systolic blood pressure} + \frac{2}{3}\,\text{Diastolic blood pressure}$$

For example, a blood pressure of 120/90 mmHg gives a mean arterial pressure of 100 mmHg.

Measuring blood pressure

There are two overall methods for measuring blood pressure; direct and indirect. Direct methods are considered more accurate, however these involve the placement of a pressure transducer (sensor) into an artery to directly measure the blood intra-arterial pressure. This method is commonly used in critical care areas such as intensive care units where patients require continuous and accurate monitoring. However this is not practical outside of these areas. Indirect blood pressure monitoring uses external cuffs to assess blood pressure either through auscultation or changes in cuff pressure. Wherever the environment, blood pressure measurements should be undertaken by trained healthcare professionals using equipment that is accurate, validated and well maintained. Failure to achieve this may result in errone-ous or inaccurate readings being obtained.

The auscultatory method of measurement using mercury sphygmomanometers (a sphygmomanometer is a blood pressure measuring device) has been the mainstay of blood pressure measurement since blood pressure has been measured. However with an anticipated withdrawal of mercury devices for health and safety reasons alternative devices are required.[27]

Mercury sphygmomanometers

The mercury sphygmomanometer has been the perceived gold standard equipment for blood pressure measuring for many years. The simplistic design of these devices makes them easy to use and maintain. However there is a risk of chemical spillage, therefore special precautions are required in areas where they are used.[26] Despite the simplistic design this equipment requires maintenance with studies finding that many devices are often inaccurate or defective due to poor maintenance schedules.[28,29] This system relies upon the pressure created by a column of mercury within the device to provide a measurement.

Aneroid sphygmomanometers

In these devices the pressure is registered by a series of metal bellows that expand as the cuff pressure increases and a series of levers that register pressure on a circular scale.[26] This device is however susceptible to damage from rough handling and poor maintenance.[30] The accuracy of these monitors does appear questionable with variations between manufacturer and mercury devices.[31]

Non-invasive automated sphygmomanometers

The use of automated devices has been common place for many years, with many ambulance services and acute care settings opting for the ease of use to reduce staff workload and to allow for measurement in a variety of settings. The majority of these devices are based upon a technique known as oscillometry. This relies upon oscillations of pressure being felt in the cuff being maximal at mean arterial pressure.[32] The oscillations begin well above systolic blood pressure and continue below diastolic blood pressure. This requires the blood pressure to be estimated from an algorithm. This method has the benefit of not requiring the cuff to be placed on specific points over the brachial artery as there is no transducer as with the mercury and aneroid sphygmomanometer.

The sphygmomanometer

A sphygmomanometer consists of a compression bag or bladder within a non-elastic cuff and an inflation bulb, pump or other device that is linked to the bag by durable tubing. In addition there is a measurement scale for reading the value and a control valve to release the pressure within the cuff.

Measuring blood pressure (manual methods)

Location of the measurement

The standard location for blood pressure measurement is the upper arm, with a stethoscope positioned over the brachial artery at the crease of the elbow. There are other sites that can be used such as the wrist, finger and leg but these have yet to fully validated for accuracy.[33,34]

Posture of the subject

Posture effects blood pressure, generally blood pressure will generally increase from the lying to the sitting or standing position. In the clinical setting the position of the patient should be based upon how they are most comfortable, however the position should be considered when documenting findings and making clinical decisions.

Arm position

The position of the arm can have a major influence upon blood pressure measurement. The upper arm should be at the level of the right atrium (mid-sternal level). If the arm is too high readings can be falsely low or if the arm is too low readings can be too high. It is suggested that the change in reading may be up to 10 mmHg or 2 mmHg for every inch above or below the heart level.[35] If the arm in which measurement is being taken is unsupported this results in isometric exercise which can increase blood pressure and heart rate. Effects of this are estimated to be as much as a 10% increase in diastolic blood pressure, therefore supporting the arm is recommended.[36]

Which arm?

This remains a controversial area as some studies have found differences in blood pressure between arms in same subject simultaneous measurements.[37] At present there appears no agreed reason for this, although a consensus of opinion suggests any marked difference (>20 mmHg systolic or >10 mmHg diastolic pressure) between arms should be investigated further as they may indicate pathology of the aorta or upper extremity arterial obstruction.[26] It is recommended that blood pressure should initially be checked in both arms and the arm with the higher blood pressure should be used for subsequent measurements.[26,38,39]

The cuff and bladder

The sizing of the cuff and bladder in blood pressure measuring is paramount to accurate findings. The estimation of intra-arterial pressure by indirect means such as sphygmomanometry is predicated on a proper relationship between cuff size and the extremity. However sophisticated the measuring device used if it is dependent upon cuff occlusion of the arm, it will be prone to inaccuracy due to miscuffing. Several dated studies noted that undersized cuffs cause falsely high reading and oversized cuffs produced falsely low readings.[40,41] With more recent studies suggesting that a cuff that is too small produces larger errors in blood pressure recording than a cuff that is too large.[42-45] The optimal size of cuff that should be used should have a bladder length that is 80% of the arm circumference and a width that is at least 40% of arm circumference.[26,46]

The stethoscope (auscultation)

Using a stethoscope placed over the brachial artery it is possible to identify a series of five stages as the blood pressure reading falls from the systolic to the diastolic.[1,26] These sounds are known as Korotkoff's sounds. During the raising of the pressure in the cuff and bladder the blood flow through the brachial artery is cut occluded, as it is gradually deflated pulsatile blood flow is restored though the artery, resulting in a series of sounds. These sounds have been classified as phases as seen below:

Phase 1: A clear tapping sound corresponding with the return of a palpable pulse. The onset of phase 1 corresponds with systolic blood pressure.
Phase 2: Sounds become softer and longer.
Phase 3: Sounds become crisper and louder.
Phase 4: Sounds become softer and muffled.
Phase 5: Sounds disappear completely. This is considered to be the diastolic blood pressure value.

The Korotkoff sounds method tends to give lower systolic values than that of intra-arterial methods and diastolic values that are higher.[47-50] There has been disagreement over the reliability of using phase 4 or 5 to determine diastolic value as it is often difficulty in differentiating when phase 4 commences, in addition this tends to give an inaccurately high diastolic value. It is now considered appropriate to use phase 5 sounds for diagnostic accuracy as they are easier to determine. This method is not however possible in all patients, as in some patients, the disappearance of sounds does not occur despite complete deflation of the cuff. In this scenario the 4th phase sound should be used.[37,51] Patients who are prone to the continuation of the Korotkoff sounds include pregnant women, those with aortic insufficiency and patients with arterio-venous fistulas (for haemodialysis).

In older patients with a wide pulse pressure the Korotkoff sounds may disappear between the systolic and diastolic pressures and reappear as the cuff is deflated, this is known as the auscultatory gap.[26] The auscultatory gap is thought to be a result of fluctuating intra-arterial pressures or organ damage.[52]

Palpatory estimation of blood pressure

In some situations such as a noisy road traffic collision site it can be difficult to achieve a valid blood pressure based upon auscultatory techniques. This is also the case with those patients in whom it is difficult to determine the Korotkoff sounds. In these situations it is possible to estimate systolic blood pressure by palpation of the brachial artery when deflating the cuff.[53] The cuff should firstly be inflated to approximately 30 mmHg above where the brachial pulse can no longer be felt and then as the cuff is deflated the return of the pulse should be noted. This is suggested to be the approximate value of the systolic blood pressure.

Advanced Trauma Life Support principles[54] suggest that if the patient has a carotid pulse that the systolic blood pressure is 60-70 mmHg; if carotid and femoral pulses are present the systolic blood pressure is 70-80 mmHg and if the radial pulse is present the systolic blood pressure is greater than 80 mmHg. However there is little support provided for these broad estimations, Deakin and Low (2000)[55] found these figures to be an overestimate of actual intra-arterial blood pressure in a small scale study. It appears that the suggested ATLS estimations may not be reliable and management should not be based solely upon information gained by this technique until further evidence has been provided to either support or dispel the proposal.

THINK

How will you assess the blood pressure or circulatory assessment in a trapped patient at a noisy RTC? What else can you do to assess your patient?

Technique for blood pressure measurement (auscultatory measurement)

A step-by-step guide to blood pressure measurement

Procedure	Rationale
1. Explain to the patient the procedure and gain informed consent.	To reduce the likelihood of 'white coat' hypertension and gain a more accurate measurement.
2. Allow the patient to rest if possible.	To reduce anxiety and orthostatic changes can be eliminated.
3. Ensure that the upper arm is exposed, supported and positioned at heart level.	This allows access to the brachial artery for measurement and ensures that a true measurement is achieved as arm height can influence blood pressure.
4. Ensure that tight or restrictive clothing from the upper arm is removed.	To reduce any tourniquet effect above the measurement site as this will alter blood pressure recording.
5. Select and appropriate sized cuff (covers 80% of the circumference of the arm and width is 40% of the arm circumference).	Both overcuffing and undercuffing can influence blood pressure measurement (see earlier in this section).
6. Apply the cuff firmly around the upper arm with the indicator line or centre of the bladder of the brachial artery.	This ensures that the pressure sensor is over the site of the artery and the site for auscultation is clear.
7. Place the measurement scale where it can easily be seen.	So the reading can be clearly seen.
8. Ask the patient to remain still and not talk during the procedure.	This can cause inaccurate measurements and inhibit the ability to hear the Korotkoff sounds.

Procedure	Rationale
9. Palpate the brachial artery.	To ensure that the site for auscultation can be clearly identified.
10. Inflate the cuff, noting when the brachial pulse disappears and inflate the cuff a further 30 mmHg.	This can assist in providing an estimate of systolic blood pressure.
11. Slowly deflate the cuff noting when the brachial pulse returns.	
12. Wait for approximately 30 seconds and then re-inflate the cuff to 30 mmHg above where the brachial pulse is lost.	The previous steps allow for an estimation of when the Korotkoff's sounds are expected.
13. Place the diaphragm of the stethoscope over the brachial artery just below the cuff.	This is the ideal site for auscultating for Korotkoff's sounds.
14. Deflate the cuff slowly (approx 2 mmHg per second or per heart beat).	This will allow for a precise measurement.
15. The systolic value is taken when distinct clear tapping sounds can be heard (phase 1).	This will be expected around the identified pressure when the brachial pulse is no longer felt.
16. When all sounds disappear the diastolic value is recorded (phase 5); be aware of the auscultatory gap.	This can be problematic in certain groups; therefore the sound may not be fully lost.
17. Record all relevant details.	To monitor trends in blood pressure over time or pre- and post-treatment.

In automated blood pressure measurement the principles remain the same whereby cuff size and placement is paramount, alongside arm and patient positioning. It is recommended that the user refers to the guidance for the equipment in their workplace.

Common sources of error

Errors in blood pressure measurement are often the result of incorrect technique or faulty equipment.[56] Whilst equipment failure can be limited by regular checks and maintenance, observer error is more widely prevalent.[54] Observer error can be classified into three broad areas.[57]

- Systematic error – This may be caused by lack of concentration, poor hearing, poor technique and failure to interpret Korotkoff's sounds.
- Terminal digit preference – This refers to the notion that observers will commonly 'round up' or 'round down' to the nearest 0 or 5. Studies into this area report high levels of reporting for the figures ending in 0 or 5, suggesting that this may be a common occurrence.[58,59]

- Observer prejudice or bias – This is the practice whereby the observer adjusts a blood pressure measurement to meet a perceived notion of what the blood pressure should be. This is most evident when an arbitrary figure is placed against what a blood pressure should be, for example to justify a treatment.[60]

Utilising the suggested blood pressure measuring technique will assist in the reduction of such observer error and lead to more accurate recording of blood pressure parameters.

Blood pressure measurement in special situations

Arrhythmias can be a cause of considerable variation in blood pressure. When the cardiac rhythm is very irregular the cardiac output and blood pressure can vary greatly from beat to beat.[26] This can make the interpretation of Korotkoff sounds virtually impossible, with evidence suggesting that the presence of major arrhythmia can cause a high level of observer error.[60] There are no set guidelines for the measurement of blood pressure in patients with arrhythmias, therefore it is suggested that blood pressure should be measured several times and an average value used. Automated devices are also of questionable benefit in the patient with a significant arrhythmia, with frequent inaccuracies reported; therefore any device used should be validated for that patient group.[61] If severe bradycardia is present (i.e. under 50 beats per minute) deflation of the cuff should be slower to prevent underestimation of systolic blood pressure and over estimation of diastolic blood pressure.

Key Point

The position of the patient, the arm and inappropriate use of equipment may all lead to erroneous blood pressure measurements; therefore careful adherence to the detailed procedure is essential for accurate blood pressure measurement. Ensure the cuff is the correct size and that the arm is supported at the level of the heart.

The electrocardiogram

Contraction of muscle is secondary to depolarisation of cells whereby ionic movements within the sodium, potassium and calcium channels cause a shift in the electrical balance. These electrical currents that are generated in and transmitted through the heart can be detected throughout the body by electrodes, using a machine known as an electrocardiograph.[1] This technology allows for the collection of a graphic record of the electrical activity of the heart, referred to as an electrocardiogram (ECG). It is not the intention of this chapter to provide the reader with the ability to interpret the ECG but to provide the reader with techniques and understanding of how to prepare the patient and collect an ECG tracing.

Indications for ECG recording

There are a variety of situations when an ECG is required including:

- Electively prior to surgery or drug treatments.
- As an investigation into the acutely unwell patient usually in the presence of indicators such as chest pain, cardiac rhythm changes or haemodynamic disturbance.
- In the assessment of the collapsed patient or in cardiac arrest.

Types of ECG

There are two common types of ECG tracing that are undertaken. These are the 3-lead ECG and the 12-lead ECG. Both types of ECG have specific areas of value, with the 3-lead ECG being commonly used for gross rhythm abnormality assessment in cardiac arrest and for continuous monitoring. However the 12-lead ECG is more commonly used for its diagnostic capability in acute coronary syndromes and cardiac assessment. Whilst the each procedure will be discussed individually, the general principles of patient preparation will be discussed as a whole as it does not markedly differ between the two types of ECG recording. It is important to note that the term lead does not refer to the number of cables running from the ECG machine to the patient but to the number of 'views' of the electrical activity that these leads provide.

Basic principles of electrocardiography

The ECG is a non-invasive procedure that records all action potentials and electrical activity within the heart, not just a tracking of a single action potential through the heart.[1] The electrocardiograph is a galvanometer (a sensitive electromagnet) which can detect and record changes in electromagnetic potential. It has a positive pole and a negative pole. The wire extensions from these poles have electrodes at each end; a positive electrode at the end of the extension from the positive pole, and a negative electrode at the end of the extension from the negative pole. The paired electrodes together constitute an electrocardiographic lead. Recording electrodes (leads) are placed at various sites of the body to ensure that a variety of 'views' of the conduction system of the heart are obtained. An electrode is normally attached to the skin using a sticky pad that has a layer of conductive gel on the skin surface side to allow for transmission of action potentials through the skin to the electrocardiograph.

A typical 3-lead ECG will comprise of 3 bipolar leads that measure the voltage difference between two electrodes, either between the arms or between an arm and a leg as seen in Figure 5.1. These lead are referred to as standard leads I, II, and III and measure the voltage between two distinct pints for each lead.

Lead I: Right arm to the left arm
Lead II: Right arm to the left leg
Lead III: Left arm to the left leg.

The relationship between these leads is known as the principle of Einthoven's Triangle and is used in the determining the electrical axis of the heart. As an action potential is generated within the heart and moves along the conduction pathways it will move away from one electrode to be nearer to another. When this current is moving toward an electrode it will cause a positive (upward) deflection on the electrocardiogram; if the current moves away from the electrode it will result in a negative (downward) deflection. In the event that the current moves at an equidistant point between two electrodes or there is no electrical activity the electrocardiogram will see neither a positive or negative deflection (isoelectric). Typically patients will be monitored using standard lead II as this provides the most electrical information regarding the electrical conduction pathways of the heart.

The development of the 12-lead ECG as an improved diagnostic tool saw the inclusion of 9 further views of the heart from the placement of additional unipolar leads (using a further 7 not 9 extra electrodes). These leads take a view of the electrical activity of the heart from a single electrode; these electrodes are designed to measure the voltage that passes towards it. Again electrical activity towards the electrode will result in a positive deflection, and away from the electrode will produce a negative deflection. These leads include three limb leads (aVR, aVF and aVL) and six chest (or pre-cordial) leads (V1–V6).

The limb leads are unipolar and are placed on the limbs, they are often referred to as the augmented limb leads (thus prefixed with the letter 'a'). This means that the voltage (V) is amplified (by approximately 50%) to make it more readable. These leads are derived from the standard leads (I, II, III), however they look at the heart from a different angle to the standard leads as shown in Figure 5.1.

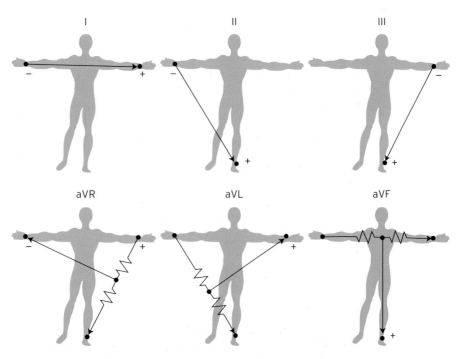

Figure 5.1 Three bipolar leads and augmented limb leads.

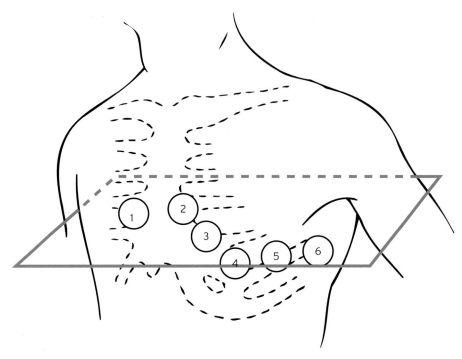

Figure 5.2 The horizontal plane of the precordial leads. From Petersen O. *Human Physiology Lecture Notes*, 5th edn, copyright 2007, with permission of Blackwell Publishing.

The pre-cordial or chest leads (V1-6) are not augmented as they are near enough to the heart for a strong electrical signal to be obtained. These leads view the hearts electrical activity from the horizontal plane and measure anterior voltage change (Figure 5.2).

Each pre-cordial lead has a view and section of the heart that it views the best:

V1-V2: The right side of the heart
V3-V4: The interventricular septum and apex
V5-V6: The left side of the heart.

ECG settings

A standard electrocardiograph is set to run at a paper speed of 25 mm/second although some machines are set to run at different speeds. In the ECG paper the vertical lines are set to show time, these show small boxes that equate to 0.04 seconds and larger boxes (made up of 5 small boxes that equates to 0.2 seconds (hence there are 5 large boxes per second). The horizontal lines show amplitude, in a standard electrocardiograph the paper is set to record 1cm (10 mm) per millivolt (mV). A standard ECG recording will provide a calibration signal of 1mV prior to the recording to ensure that the machine is correctly calibrated for interpretation. An example of ECG standard paper setting can be seen in Figure 5.3.

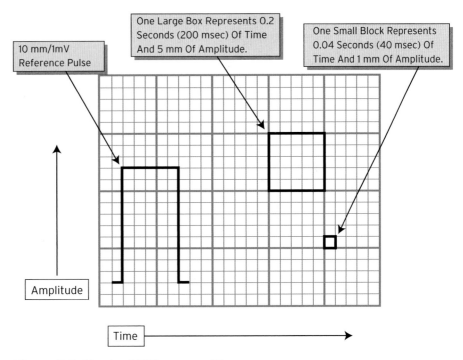

Figure 5.3 Standard ECG paper settings.

Patient preparation

Unrestricted access to the skin in the chest area, arms and legs is required to allow for the correct placement of ECG electrodes.[62] The practitioner should ensure that the patient is relaxed and dignity is maintained at all times to ensure that minimal artefact is present on the recording. The appearance of the ECG can vary depending upon the position of the body at the time of recording; therefore current guidance suggests that the patient should be in a recumbent position with any variation upon this position documented upon the ECG.[63] Ideally the patient should be upon a comfortable surface and relaxed to reduce motion and muscular artefact as this can aid in the collection of a clinically accurate recording.

Skin preparation is often required to help produce an artefact free accurate ECG, as such there are a variety of methods available that are designed to reduce the impedance between the skin and the electrode.[63] The American Heart Association and British Cardiovascular Society suggest the following methods can be used.[63]

- The removal of chest hair using a razor to allow for greater contact between the electrode and the skin. This requires consent, a clean razor and sharps disposal box.
- Exfoliation of the skin may be required and should be undertaken gently using a paper towel, gauze swab or specifically designed abrasive tape. This can further reduce impedance between the skin and the electrode.
- It may be necessary to cleanse the skin to remove excess contaminants or sweat, a variety of methods can be used such as soap and water or alcohol wipes. However care should be taken if there is broken or sensitive skin.

Positioning of the electrodes

General principles

There are a few principles that are applied relating to general placement in both 3- and 12-lead ECGs, adherence to these principles can significantly improve ECG recording and subsequent interpretation.

Procedure	Rationale
1. Make the patient at ease.	A tense or anxious patient is likely to have increased movement and subsequently increased artefact. If the patient is not relaxed the ECG will record somatic muscle action potentials as well as cardiac thus making the ECG more difficult to interpret; a common example of this is clenched fists.
2. Place the electrode over bone not muscle.	This will reduce the likelihood of muscle movement interfering with the recording.
3. Place the patient in a recumbent position.	Other positions may alter the trace by increased muscle activity in sitting or by altering the anatomic position of the heart.
4. The patient should be on a surface (i.e. couch) that can support the limbs.	This will again reduce muscle movement and artefact. If the patient is not in a recumbent position this should be noted upon the trace as it may affect comparison with subsequent ECG recordings.

THINK

Are you able to achieve this with all patients? When might it be difficult to achieve a high quality ECG? What can you do to improve the tracing?

The positioning of the electrodes is primarily determined by the type of ECG being recorded with the 3-lead ECG differing from the 12-lead ECG.

The 3-lead ECG

Due to the 3-lead ECG being non-diagnostic, there are often differing derivations of lead placement used in clinical practice.[64] However the alteration of lead placements can lead to changes in the amplitude of an ECG and subsequent interpretation, therefore it is important that a standardised approach is used. This is especially important in 12-lead electrocardiography due to the diagnostic quality of the tracing.

In a 3-lead ECG there are naturally, 3 electrodes; these electrodes are commonly colour coded to allow for easy recognition or are labelled to identify their position. The leads are:

- Right arm limb lead (RA/or red electrode) – right forearm, proximal to the wrist.
- Left arm limb lead (LA/or yellow electrode) – left forearm, proximal to the wrist.
- Left leg limb lead (LL/or green electrode) – left lower leg, proximal to ankle.
- Some machines may have a fourth lead (right leg lead [RLL]/or black electrode), this lead acts as an 'earth' and is neutral to prevent current interference – right lower leg, proximal to the ankle.

The 12-lead ECG

The 12-lead ECG is a diagnostic tool and therefore the placement of the leads is paramount. Small changes in position of electrodes may lead alter the appearance of the ECG and evidence suggests that such variations may invalidate subsequent diagnosis.[65-67] To ensure consistency between recordings it is recommended that that the electrodes are placed in standardised positions.[63]

The limb leads should be placed as per the standard leads as shown with 3-lead electrocardiography. It is imperative that any recordings made from other sites (for example the upper arms for RA and LA leads in a patient with excessive limb tremor) are clearly identified as such to avoid later confusion or misdiagnosis. The correct anatomical positions for the precordial leads have been defined and are shown in Table 5.4.

This is shown anatomically in Figure 5.4.

When recording an ECG in female patients, convention suggests that the lateral chest electrodes (V4, V5, V6) should be placed below the left breast. There is recent evidence to suggest that positioning of the electrodes over the breast may not attenuate the signal,[68,69] however there is currently insufficient evidence to make an informed decision upon this.

Table 5.4 The position of the precordial leads[63]

Lead/electrode	Position
V1	Fourth intercostal space at the right sternal edge
V2	Fourth intercostal space at the left sternal edge
V3	Midway between V2 and V4
V4	Fifth intercostal space mid-clavicular line
V5	Left anterior axillary line at the same horizontal level as V4
V6	Left mid axillary line at the same horizontal level as V4 and V5

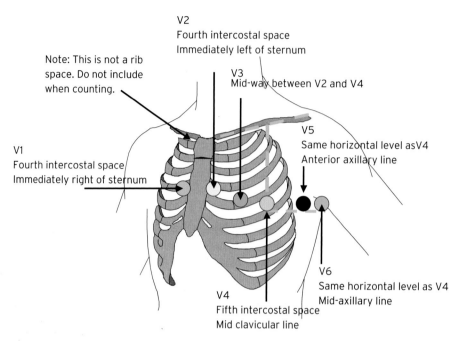

Figure 5.4 The anatomical placement of the precordial leads. Reproduced from Clinical Guidelines by Consensus, '*Recording a 12-lead Electrocardiogram: An Approved Methodology*', copyright 2006 with permission of The Society for Cardiological Science and Technology.

Recording the ECG

In order to record a good quality ECG it is imperative that the patient is relaxed and comfortable to ensure reduced muscle artefact; this may be problematic in some patients due to anxiety or pre-existing medical conditions, try to make the patient as comfortable and relaxed as possible. It may be necessary to adapt the recommended ECG recording techniques, for example the wheelchair patient or amputee. Any change from the standard position of the patient or leads should be annotated in the patient notes and on the ECG to make sure that diagnostic changes are not influenced. Patient details should be recorded upon the tracing (either inputted into the machine or hand written); failure to do so will mean that the recording is discarded as it cannot be linked to the specific patient. Ideally place the patients name and another identifier such as date of birth or hospital number on the ECG.

If the ECG complexes are of a high or low voltage the recording can be difficult to interpret, in such an event the 'gain' (scale) of the recording can be adjusted to aid interpretation. Any change to the gain should be noted on the tracing as this may alter diagnostic criteria.

Key Point

The positioning of the electrodes, especially in the case of a diagnostic 12-lead ECG are of utmost importance. The leads should be placed as described; any variation of this (if unavoidable) should be noted on the ECG tracing.

Cardiac auscultation

The recognition and interpretation of heart sounds is an infrequently used skill for prehospital care providers, however the information gathered from such an investigation can be useful in the assessment and diagnosis of many conditions. Normal heart sounds are created by the noise of the valves of the heart closing (they do not make a noise when they open). It is therefore essential to have a clear comprehension of cardiac anatomy and the cardiac cycle to understand the sounds that are produced in the normal or abnormal heart. The recognition of heart sounds is often problematic as the sound of a normal heart may well be faint and abnormalities are often very subtle, in addition prehospital care staff often have little exposure to such a skill therefore skill decay is likely.

It is not the purpose of this section to provide a detailed description of heart sounds and classification of abnormal heart sounds but to provide the practitioner with the basic skills in cardiac auscultation.

THINK

Do you understand the anatomy and physiology of the heart and cardiac cycle? If not then refer to a good anatomy and physiology text to help.

Indications for auscultation of the heart

There are a variety of reasons for cardiac auscultation that are often dependent upon your area of work. Indications include:

- The assessment of chest injury and consideration of cardiac contusion or tamponade.
- The assessment of cardiac function, especially if suspicious of cardiac murmur.
- As a part of the assessment for the confirmation of death.

General principles of cardiac auscultation

To adequately assess cardiac sounds it is essential to have a stethoscope that incorporates a bell and a diaphragm; correct use of this will enhance the quality of heart sounds.[70] The 'bell' when applied gently to the skin will pick up low frequency sounds, however the diaphragm when pressed firmly against the skin will allow for high pitched sounds to become more audible.

The normal heart has two distinct sounds heard during the a single cardiac cycle, these are described as a 'Lub' and 'Dub'.[2,4] The first heart sound (S_1) (Lub) is generated by the vibrations from the closure of the mitral valve and tricuspid valve during ventricular systole; this is usually heard as a single sound but on occasion the two distinct valve closures can be heard.[71] The second heart sound (S_2) (Dub) is produced by the closure of the aortic and pulmonary valves at the start of ventricular diastole. As the pressure of blood in the aorta is usually higher than in the pulmonary artery the aortic valve closure is often louder resulting in a potential 'split' sound whereby the two valves closing can be heard separately.

There are a variety of 'added' or abnormal sounds, it is beyond the scope of this section to describe each sound however the added sounds heard are described as one of the following categories:

- Extra heart sounds – These are classed as third and fourth heart sounds. A third heart sound (S_3) is a low pitched sound in early diastole best heard at the apices of the heart. It coincides with rapid ventricular filling immediately after the opening of the atrioventricular valves. A fourth heart sound is less common as is caused by the forceful atrial contraction against a non compliant ventricle. The fourth heart sound is actually heard before the first heart sound and is described as soft and low pitched.[2]
- Added sounds – These consist of snaps (caused by the sudden opening of a stenosed mitral valve); ejection clicks (occurs in early systole – caused by pulmonary or aortic stenosis); mid-systolic clicks (occur in mitral valve prolapse).
- Mechanical heart valves – These valve replacements make a sound both on opening and closing. They are described as high pitched and metallic sounding. They may be audible without a stethoscope.
- Pericardial rub – This is described as a superficial scratching sound that is best heard with the diaphragm of the stethoscope. It is most commonly caused by conditions such a viral pericarditis.
- Murmurs – These are caused by turbulent blow flow over an abnormal valve, septal defect, obstruction or increased blood flow over a normal valve. There are numerous causes of heart murmur ranging from innocent murmurs in a healthy heart to severe cardiac disorders. Murmurs are characterised by a number of

factors including timing; duration; character; pitch; intensity; location and radiation.

Examples of heart sounds and additional information can be found in essential reading and on-line at websites such as:
http://depts.washington.edu/physdx/heart/demo.html
http://www.merck.com/

The technique of cardiac auscultation

There is no consensus upon what constitutes a correct structure for auscultation of the heart, however it is essential to have a structured approach so that the examination is performed fully. There are four standard sites that are utilised for this procedure:

- Mitral area – The left fifth intercostal space in the mid-clavicular line. This is the best site for auscultating the mitral valve.
- Tricuspid area – The left fourth intercostal space lateral to the sternum. This location will provide the best site for auscultating the tricuspid valve.
- Pulmonary area – Second intercostal space at the left sternal border. This is noted as the best location for auscultating the pulmonary valve.
- Aortic area – Second intercostal space at the right sternal border. This is where the aortic valve sounds are best heard.

These can be seen in Figure 5.5.

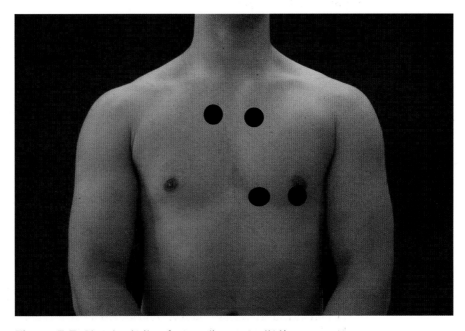

Figure 5.5 Standard sites for cardiac auscultation.

The procedure of cardiac auscultation

Procedure	Rationale
1. Explain the procedure to the patient.	To ensure that you have informed consent and a co-operative patient.
2. Whilst ensuring patient dignity, expose the patient's chest.	Patient dignity is essential; however exposure of the relevant anatomy is vital in locating the relevant auscultation areas.
3. Ensure that the environment is as quiet as possible.	The heart sounds may be difficult to hear in ideal circumstances therefore the less ambient noise present the better.
4. Position the patient in a supine position at an angle of approximately 45°.	This aligns the auscultation areas with the underlying heart.
5. Ask the patient to breathe normally.	Deep breathing or Valsalva manoeuvre in holding the breath can either interfere with auscultation or reduce venous return thus causing murmurs to become quieter.[2,71]
6. Using the diaphragm auscultate over the mitral area at the same time palpate the carotid artery.	This will allow easier determination of S1 and S2, the carotid pulse will coincide with S1.
7. Continue to auscultate using the diaphragm over the tricuspid, pulmonary and aortic areas.	Identify S1 and S2 at all points, assess for the presence of any added sounds or third/fourth heart sounds.
8. Ask the patient to roll into a left lateral position (known as left lateral decubitus), auscultate using the bell over the mitral area.	This will bring the left ventricle nearer to the chest wall making mitral valve disorders easier to hear. The sound of mitral stenosis for example is a low pitched mid-diastolic sound.
9. Note and record the presence of normal heart sounds (S1 and S2); also record the presence of any sound splitting, added sounds or murmurs.	It is essential to note any examinations undertaken and the results obtained to examine changes over time.
10. Remember that the absence of heart sounds or the muffling of sounds may be clinically significant.	

As previously stated, this is a rarely undertaken and difficult to master skill, therefore a sound understanding of cardiac auscultation is vitally important for those times when the skill is required. See References for suggested resources for this skill.

Temperature measurement

Accurate temperature measurement and monitoring is a critical component of the assessment and management of the critically ill patient and in minor illness assessment. All cell metabolism results in heat production and any illness, injury, activity or environmental change may affect the body's temperature. Generally the body's temperature is maintained between 36 and 37.5 °C.[4] Humans are described as homoeothermic which is defined as have a core temperature that is regulated despite environmental changes. The human body is generally broken down into two compartments in reference to temperature, the peripheral compartment and the core thermal compartment. The peripheral compartment is described as non-homogeneous in which temperature may vary over time and be influenced by extremes of environment and physiological challenges.[71] The core thermal compartment is well-perfused and comprises of 50-60% of the body mass including the major organs of the trunk and head. This compartment is relatively stable as it is well supplied by arterial blood and represents the balance between heat generation and heat loss well.[72] The body core generally has the higher temperature, with temperature at the exterior (skin) being the coolest. As such core body temperature is considered the most accurate and effective method of temperature assessment.[3,72]

Indications for temperature measurement

There are a variety of reasons for temperature monitoring, these include:

- To determine a set a baseline observations for the monitoring of trends over time.
- In the presence of infection or severe systemic illness.
- In extreme environmental conditions, i.e. in cold water near drowning or falls in the elderly in a cold environment, or in hot temperatures with suspected heat-related illness.

These are just a few of the indications for temperature measurement it is recommended that the practitioner considers the necessity for temperature measurement on an individual case basis.

Extremes of temperature

There are a variety of causes of temperature fluctuation including elevated temperature in the morning due to the body's circadian rhythm[3]; elevated temperature due to ovulation, exercise and eating[1] and the effects of aging. In the emergency setting there are three key concepts of temperature; normothermia; hypothermia and pyrexia.

Normothermia is the state of normal core body temperature (between 36 and 37.5 °C), this is maintained by the body's homeostatic mechanisms. A body temperature outside of this range will result in derangement of the cellular activity of the body. Hypothermia is defined as a core body temperature below 35.0 °C, at temperatures below this point the patient will deteriorate in neurological, cardiovascular and respiratory function and ultimately death will occur at temperatures below

23 °C.[72] There are a variety of causes of hypothermia, those most relevant to the prehospital care practitioner are:

- Environmental conditions.
- Medications that increase heat loss or alter cold perception (such as alcohol).
- Metabolic conditions such as hypoglycaemia.

Pyrexia (sometimes referred to as hyperthermia or fever) is defined as a significant rise in core body temperature above 37.0 °C; beyond this pyrexia may be referred to as low grade (normal – 38.0°); moderate to high-grade pyrexia (38.0–40.0 °C) and hyperpyrexia (40.0 °C and above).[3] As with hypothermia extremes, symptoms will include changes to neurological, cardiovascular and respiratory function and ultimately death.

Methods of temperature measurement

There are a variety of methods of temperature measurement each with relevant flaws and benefits. These include:

Pulmonary artery catheterisation

A pulmonary artery catheter is the passing of a probe into the pulmonary artery where it is bathed in arterial blood. This is considered the most accurate method of core temperature measurement,[73] however this method is inappropriate in the pre-hospital and non-critical care environment due the technical and invasive nature.

Tympanic thermometry

Tympanic thermometry is the preferred instrument of non-invasive temperature measurement in the majority of emergency and primary care settings, often due to the rapidity and simplicity of measurement. The tympanic thermometer works by recording temperature of the tympanic membrane, using infra-red light to detect thermal radiation, which receives blood from the internal carotid artery, which also supplies blood to the hypothalamus (the thermoregulatory centre of the brain).[74]

However, despite the appeal of tympanic thermometers there are a number of factors that may influence recording. These include operator technique, patient anatomy, calibration, accuracy and inherent error.[72,74] Values obtained from this equipment vary due to the position of the probe in the ear canal with temperature being highest nearer to the tympanic membrane and reducing with distance away from the tympanic membrane. Exposure and accessibility of the tympanic membrane may be improved with a 'tugging' technique that aligns the ear canal. By pulling back on the pinna of the ear it is proposed that the probe will be able to pass further into the ear canal.

However despite the anatomical justification of this technique little evidence exists to support the 'tug' technique over simply placing the probe in the ear.[72,74] It is recommended that whichever technique for insertion is used that a seal must be obtained around the probe to stop environmental air being sensed at the probe as this may alter the acquired reading.[3]

Mercury thermometers

Mercury thermometers were initially the mainstay of temperature recording; however they are now being phased out due to concerns over mercury safety, the time constraints of their use and efficacy of thermometers at extremes of temperature.[3] As such these thermometers are not recommended for use in the prehospital environment.

Digital analogue probe thermometers

These thermometers are growing in popularity due to ease of use and timeliness of measurements. These non-disposable probes are used alongside disposable covers to ensure infection control measures are adhered to and may be placed either orally (in the sub-lingual pocket), rectally or in the axilla (armpit). Whilst the measurements acquired from these methods appear to be reliable and accurate, evidence suggests for accurate measurements to be obtained the probe should be in place for between 6-10 minutes.[75]

Chemical thermometry

Chemical thermometers rely upon a chemical reaction to heat to provide a readable measurement. These disposable probes are increasing in use within the prehospital field as they provide a cheap alternative to other methods. These probes can be placed orally, in the axilla or rectally (dependent upon manufacturer), however they are restricted in temperature range (35.5-40.4 °C).[76]

Temporal artery thermometers

These thermometers use radiation sensors to capture the infra-red heat from the temporal artery by scanning the forehead. The temporal artery branches from the carotid artery, therefore is suggested to be a reliable indicator if core body temperature. Recent studies suggest that this method is a reliable measure in children, however there is little evidence at present to support the use in adults.[74]

Which thermometer and site is most accurate?

There is little conclusive data to suggest that one site of temperature recording is more accurate and reliable than another. The rectal route is not recommended for prehospital care due to issues of privacy and the duration of such a procedure. Comparison of oral temperature sites and tympanic sites suggest that the oral route is preferred due to decreased variability of results[74] yet data also suggest that the tympanic route is reliable. Overall there is insufficient evidence to support one particular method, placing the onus upon the user to understand the limitations of all devices and subsequent clinical decision making. There is a growing body of evidence that the side (i.e. left versus right ear) of temperature recording may cause fluctuations of between 0.1-1.0 °C.[3,77]

There is little evidence to support the use of one thermometer over another (excluding the impractical pulmonary artery catheter), therefore no specific guidance can be issued at this point.[74-76] It is recommended that the practitioner ensure that they are suitably knowledgeable about the instrument of use in their own clinical area and apply caution in all temperature measurement interpretations. The use of digital thermometers and chemical thermometers may be limited in application due to the time constraints associated with their use.

The procedure of temperature assessment

Due to the common use of both tympanic and digital thermometers a procedure for each will be discussed.

Tympanic thermometer: A step-by-step guide to tympanic temperature recording

Procedure	Rationale
1. Explain and discuss the procedure with the patient.	To ensure that informed consent is gained.
2. Wash your hands.	To minimise the risks of cross infection.
3. Remove the thermometer from the base and ensure it is clean and the probe is clear. Use a dry wipe if required.	Alcohol based wipes can lead to low measurement and degrade the instrument.
4. Place a disposable probe cover on the instrument as per manufacturer guidelines.	This protects the probe and minimises infection risk.
5. Carefully place the probe into the ear canal ensuring a snug fit. Tugging of the pinna may align the ear canal making this easier to place the probe.	A snug fit is required to reduce the flow of ambient air to the probe tip.
6. Press the scan button (as per manufacturer guidance).	To commence scanning.
7. Remove the probe as soon as the measurement is complete.	This procedure can be uncomfortable.
8. Read the recording and document, include which ear is measured.	The reading may vary between ears therefore a baseline is essential.
9. Remove and dispose of the probe cover.	To ensure infection risk is minimised.

Digital thermometer: A step-by-step guide to digital temperature recording

Procedure	Rationale
1. Repeat steps 1 to 4 above.	
2. Place the thermometer in the axilla or sub-lingual pocket (as appropriate).	There appears to be no link between oxygen or medical gases and reducing oral temperature; the axilla is less invasive for the patient and enables them to talk during measurement.
3. Leave the probe in place for between 5-10 minutes.	Peak measurement occurs at approximately 9 minutes.
4. When a peak reading is reached remove the thermometer and record the reading.	

Chapter Key Points

1. The process of cardiovascular assessment is complex and altered by a large number of variables.
2. It is advisable to further research this area and take up any opportunities to gain experience to gain confidence and proficiency of skills. It is important to note the process of assessment of cardiovascular observations as slight changes in technique may cause significant changes in findings.

References and Further reading

1 Marieb E, Hoehn K. *Human Anatomy and Physiology*, 7th edn. San Francisco: Pearson Education, 2007.
2 Douglas G, Nicol F, Robertson C. *MacLeod's Clinical Examination*. London: Elsevier, 2005.
3 Boon N, Colledge N, Walker B (Eds) *Davidson's Principles and Practice of Medicine*, 20th edn. London: Churchill-Livingstone, 2006.
4 Thomas J, Monoghan T. *Oxford Handbook of Clinical Examination and Practical Skills* 5. Oxford: Oxford University Press, 2006.
5 Cox L, Roper T (Eds) *Clinical Skills*. Oxford: Oxford University Press, 2006.
6 Swash M (Ed) *Hutchinson's Clinical Methods*. Edinburgh: W.B. Saunders, 2002.
7 Hwu Y. Coates V, Lin F. A study into the effectiveness of different measuring times and counting methods of human radial pulse rates. *J Clin Nurs* 2000;9:146-152.
8 Sneed N, Hollerbach A. Measurement error in counting heart rate: potential sources and solutions. *Crit Care Nurse* 1995;15(1):36-40.

9 Sneed N, Hollerbach A. Accuracy of heart rate assessment in atrial fibrillation. *Heart and Lung* 1992;21(5):427-433.

10 Jevon P. Measuring capillary refill time. *Nurs Times* 2007;103(12):26-27.

11 Anderson B, Kelly A *et al.* Impact of patient and environmental factors on capillary refill time in adults. *Am J Emerg Med* 2008;26:62-65.

12 Schriger D, Baraff L. Defining normal capillary refill: variation with age, sex and temperature. *Ann Emerg Med* 1988;17:932-935.

13 Gorlick M *et al.* Effect of ambient temperature on capillary refill in healthy children. *Paediatrics.* 1993;92(5):699-702.

14 Holcomb JB, Niles SE, Miller CC *et al.* Prehospital physiologic data and life saving interventions in trauma patients. *Military Med* 2005;170:7-13.

15 Shriger DL, Baraff LJ. Capillary refill - is it a useful predictor of hypovolaemic states? *Ann Emerg Med* 1991;20:601-605.

16 Klup, NL, Keenan A. An evaluation of the reliability and validity of the capillary refill time test. *Foot* 2007;17(1);15-20.

17 Lewin J, Maconochie I. Capillary refill time in adults. *Emerg Med J* 2008;25:325-326.

18 Strosik KS, Pieper CH, Cools F. Capillary refilling time in newborns - optimal pressing time, sites of testing and normal values. *Acta Paed* 1998;87(3):310-312.

19 O'Brien E, Asmar R, Beilin L *et al.* European Society of hypertension recommendations for conventional, ambulatory and home blood pressure measurement. *J Hypertens* 2003; 21(5):821-848.

20 Beevers G, Lip G, O'Brien E. ABC of hypertension; Blood pressure measurement. *BMJ* 2001;322, 981-985.

21 Ben-Dov I, Perk G, Ben-Arie L, Mekler J, Bursztyn M. Pulse pressure is more susceptible to the white coat effect than is systolic blood pressure. *Am J Hypertens* 2004;17:535-539.

22 Joint British Societies. Joint British Societies Guidelines on Prevention of Cardiovascular Disease in Clinical Practice. *Heart* 2005;91(suppl 5):v1-v52.

23 National Institute for Clinical Excellence. Hypertension: *Management of primary hypertension in adults in primary care.* Clinical Guideline 34. London: NICE, 2006.

24 Hinckley P, Walker S. Measuring blood pressure. *New Pract Nurse* 2005;29(9):54-61.

25 Pickering T, Hall J, Appel L *et al.* Recommendations for blood pressure measurement in humans and experimental animals: Part 1: Blood pressure measurement in humans: A public statement for professionals from the sub-committee of professional and public education of the American Heart Association council on high blood pressure. *Circulation* 2005;111:697-716.

26 Jevon P, Holmes J. Blood pressure measurement: Part three: lying and standing blood pressure. *Nurs Times* 2007;103(20):24-25.

27 Williams B. Poulter N. Brown M *et al.* Guidelines for management of hypertension: report of the fourth working party of the British Hypertension Society, 2004-BHS IV. *J Hum Hypertens* 2004;18:139-185.

28 Mion D, Perrin A. How accurate are sphygmomanometers? *J Hum Hypertens* 1998;12:245-248.

29 Markandu N, Whitcher F, Arnold A, Carney C. The mercury sphygmomanometer should be abandoned before it is proscribed. *J Hum Hypertens* 2000;14:31-36.

30 Yarows S, Qian K. Accuracy of aneroid sphygmomanometers in clinical usage. *Blood Press Monit* 2001;6:101-106.

31 Canzanello V, Jensen P, Schwartz G. Are aneroid sphygmomanometers accurate in hospital and clinic settings? *Arch Intern Med* 2001;161:729-731.

32 Mauck G, Smith C, Geddes L, Borland J. The meaning of the point of maximum oscillations in cuff pressure in the indirect measurement of blood pressure. *J Biomechan Engin* 1980;102:28-33.

33 Wonka F, Thummler M, Schoppe A. Clinical test of a blood pressure measurement device with a wrist. *Blood Press Monit* 1996;1:361-366.

34 Sesler J, Munroe W, McKenny J. Clinical Evaluation of a finger oscillometric blood pressure device. *DICP* 1991;25:1310-1314.

35 Netea, R, Lenders J, Smits P, Thien T. Arm position is important for blood pressure measurement. *J Hum Hypertens* 1999;13:105-109.

36 O'Brien E, Petrie J, Littler W *et al*. Blood Pressure Measurement: *Recommendations of the British Hypertension Society*, 3rd edn. London: BMJ Publishing, 1997.

37 Lane D, Beevers M, Barnes N *et al*. Inter-arm differences in blood pressure: when are they clinically significant? *J Hypertens* 2002;20:1089-1095.

38 Beevers G, Lip G, O'Brien E. Blood pressure measurement - Part one: sphygmomanometry; factors common to all techniques. *BMJ* 2001;322;981-985.

39 Medicines and Healthcare Regulatory Agency. *Measuring Blood Pressure - Top Ten Tips*. London: MHRA, 2006.

40 Ragan C, Bordley J. The accuracy of clinical measurement of arterial blood pressure. *Bull John Hopkins Hosp* 1941;69:504.

41 Berliner K, Fujiy H, Lee D, Yildiz M, Garnier B. Blood pressure measurements in obese persons; comparison of intra-arterial and auscultatory measurements. *Am J Cardiol* 1961;8:10-17.

42 Linfors E, Feussner J, Blessing C *et al*. Spurious hypertension in the obese patient. Effect of sphygmomanometer cuff size on prevalence of hypertension. *Arch Intern Med* 1984;144:1482-1485.

43 Bovet P, Hungerbuler P, Quilindo J *et al*. Systematic difference between blood pressure readings caused by cuff type. *Hypertension* 1994;24:786-792.

44 Arcuri E, Santos J, Silva M. Is early diagnosis of hypertension a function of cuff width? *J Hypertens* (Suppl) 1989;7:s60-s61.

45 Russell A, Wing L, Smith S *et al*. Optimal size of cuff bladder for indirect measurement of arterial blood pressure in adults. *J Hypertens* 1989;7:607-613.

46 Wallymahmed M. Blood pressure measurement. *Nurs Stand* 2008;22(19):45-48.

47 Hunyor S, Flynn J, Cochineas C. Comparison of performance of various sphygmomanometers with intra-arterial blood pressure readings. *BMJ* 1978;2:159-162.

48 Roberts L, Smiley J, Manning G. A comparison of direct and indirect blood pressure determinations. *Circulation* 1953;8:232-242.

49 Breit S, O'Rourke M. Comparison of direct and indirect arterial pressure measurements in hospitalised patients. *Austral NZ J Med* 1974;4:485-491.

50 Holland W, Hummerfelt S. Measurement of blood pressure; comparison of intra-arterial and cuff values. *BMJ* 1964;2:1241-1243.

51 Perloff D, Grim C, Flack J *et al*. Human blood pressure determination by sphygmomanometry. *Circulation* 1993;88:2460-2470.

52 Cavallini M, Roman M, Blank S, Pini R, Pickering T, Deveraux R. Association of the auscultatory gap with vascular disease in hypertensive patients. *Ann Intern Med* 1996;124:877-883.

53 Beevers G, Lip G, O'Brien E. ABC of hypertension: blood pressure measurement. *BMJ* 2001;322:1043-1047.

54 American College of Surgeons Committee on Trauma. *Advanced Trauma Life Support*, 7th edn. Chicago: American College of Surgeons, 2004.

55 Deakin C, Low L. Accuracy of the advanced trauma life support guidelines for predicting systolic blood pressure using carotid, femoral and radial pulses: observational study. *BMJ* 2000;321:673-674.

56 Parati G, Faini A, Castaglioni P. Accuracy of blood pressure measurement: sphygmomanometer calibration and beyond. *J Hypertens* 2006;24:1915-1918.

57 Rose G. Standardisation of observers in blood pressure measurement. *Lancet* 1965;1:673-674.

58 Wingfield D, Cooke J, Thijs L *et al*. Terminal digit preference and single number preference in the Syst-Eur trial: influence of quality control. *Blood Press Monit* 2002;7:169-177.

59 Wen S, Kramer M, Joey J, Hanley J, Usher R. Terminal digit preference, random error and bias in routine clinical measurement of blood pressure. *J Clin Epidemiol* 1993;46:1187-1193.

60 Sykes D, Dewar R, Mohanaruban K *et al*. Measuring blood pressure in the elderly: does atrial fibrillation increase observer variability? *BMJ* 1990;300:162-163.

61 Stewart M, Gough K, Padfield P. The accuracy of automated blood pressure measuring devices in patients with controlled atrial fibrillation. *J Hypertens* 1995;13:297-300.

62 The Society for Cardiological Science and Technology. *Clinical Guidelines by Consensus: Recording a Standard 12-lead Electrocardiogram*. London: British Cardiovascular Society, 2006.

63 Kligfield PD *et al*. Recommendations for the standardisation and interpretation of the electrocardiogram – American Heart Association. *J Am Coll Cardiol* 2007;49(10): 1109-1127.

64 Jevon P. Cardiac monitoring. *Nurs Times* 2007;103(1):26-27.

65 Pahlm P *et al*. Evaluation of changes in standard electrocardiographic QRS waveforms recorded from activity-compatible proximal limb lead positions. *Am J Cardiol* 1992;69:253-257.

66 Sevilla DC *et al*. Invalidation of the resting electrocardiogram obtained via exercise electrode sites as a standard 12-lead recording. *Am J Cardiol* 1989;63:35-39.

67 August T. *et al*. Positional and respiratory changes in precordial lead patterns simulating acute myocardial infarction. *Am Heart J* 1958;55:706-714.

68 Colaco C *et al*. False positive ECG reports of anterior myocardial infarction in women. *J Electrocardiol* 2000;33:239-244.

69 Macfarlane PW *et al*. Precordial electrode placement in women. *Neth Heart J* 2003:11;118-122.

70 Chizner M. Cardiac auscultation: rediscovering the lost art. *Curr Probl Cardiol* 2008;33:326-408.

71 Hooper V. Thermoregulation. In: Quinn D, Schick L (Eds) *Perianaesthesia Nursing Core Curriculum*. St. Louis: Saunders, 2004.

72 Greaves I, Porter K, Hodgetts T *et al*. *Emergency Care: A Textbook for Paramedics*. Edinburgh: Saunders, 2006.

73 Hooper V, Andrews J. Accuracy of non-invasive core temperature measurement in acutely ill adults: The state of the science. *Biol Res Nurs* 2006;8;1;24-34.

74 Pullen R. Using an ear thermometer. *Nursing* 2003;33(5):24.

75 Latman N, Hans P, Nicholson L *et al*. Evaluation of clinical thermometers for accuracy and reliability. *Biomed Instrument Technol* 2001;35:259-265.

76 Farnell S, Maxwell L, Tan S *et al*. Temperature measurement: comparison of non-invasive methods used in adult critical care. *J Clin Nurs* 2005;14:632-639.

77 Heusch A, Suresh V, McCarthy P. The effect of factors such as handedness, sex and age on body temperature measured by an infrared 'tympanic' thermometer. *J Med Engin Technol* 2006;30(4);235-241.

Chapter 6

Respiratory observations and examination techniques

Content

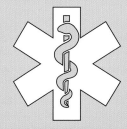

The respiratory system has two primary functions – to supply the body with oxygen and dispose of carbon dioxide.[1] To achieve these four processes, collectively known as respiration must occur:

- Pulmonary ventilation – Movement of air into and out of the lungs, usually referred to as breathing.
- External respiration – Movement of oxygen from the lungs into the blood and movement of carbon dioxide from the blood into the lungs.
- Transport of respiratory gases – Oxygen and carbon dioxide must travel from the lungs to the tissues and from the tissues to the lungs respectively.
- Internal respiration – Movement of oxygen from the blood to the tissues and movement of carbon dioxide from the tissues to the blood.

The respiratory system comprises of the nose, nasal cavity, pharynx, larynx, trachea, bronchi, smaller airways (bronchi and bronchioles) and the alveoli.[1] Due to the location of the lungs a major proportion of respiratory assessment requires an assessment of the anterior and posterior chest as well as the axillae. The lungs are situated within the thoracic cage with the apex sitting above the level of the clavicle and the anterior portion of the base at approximately the sixth rib. However due to the conical shape of the lungs the posterior base of the lung sits much lower at approximately the level of the eleventh rib. This is reflected in some of the examination techniques used in respiratory assessment.

The control of ventilation occurs through voluntary mechanisms regulated by the central nervous system and involuntary mechanisms controlled by the respiratory centre in the medulla oblongata and pons in the brain stem.[2] Breathing consists of two distinct phases, the inspiratory phase – lasting for approximately 2 seconds as the lungs fill; and the expiratory phase – a passive phase lasting approximately 3 seconds where air is expelled from the lungs.[1] The volume of air that is moved in and out of the lungs per minute is termed minute volume, this is determined by the respiratory rate and the tidal volume (volume of air moved by each breath), and therefore changes in either of these values can significantly change minute volume and the subsequent delivery of oxygen to the alveoli and carbon dioxide from the lungs to the environment.

The deterioration of breathing is one of the major causes of critical illness in the UK,[3] therefore the accurate assessment and management of respiratory function is paramount in patient care.

Indications for respiratory assessment

There are a variety of conditions that require respiratory assessment of varying levels, the level of assessment and observation should be based upon clinical judgement; however a basic assessment should be undertaken in any patient contact. Common indications for respiratory assessment are:

- To determine a baseline level of respiratory function and adequacy for future assessment.
- To provide diagnostic information in respiratory conditions such as asthma and COPD.
- To provide assessment of the efficacy of treatments/interventions.

Respiratory rate

Respiratory rate is the number of times per minute that a person breathes. There is some disagreement over what constitutes a 'normal' rate or Eupnoea in adults, with normal rates varying from 10 breaths per minute to 25 breaths per minute.[1,2,4,5] It is agreed however that breathing rates rise in the young and in the elderly,[6] as can be seen below. The ratio of respiratory rate to pulse rate is suggested to be approximately 1:5,[6] with some authors suggesting a ratio of 1:4.[7] As there is little consensus as to what constitutes a normal rate, it is therefore difficult to ascertain what is abnormal rate, therefore consideration of respiratory rate should be taken as an overall picture using other observations of the patient, such as level of consciousness or colour, as a guide.

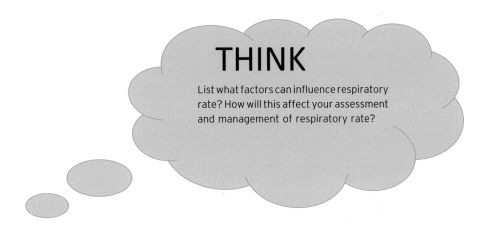

THINK

List what factors can influence respiratory rate? How will this affect your assessment and management of respiratory rate?

Tachypnoea

Tachypnoea is an abnormally fast respiratory rate based upon norm values (>20 breaths per minute),[8] and can be one of the first indications of respiratory distress. There can be numerous causes of tachypnoea such as anxiety, fever, exercise, hypoxia and pain.[1,4,9] The British Thoracic Society (2007) suggest that respiratory rate is a major indicator in severity of respiratory illness, with respiratory rates of over 25 breaths per minute indicative of acute severe exacerbation of conditions such as asthma (in adults).[10]

Table 6.1 Respiratory rates by age[8]

Age	Respiratory rate (range)
<1 year	30-40 (breaths/min)
1-2 years	26-34 (breaths/min)
2-5 years	24-30 (breaths/min)
5-12 years	20-24 (breaths/min)
>12 years	12-20 (breaths/min)

Bradypnoea

Bradypnoea is an abnormally slow respiratory rate (<12 breaths per minute),[8] that can indicate a severe deterioration of a patients condition.[10] Causes include fatigue, hypothermia, central nervous system depression and certain drugs such as opiates.[11]

Measuring respiratory rate

There is little evidence of how to measure respiratory rate, however consensus suggests that rate should be counted over a minute with the patient at rest and ideally without the patients knowledge it is being counted so as not to make them conscious of their respiratory rate.[2,5] There are a variety of methods that can be used to identify respiratory rate as seen below:

- Direct vision of chest movement.
- Use of specialist oxygen masks that incorporate respiratory rate indicators. The accuracy of these has been validated within the Emergency Department; however large scale studies have not been undertaken.[12]
- Counting of respiratory rate during auscultation.

Other methods have been suggested such as the visualisation of condensation on the inside of an oxygen mask; however the use of such techniques has not been validated and cannot be recommended.

Respiratory depth assessment

Respiratory depth is the volume of air inhaled and exhaled from the lungs with each respiration. The volume of air moved in a normal breath is termed tidal volume, in the average adult tidal volume is considered to be 500 mL.[1] This is typically measured with a spirometer, however a spirometry is not commonly utilised in prehospital care, and therefore the estimation of respiratory depth is undertaken by reviewing chest expansion or through the use of ventilatory methods discussed in other chapters such as the bag-valve-mask. However the assessment of the depth of respiration is important when considering the respiratory status of any patient.

THINK

What is more important respiratory rate or depth? Or are they equally important? Can you assess depth of breathing accurately? If not what can you do to make this estimation more accurate?

Chest and respiratory inspection

Whilst there is no scientific evidence to support the visualisation and inspection of the respiratory system, it is an inherent consideration for all patients with respiratory disease and related injury as visual indicators can emphasise the level of effort required for the patient to breathe, highlight the presence of injury, and provide clues in the formulation of a diagnosis. A thorough inspection of the airways, the neck (larynx and trachea), and the chest (for signs such as bruising, deformity, accessory muscles and equality of chest movement) can aid the practitioner and should form a part of every respiratory assessment. It is recommended that a thorough understanding of the underlying anatomy, physiology and pathophysiology of illness and injury be achieved so that the presence of and importance of visual indicators can be fully understood.

Chest compliance

Healthy lungs are stretchy and distensible; this is known as lung compliance. Lung compliance is determined by two factors, the distensibility of the lung tissue and alveolar surface tension.[1] However since the lungs are contained within the thoracic cage the compliance of the thoracic wall is also a key factor in lung compliance. Within the prehospital setting it is not possible to measure lung compliance, however thoracic wall compliance can be considered using a simple technique. In the healthy adult both sides of the thorax should expand symmetrically. Failure of the chest wall to expand either unilaterally or bilaterally may indicate disorders such as fibrosis, lung collapse or pleural effusion.

Assessing chest compliance

There is little evidence regarding the use of chest compliance as a measurement of respiratory function, however it can be a useful tool in the assessment of respiratory illness or injury. The method described below is a simple technique to assess the equality and depth of respiration.

Step-by-step procedure for assessing chest compliance

Procedure	Rationale
1. Gain informed consent from the patient and explain the procedure.	This procedure involves placing the hands upon the chest and back; therefore consent is vital.
2. To assess the function of the lower lobes place the hands firmly upon the chest with the fingers spread around the sides of the chest and extended thumbs meeting at the midline of the chest as seen in Figure 6.1 below.	This will provide an assessment of the expansion of the lower ribs and anterior chest wall.

Procedure	Rationale
3. The thumbs should be lifted slightly off of the chest.	This will allow easier movement of the hands upon the chest wall with inspiration and exhalation.
4. Ask the patient to inhale deeply (take a deep breath).	A normal inhalation may not provide enough movement to give an adequate assessment of the movement of the chest wall.
The thumbs should move apart symmetrically at least 5 cm.[14]	This is the expected norm for chest expansion in a healthy adult.
This technique may also be performed upon the back with the hands placed below the scapula (Figure 6.2 below).	This will provide an indication of the movement and expansion of the posterior chest wall.

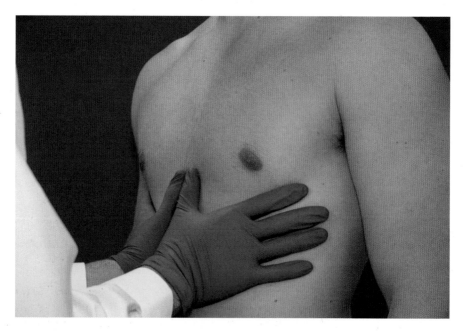

Figure 6.1 Expansion of the lower anterior chest.

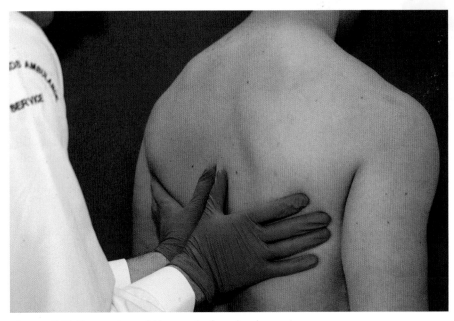

Figure 6.2 Expansion of the posterior chest.

Respiratory pattern/rhythm assessment

The normal respiratory rhythm has regular cycles co-ordinated by the central nervous system, with the expiratory phase slightly longer than the inspiratory phase. However, variations exist in the presence of underlying disorders. It is therefore important to note the rhythm of breathing during the measurement of respiratory rate.

Definitions

There is a variety of recognised breathing patterns that have clinical significance and should be noted if present.

- Apnoea is a loss of all respiration,[1] therefore it is an indication of critical illness or injury and death.
- Hypopnoea is a severe reduction of respiratory rate and depth that differs from bradypnoea due to the severity.
- Biot's breathing is an irregular breathing pattern that is differentiated from Cheynes–Stokes breathing (below) by the equal depth of respiration. It is commonly a result of central nervous system disorders.[6]
- Cheyne–Stokes breathing is a periodic breathing pattern in which there is a gradual increase in depth of breathing, followed by diminished respiratory effort, often associated with a brief period of apnoea.[13] This is often seen in patients with severe illness and most noticeably seen in cardiac failure, narcotic poisoning and neurological disorders.

- Kussmauls breathing is described as an increase in the depth and rate of breathing often resulting in a sighing pattern. This is commonly a result of metabolic acidosis secondary to conditions such as renal failure, salicylate poisoning and diabetic ketoacidosis.[14] Kussmauls breathing is a variation of hyperventilation that is also an increase in respiratory rate and depth.[1]

Measuring respiratory rhythm

There are no set guidelines or evidence for the observation of respiratory patterns; however consensus of opinion suggests that observing breathing for a period of one minute is best practice to allow for any changes to be noted and evaluated.[6,13]

Oxygen saturation/pulse oximetry

Oxygen is transported to the tissues in the blood, with approximately 3% transported in the blood plasma and 97% transported on haemoglobin creating oxyhaemoglobin.[1,15] Oxygen saturation is defined as the ratio of oxyhaemoglobin to the total concentration of haemoglobin.[15] Disease and injury processes can alter the ability of blood to carry or receive oxygen. Therefore the ability to measure oxygen levels in the blood can be a useful indicator of respiratory function. Oxygen saturations can be measured invasively via arterial blood gases (SaO_2) and non-invasively via pulse oximetry (SpO_2). Prior to the introduction of methods such as pulse oximetry detection of hypoxaemia (lack of oxygen in the blood) was reliant upon observation methods such as cyanosis at the lips (circumoral cyanosis). However this is considered to be a late sign with high levels of subjectivity due to eyesight differences and experience of the examiner.[16] The ability to undertake arterial blood gas sampling for SaO_2 levels is impractical in the prehospital; setting, therefore pulse oximetry is the routinely utilised method.

Pulse oximetry

The pulse oximeter measures the pulse rate and the saturation of haemoglobin in arterial blood. Through the use of two light sources (red and infrared) and a sensor, light absorption is measured. Pulse oximeters utilise the physiological difference in light absorption between oxygenated haemoglobin and reduced (deoxygenated) haemoglobin to provide a ratio reading displayed as a percentage of total haemoglobin.

There are a wide variety of products available within healthcare settings, providing pulse oximetry probes that are designed for differing areas of the body including the finger, forehead and the ear-lobe. Each practice area will have a preferred pulse oximeter manufacturer and probe configuration, however the principles remain the same regardless of make and model.

Indications for pulse oximetry

There are numerous reasons for the undertaking of pulse oximetry; examples of these are shown below:

- To assess respiratory function in respiratory illness or injury.
- To review the efficacy of respiratory interventions such as oxygen therapy.
- To gain a baseline measurement of oxygen saturation prior to interventions such as sedation and anaesthesia.

Limitations of pulse oximetry

The use of a pulse oximeter is not without limitations and sources of error. A variety of potential limitations have been identified and call into question measurements achieved through pulse oximetry:

- Nail polish - there has been growing concern over the validity of SpO_2 measurements achieved in patients who are wearing nail polish. Common practice as a result has been to remove nail polish prior to measurement[17] which obviously has time and expense implications. However recent large-scale studies have noted that whilst small differences (<1.6%) occur with dark colour nail polishes (brown and blue), that these changes are not clinically significant.[17,18] However it is noted that a difference in measurement can be caused by nail polish.
- Carbon monoxide poisoning - due to the affinity of carbon monoxide (CO) and haemoglobin, the presence of CO will result in the formation of carboxyhaemoglobin. However pulse oximeters are unable to detect the difference between oxyhaemoglobin and carboxyhaemoglobin, therefore in the presence of carbon monoxide (for example in smoke inhalation) pulse oximeters can provide a falsely elevated reading. In these situations SpO_2 should not be relied upon.[2,16,19]
- Poor peripheral circulation - as the pulse oximeter is reliant upon pulse waves, poor perfusion due to conditions such as cold or hypotension can result in inadequate readings.[16] Pulse oximetry has been found to be reliable with systolic blood pressures of >80 mmHg; however blood pressure readings below this level can lead to inaccurate or unreliable detection of the pulse waves and subsequent erroneous readings.[20,21] This is supported by findings in critically ill patients in two studies reviewing centrally sited SpO_2 probes (ear lobe/forehead) versus peripheral fingertip probes, with greater reliability and sensitivity found in more centrally sited probes.[22,23]
- Motion artefact - the excessive motion of digits from tremor, seizure or shivering can interfere with signal detection or interpretation. Therefore the placement of the probe is vital, alongside calming of the patient wherever possible.[16,24]
- High intensity lighting - this can lead to false readings due to the infiltration of light into the probe. This can be limited by correct application of the probe and by reducing bright light sources.[16]
- Age, sex and dark skin have not been shown to interfere with SpO_2 monitoring in previous studies[25] however a recent study suggests that dark skin can decrease the accuracy of pulse oximetry at low levels of oxygen saturation (<80%). Further research is required to clarify this situation before practice can be changed.
- High bilirubin levels in hepatitis and cirrhosis of the liver and some blood dyes used in angiography may reduce the accuracy of monitoring as they alter the colour of the blood.[26]

● Oximeters require a steady pulse signal, therefore conditions that affect the consistency of a pulse may reduce accuracy. One common example is the presence of cardiac arrhythmias such as atrial fibrillation.

Technique of pulse oximetry

A standardised approach to pulse oximetry can aid accuracy of results, and a step-by-step procedure is given below.

A step-by-step approach to pulse oximetry

Procedure	Rationale
1. Gain informed consent from the patient and explain the procedure.	This should be gained in all procedures as it is a legal requirement in any patient who can consent.
2. Ensure that the patient is warm and relaxed.	To reduce muscular artefact and anxiety related movement. Also consider bright lighting and rectify if safe and practical to do so.
3. Ensure that the equipment is clean and in good working order.	To minimise cross infection risk and ensure an accurate reading.
4. Select a suitable site for the probe, avoiding cold or shaking extremities, this is usually a finger tip. If there is nail varnish on the finger nail this may be removed to aid accuracy.	Shaking or cold extremities can affect the reading.
5. Turn on the pulse oximeter.	Naturally this is essential; turning on the probe prior to the procedure can cause noise alarms on the probe to be activated which may increase patient anxiety.
6. Ensure that the pulse oximeter is registering the pulse, and ensure that the pulse registered matches the patient pulse.	Artefact may alter the pulse reading and result in erroneous readings.
7. Take the reading. Some pulse oximeters can take a few seconds to register a true level so do not rush the procedure. It is recommended that an oximeter is given five minutes to 'settle' prior to taking a reading.[26]	Taking the reading too early may produce a false result and alter the clinical impression or management plan.
8. Consider external factors and limitations of pulse oximetry when interpreting readings.	A variety of factors may influence readings, therefore place the reading in context with other examination findings.

THINK

There are limitations in the accuracy of oximetry. What other factors should you assess when considering the oxygen saturation levels in any patient?

Key Point

Pulse oximetry has a number of potential flaws and limitations, therefore reliance upon such measures should be avoided and oxygen saturations used to compliment a full patient assessment.

Peak flow measurement

Peak expiratory flow rate measurement (PEFR) or peak flow is a simple and commonly used test of lung function. It is defined as the highest flow achieved from a maximal forced expiration started without hesitation from a maximal inhalation.[27] PEFR is measured in litres per minute, occurring early in forced expiration, within the first tenth of a second.[28] PEFR can be used as an indicator of airflow obstruction and restriction. It is a single measure of lung function and therefore should be utilised alongside other measures.

Measurements obtained should be considered against a set of norm values which can be acquired from a variety of sources such as:
The British Thoracic Society: www.brit-thoracic.org.uk/
Asthma UK: www.asthma.org.uk

A PEFR measurement is commonly obtained with a mini Wright peak flow meter. This device is a plastic tube with a plastic mouthpiece leading to the tube, along the barrel of the meter runs a scale that allows for the measurement. At the far end of the device is an air exhaust that allows exhaled air to be vented.

Indications for the use of PEFR

The PEFR reading is commonly used for the monitoring and assessment of asthma and COPD,[29] however it can be used in any respiratory condition. The common indications for PEFR assessment are:

- Confirmation of diagnosis of asthma.
- Measurement of severity of respiratory illness.
- Monitoring of treatment for respiratory conditions.

Whilst the British Thoracic Society (2007)[10] suggest that PEFR can be a useful tool in the assessment of severity of illness, further studies question the reliability of PEFR as a single indicator for illness severity.[30,31] However these studies are not without flaws suggesting that further research is required to fully evaluate the use of PEFR for indication of severity.

Technique of PEFR measurement

Procedure	Rationale
1. Gain informed consent from the patient and explain the procedure.	This should be gained in all procedures as it is a legal requirement in any patient who can consent.
2. Establish patient's best known PEFR or Norm value.	Whilst standardised charts are useful, patients with a respiratory illness history will have different normal value based upon their previous attempts.
3. Ensure that the equipment is clean and in good working order.	To minimise cross-infection risk and ensure an accurate reading.
4. Instruct the patient on the procedure and the flowing steps that must be taken.	A prior understanding of what is expected from the patient will provide a more fluent and accurate attempt.
5. Ask the patient to take a deep breath (maximum inhalation).	The reading is based upon maximal exhalation, therefore maximal inhalation is required first.
6. Immediately place the mouthpiece of the meter between the teeth so that the teeth and tongue do not obstruct the mouthpiece.	Obstructing the mouthpiece will reduce the acquired measurement.
7. The patient is then required to undertake a maximal exhalation without delay. This should be described as a short sharp 'huff'.	The first tenth of a second is key in PEFR measurement, delay in exhalation will reduce the maximal flow produced.

Procedure	Rationale
8. Note the reading on the meter and document.	Changes over time are important in assessing condition and efficacy of treatment.
9. This process should be undertaken three times to provide a best of three recording. However it important that sufficient recovery time is given between attempts.	More than five efforts are not likely to be beneficial as exhaustion and fatigue can occur.[27]

PEFR measurements in asthma can induce bronchoconstriction, therefore if repeated measurements produce lowering results testing should be ceased to prevent deterioration.[27] Consideration should also be given as to whether the patient is able to undertake testing, as severe reduction of respiratory function may inhibit the ability to record a PEFR reading.

Factors affecting PEFR measurement

As with any measurement technique in health assessment there is always potential for error in measurement. Common errors noted in PEFR measurement include:

- Failure to take a maximal inhalation – this will result in a sub-maximal exhalation.
- Holding the breath at the point at maximal inhalation – thus reducing the ability to provide a maximal exhalation.
- Blocking the mouthpiece with the tongue or the teeth – thus reducing the airflow through the meter.
- Failure to make a maximal exhalation – thus providing a falsely low reading.
- Leaks within the PEFR meter – thus reducing airflow through the device resulting in a falsely low reading.
- Blocking of the pointer – thus stopping an accurate reading.

Adapted from Booker (2007).[28]

There are no studies that investigate the extent of these sources of error; however a consensus of opinion suggests that they do commonly occur.[6,28]

Chest percussion

Percussion is a technique of physical examination that allows for the recognition of differing sounds resulting from vibrations through differing types of tissue potentially differentiating between air filled, fluid filled or solid areas beneath. It can be undertaken on either the chest for respiratory percussion or the abdomen to assess intra-abdominal injury and illness. Percussion of the chest will only penetrate tissues approximately 5-7 cm into the chest; therefore not all lesions and respiratory disorders can be recognised using this technique,[32] but in the absence of chest X-ray facilities in the field percussion is still a major tool within prehospital care.[5]

The aim of chest percussion is to compare the percussion note of the right and left sides of the chest. There are five typical percussion sounds that can be heard,

Table 6.2 Percussion note characteristics. Adapted from *Bates' Guide to Physical Examination and History Taking*[32] Bickley and Szilagyi (2003)

	Relative intensity	Relative pitch	Relative duration	Example location
Flatness	Soft	High	Short	Thigh or over areas of pleural effusion
Dullness (hyporesonant)	Medium	Medium	Medium	Liver or over consolidated lung tissue/lung collapse. This can be heard whenever fluid or solid tissue replaces air containing lung tissue
Resonance	Loud	Low	Long	Normal lung
Hyperreso-nance	Very loud	Lower	Longer	None normally – may be present in pneumo-thoraces, emphysema and exacerbations of asthma
Tympany	Loud	High (a musical timbre)	Distinguished by its musical timbre	Gastric air bubble or puffed out cheek

as seen in Table 6.2. These can be simply examined and recognised (even on your own chest) using the technique explained later.

Indications for chest percussion

The percussion of the chest should be performed as an aid to diagnosis when there is suspicion of an underlying respiratory illness or injury, such as those listed below:

- Pneumothoraces and haemothoraces
- Pneumonia and chest infections
- Pleural effusion
- Lung lesions
- Asthma, emphysema and chronic bronchitis.

The technique of chest percussion

A step-by-step guide to chest percussion

Procedure	Rationale
1. Gain informed consent from the patient and explain the procedure.	This should be gained in all procedures as it is a legal requirement in any patient who can consent.
2. Place your left hand palm down firmly against the chest, ensuring that the middle finger is aligned between the ribs and the fingers are spread slightly apart (Figure 6.3 below).	Sound conduction through bone can be reduced.
3. Press the left middle finger firmly against the chest wall.	To allow for transmission of the pressure wave when the finger is struck.

Procedure	Rationale
4. Flex the right hand at the wrist with the middle metacarpophalangeal joint slightly flexed.	This will ensure that a fluid motion is used and the force applied is appropriate.
5. Hyperextend the wrist further then briskly flex the wrist using the pad of the middle finger of the right hand to strike the middle phalanx or distal interphalangeal joint of the left middle finger (see Figure 6.4 below).	
6. Immediately remove the percussing finger (the right hand).	Maintaining the percussion finger on the struck finger will dull the sound wave produced.
7. This procedure can be repeated swiftly to provide a second sound.	This is only necessary if you wish to confirm the first sound.
8. As you strike the two fingers listen and feel the percussion note.	Try to identify the quality of the percussion note.
9. Percussion should be undertaken upon a minimum of four areas on each side (left and right) of the anterior chest – including over the clavicles; the axillae should also be percussed at this time.	A thorough examination should be undertaken to ensure no areas of lung are omitted.
10. Further percussion should be undertaken on a minimum of four sites on each side of the posterior chest, excluding over the scapulae.	The thickness of muscle and bone alters the percussion note from the tissue. This is to ensure that all lung fields are percussed for findings. An example pattern of percussion can be seen in Figures 6.5–6.7 below.
11. If the upper posterior chest is percussed the patient should be encouraged to fold their arms.	This will move the scapulae laterally for ease of percussion.

Scenario

You are called to a patient in severe respiratory distress following being struck in the chest by a piece of machinery. You notice that the patient has severe bruising to the left side of his chest and has poor oxygenation (SpO_2 = 82%) recorded, alongside a marked tachycardia (140 bpm). On auscultation and percussion you are unable to hear any sounds due to the noisy environment. What are the likely diagnoses for this patient? How can you assess the patient further? What actions may you need to take in treating this patient?

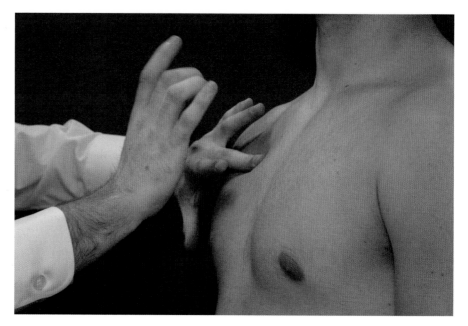

Figure 6.3 The initial hand position for chest percussion.

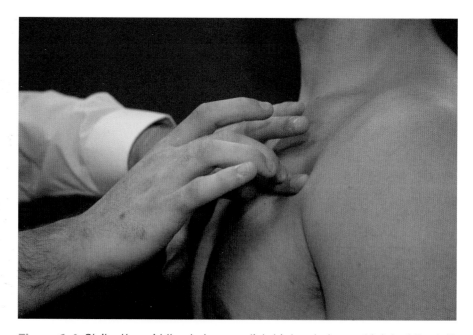

Figure 6.4 Strike the middle phalanx or distal interphalangeal joint of the left middle finger.

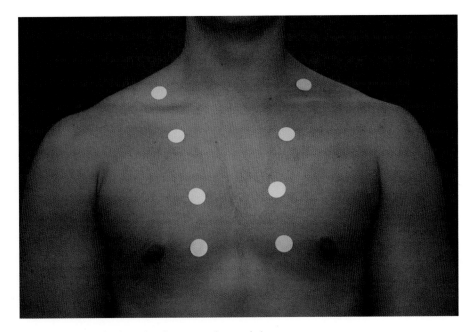

Figure 6.5 Anterior chest percussion points.

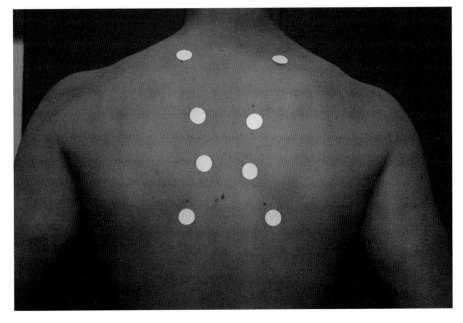

Figure 6.6 Posterior chest percussion points.

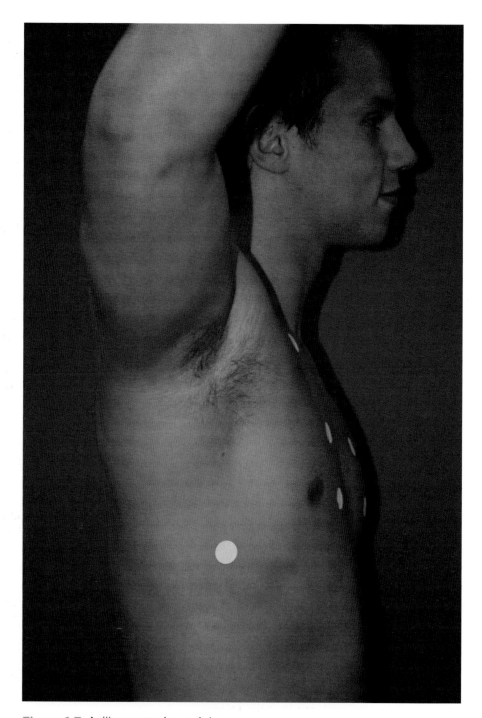

Figure 6.7 Axilla percussion points.

If a difference in percussion tone is noted between sides the area should be re-percussed to confirm findings. The skill of percussion does take some practice to attain competence therefore practice is necessary. This technique can be practiced on both yourself, colleagues and even on inanimate objects such as walls.

> You can use surfaces such as walls or boxes to practice. Each surface will produce a different sound. Percussing the right side of the abdomen will also produce differing sounds ranging from resonance over the lung to a dull note over the liver. Practise on willing colleagues or friends to get used to identifying differing notes.

Tactile vocal fremitus

Tactile vocal fremitus is a vibration test felt upon the chest when the patient speaks. It is a technique that is seldom used by practitioners due to lack of sensitivity, however this test can be useful in the assessment of suspected effusion and con-solidation. Human speech is generally at a low frequency that can be detected as vibration upon the chest wall. At times of consolidation vibrations will increase due to transmission of sound waves through thicker tissue. However in cases such as lung collapse, pneumothorax and pleural effusion vibrations are reduced.

Technique of tactile vocal fremitus

A step-by-step guide to tactile vocal fremitus assessment

Procedure	Rationale
1. Gain informed consent from the patient and explain the procedure.	This should be gained in all procedures as it is a legal requirement in any patient who can consent.
2. Place the ulna border of the hand horizontally against the chest.	This side of the hand is sensitive to movement beneath.
3. Ask the patient to say 'ninety nine', whilst the patient is speaking concentrate upon the vibrations felt in the hand.	The vibration caused by saying 'ninety nine' is accentuated by effusion and consolidation in the lung.
4. This should be repeated in all fields of the anterior/posterior chest and the axilla in the areas highlighted in Figures 6.5-6.7.	A thorough examination should be undertaken to ensure no areas of lung are omitted.

This is a test that requires skill and experience to utilise fully therefore practice is highly recommended. As an uncommonly used skill this is not expected to be used frequently but can be a useful addition in the assessment of respiratory disorders.

Chest auscultation

Auscultation of the lungs is the most important assessment of airflow through the trachea-bronchial tree. It allows the practitioner to assess the quality of airflow to the lungs and the condition of the lungs. Auscultation is the technique of listening to the sounds generated by airflow in breathing; in addition the examiner should listen for added (adventitious) sounds produced during the respiratory cycle. Despite the frequency of auscultation in patient assessment there is little evidence to support current techniques therefore a general consensus of expert opinion is most commonly considered.

Most sounds that reach the chest wall are low frequency and are theoretically more easily heard by using the bell of the stethoscope despite little consensus over this, the diaphragm is most commonly used in clinical practice.[5,14,31] The use of the diaphragm can lead to the stretching of the skin and trapping of hairs beneath, thus producing sounds similar to crackles (an adventitious sound); it may also be difficult in the thin patient to achieve full contact between the diaphragm and the chest wall.

Breath sounds

Breath sounds are differentiated by their intensity, pitch and duration of their inspiratory and expiratory phases.

- Normal breath sounds: These are described as vesicular and are produced by airflow in the large airways and larynx and altered by passing through the smaller airways. The sounds are soft and low pitched; described as a rustling sound. They start at the beginning of inspiration and continue through until about one third of the way through expiration where they fade away.
- Bronchial breath sounds: This is caused by increased density of matter in the peripheral lung fields allowing for the transmission of sound unchanged from the larger airways. These sounds are louder and higher in pitch, often described as hollow and blowing, often having a pause between inspiration and expiration, the expiratory phases tends to last longer than the inspiratory phase. These sounds are commonly heard in conditions such as pneumonia where air filled tissue is filled with fluid or solid lung tissue.
- Bronchovesicular: These sounds have an inspiratory and expiratory phase of an even length, there may be a pause between inspiration and expiration. These sounds are again found in conditions that alters the air filled lung tissue by fluid, fibrosis or collapse.
- Reduced breath sounds: The intensity of breath sounds relates to the airflow through the tissues, therefore reductions in airflow will from causes such as obesity, pleural effusion, fibrosis, pneumothorax and asthma to name a few can result in reduced ability of air to flow into the tissues. A silent or quiet chest is not a sign that the lung fields are clear. In some cases asking the patient to cough can ease a bronchial obstruction and make breath sounds easier to hear.[14]

Added sounds (adventitious)

There are a variety of additional breath sounds that can have a clinical significance, therefore practitioners should be able to recognise and describe adventitious sounds. A selection of common additional sounds can be seen below:

- Wheeze: These are musical sounds and should be timed with the respiratory cycle. They are caused by narrowing of the airways. A wheeze tends to be louder on expiration as the airways naturally dilate on inspiration and narrow on expiration. High pitch wheezes emanate from the smaller airways such as the bronchioles, whereas lower pitch wheezes come from larger airways such as the bronchi. A wheeze however is a poor discriminator of airway narrowing as severely restricted airways will produce a quieter wheeze due to limited air flow. Wheezes are commonly seen in asthma and COPD.
- Crackles (rales/crepitations): Crackles are usually a result of collapsed airways and alveoli being filled with air at high pressure causing an opening 'snap'. It is important to note when the crackles occur within the respiratory cycle as this can aid diagnosis. Early inspiratory crackles are indicative of small airway disease such as bronchiolitis. In pulmonary oedema crackles occur in mid inspiration. Late phase inspiratory fine crackles are suggestive of conditions such as pulmonary fibrosis and bronchial secretions in COPD, these sounds are commonly described as like rubbing hair between your fingers. Crackles may also be heard when air passes through secretions in the larger airways, these sounds are commonly more coarse and have a gurgling quality.
- Pleural rub: These sounds are produced by the inflammation of the parietal and visceral pleura that surround the lungs. The sound is likened to creaking such as bending a new leather belt or the sound of a footstep in fresh snow. It is best heard with the diaphragm of the stethoscope due to the high pitched nature of the sound and is commonly heard at the end of inspiration and the beginning of expiration. Pleural rub is often difficult to hear unless the patient is breathing deeply, so is therefore normally sought when a pleuritic type pain is presented.

Examples of breath sounds can be found on-line at sites such as:
http://www.merck.com/
http://www.rale.ca
http://www.emsvillage.com
They may also be found on CD at most medical libraries.

Technique of Auscultation

A step-by-step guide to chest auscultation

Procedure	Rationale
1. Gain informed consent from the patient and explain the procedure.	This should be gained in all procedures as it is a legal requirement in any patient who can consent.
2. Ask the patient to take deep breaths in and out through the mouth.	This increases the turbulent airflow to allow for easier recognition of sounds.
3. Place the diaphragm of the stethoscope (or bell if the patient is very slim or has a hairy chest) over the chest, commencing above the clavicle.	The apex of the lung can be heard in the supra-clavicular notch.
4. Listen to both inspiration and expiration.	Adventitious sounds may be heard on both inspiration and exhalation.
5. After each breath move the stethoscope from side to side covering all lung fields both anteriorly, posteriorly and in the axillae. It is suggested that for a thorough assessment the sites shown in earlier in the chapter for percussion sites should be used.	A thorough examination should be undertaken to ensure no areas of lung are omitted.
6. It may be useful to coach the patient's breathing by saying 'in ....and out'.	This will allow you to control the procedure.
7. Be aware of the patient's physical condition as long periods of deep breathing may cause dizziness or not be achievable in the dyspnoeic patient.[31]	It may be necessary to stop and allow the patient to breathe normally.
8. Take note of the breath sounds and presence of adventitious sounds in each lung field auscultated. If abnormality is noted then listen for longer over each lung field.	To ensure that the quality of the sound is fully assessed.

Vocal resonance

Also referred to as transmitted voice sounds, this is an assessment tool not commonly used in prehospital care; however it has a significant diagnostic benefit when combined with other examination techniques. Vocal resonance is the auscultatory equivalent of tactile fremitus, whereby sounds are transmitted through the chest wall when the patient speaks. Normally when auscultation is performed, whilst the patient is speaking, muffled indistinct sounds will be heard. However over an area of consolidation sound transmission is increased so sounds become more distinct or more resonant. In cases such as pleural effusion, lung collapse and pneumothoraces, sound transmission is reduced thus making sounds less intelligible.

Technique of vocal resonance

A step-by-step guide to vocal resonance

Procedure	Rationale
1. Gain informed consent from the patient and explain the procedure.	This should be gained in all procedures as it is a legal requirement in any patient who can consent.
2. Place the diaphragm of the stethoscope upon the chest, it is suggested that the same areas are used as with auscultation (Figures 6.5-6.7).	To ensure that all lung fields are examined.
3. Ask the patient to say 'ninety nine'. Normally the sound will be muffled and indistinct.	These procedures will elicit differing sounds that are required to assess for consolidation or effusion.
4. Ask the patient to say 'ee'. Normally a muffled long 'ee' will be heard. If 'ee' is heard as 'ay' this is known as egophony and can indicate consolidation within the affected area.	
5. Ask the patient to whisper 'ninety-nine', the voice is normally faint and indistinct if heard at all. However in the consolidated lung the whispered voice may be heard. This is known as whispering pectoriloquy.	

Due to the complexity of this examination skill, it is not routinely recommended or required.

Chapter Key Points

1. Respiratory examination requires experience and knowledge of signs and symptoms present in differing conditions.
2. There are a number of steps in undertaking a full respiratory assessment; these procedures form only the core of assessment and are part of a fuller holistic assessment. Physical assessment must be considered alongside careful history taking and visual assessment.

References and Further reading

1 Marieb E, Hoehn, K. *Human Anatomy and physiology*, 7th edn. San Francisco: Pearson Education, 2007.

2 Moore T. Respiratory assessment in adults. *Nurs Stand* 2007;21(49):48-56.

3 Department of Health. *Comprehensive Critical Care:* A Review of Adult Critical Care Services. London: The Stationary Office, 2000.

4 Torrance C, Elley K. Respiration technique and observation. *Nurs Times* 1997;93(43)(Suppl):1-2.

5 Cox N, Roper T. *Clinical Skills*. Oxford: Oxford University Press, 2005.

6 Dougherty L, Lister S. (Eds) *The Royal Marsden Hospital Manual of Clinical Nursing Procedures*, 6th edn. Oxford: Blackwell Publishing, 2006.

7 Moore T. Respiratory assessment. In: Moore T, Woodrow P (Eds) *High Dependency Nursing Care: Observation, Intervention and Support*. London: Routledge, 2004.

8 European Resuscitation Council. *European Paediatric Life Support Course*. London: Resuscitation Council, 2006.

9 Boon N, Colledge N, Walker B. (Eds) *Davidson's Principles and Practice of Medicine*, 20th edn. London: Churchill-Livingstone, 2006.

10 British Thoracic Society. *British Guideline on the Management of Asthma*. London: British Thoracic Society, 2007.

11 Jevon P, Ewens B. Assessment of the breathless patient. *Nurs Stand* 2001;15(16):48-53.

12 Breakell A, Townsend-Rose C. The clinical evaluation of the Respi-Check mask: a new oxygen mask incorporating a breathing indicator. *Emerg Med J* 2001;18:366-369.

13 Swash M. (Ed) *Hutchinson's Clinical Methods*. Edinburgh: W.B. Saunders, 2002.

14 Douglas G, Nicol F, Robertson C. *MacLeod's Clinical Examination*. London: Elsevier, 2005.

15 Barker S. Motion Resistant pulse oximetry: a comparison of new and old models. *Anaesthet Analges* 2002;95(4):967-972.

16 DeMeulenaere S. Pulse oximetry: uses and limitations. *J Nurse Pract* 2007; May:312-317.

17 Rodden A, Spicer L, Diaz V, Steyer T. Does fingernail polish affect pulse oximeter readings? *Intens Crit Care Nurs* 2007;23:51-55.

18 Hinkelbein J, Genzwuerker H, Sogl R, Fiedler F. Effect of nail polish on oxygen saturation as determined by pulse oximetry in critically ill patients. *Resuscitation* 2007;72: 81-91.

19 Moyle J. *Pulse Oximetry*. London: British Medical Journal Books, 2002.

20 Hakemi A, Bender J. Understanding pulse oximetry, advantages and limitations. *Home Health Care Manage Pract* 2005;15(5):416-418.

21 Hill E, Stoneham M. Practical applications of pulse oximetry. *Update Anaesthes* 2000;11:4.

22 Lindholm P, Blogg S, Gennser M. Pulse oximetry to detect hypoxemia during apnea: comparison of finger and ear probes. *Aviation, Space Environment Med* 2007;78(8):770-773.

23 Schallom L, Sona C, McSweeney M, Mazuski J. Comparison of forehead and digit oximetry in surgical/trauma patients at risk for decreased peripheral perfusion. *Heart Lung* 2007;36(3):188-194.

24 Petterson M, Begnoche V, Graybeal J. The effect of motion on pulse oximetry and its clinical significance. *Anaesthes Analges* 2007;105(6)Suppl:S78-S84.

25 Louw A, Cracco Cerf C *et al.* Accuracy of pulse oximetry in the intensive care unit. *Intens Care Med* 2001;27(10):1606-1613.

26 Booker R. Pulse Oximetry. *Nurs Stand* 2008;22(30);39-41.

27 Miller MR, Hankinson J, Brusasco V *et al.* ATS/ERS Task force: standardisation of spirometry. *Eur Resp J* 2005;26(2):319-338.

28 Booker R. Peak expiratory flow measurement. *Nurs Stand* 2007;21(39):42-43.

29 Ruffin R. Peak expiratory flow monitoring. *Thorax* 2004;59:913-914.

30 Sly P, Cahill P, Willet K, Burton P. Accuracy of mini peak flow meters in indicating changes in lung function in children with asthma. *BMJ* 1994;308:572-574.

31 Emerman C, Cydulka R. Use of peak expiratory flow rate in emergency department evaluation of acute exacerbation of chronic obstructive pulmonary disease. *Ann Emerg Med* 1996;27(2):159-163.

32 Bickley L, Szilagyi P. *Bates' Guide to Physical Examination and History Taking*. Philadelphia: Lippincott Williams & Wilkins, 2003.

Chapter 7

Neurological observations and examination techniques

Content

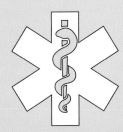

The importance of undertaking a reliable and timely neurological assessment of acutely ill patients cannot be overestimated. However evidence suggests that the neurological assessments undertaken by healthcare professionals may not always be consistent and appropriate.[1] There are numerous presentations that the practitioner may experience which require neurological assessment to establish treatment or diagnosis; these can include conditions such as hypoglycaemia, cerebro-vascular accident (or stroke) and the head injured patient. It is the intention of this chapter to provide the practitioner with an evidence based approach to standardised neurological observations that can be utilised in dealing with such patient groups.

Definitions

Neurological observations are those investigations and examination that relate to the assessment of the nervous system. These commonly focus upon six key areas:

- Level of consciousness
- Pupillary activity
- Motor function
- Sensory function
- FAST (stroke recognition)
- Vital signs.

One observation that is commonly part of a neurological assessment (although primarily an endocrine function) is blood sugar analysis. This will also be discussed as a part of this chapter.

Indications

There are a variety of indications for neurological assessment and observations that relate to any condition or presentation that could or does exhibit altered neurological status. Neurological observations should be aimed at:

- Detecting abnormality
- Detecting deterioration
- Detecting improvement.

A systematic approach to neurological assessment can assist in the detection of changes over time.

Level of consciousness assessment

Consciousness encompasses a conscious perception of sensations, voluntary initiation and control of movement, and capabilities associated with higher mental function (such as memory, logic or judgement).[2] Clinically, consciousness is graded upon a four-point scale relating to response to stimuli running on a continuum from the highest level of awareness to the most depressed, as seen below:

1. Alertness
2. Drowsiness or lethargy

3. Stupor
4. Coma.

From Marieb E, Hoehn K. (2007) *Human Anatomy and Physiology.*[2]

There are two common methods used in the assessment of levels of consciousness by healthcare professionals, the AVPU score and Glasgow Coma Scale.

AVPU score

The AVPU score is a brief examination of responsiveness that is initiated in the primary survey.[3] The scale was introduced as a method for rapid neurological assessment in the trauma patient[4] with the use of scoring based upon a grading of initial response upon the following stimuli:

A   Alert (no stimulus required).

V   Verbal stimulus required to elicit a response.

P   Painful stimulus required to elicit response.

U   Unresponsive to all stimuli.

The method for eliciting pain response will be discussed later (see GCS section). Anecdotal evidence suggests that AVPU is simpler and quicker to use than the Glasgow coma score,[5] however studies have suggested that the AVPU score may not provide the sensitivity to detect subtle changes in neurological status that result from non traumatic causes of neurological derangement.[5,6]

The Glasgow Coma Scale

This scale was introduced in 1974 by Teasdale and Jennett[7] as a standardised tool to aid physicians in the assessment and comparison of patients with altered levels of consciousness. This scale, following modifications, has been in use by healthcare professionals ever since.[8] Whilst this method is commonly accepted as the technique of choice within health services, studies have suggested that the scale may not always be reliably used in comparison to other methods such as AVPU.[9,10]

The Glasgow Coma Score (GCS) evaluates three key categories of behaviour that closely reflect activity in the higher centres of the brain; eye opening, verbal response and motor response.[11] Within each category a score is given for the level of response, with the lower the score the greater the deterioration of neurological function. The lowest score a patient can receive is 3 and the highest value is 15 (indicating a fully alert state). The GCS chart for adults can be seen in Box 7.1.

The GCS table is applicable for adolescents and has been adapted for paediatrics as seen in Box 7.2; however the use in children under the age of 3 is questionable due to developmental issues.[13]

Best eye response

Eye opening is closely linked with being awake and alert and as such is easily identified. Eye opening mechanisms are controlled by a collection of neurones located in the brain stem, hypothalamus and thalamus known as the reticular activating system that is stimulated by sensory input.[2] The patient is considered to have spontaneous eye opening when the eyes are opened without any stimulation. If either a verbal or

Best eye response (4)

1. No eye opening.
2. Eye opening to pain.
3. Eye opening to verbal command.
4. Eyes open spontaneously.

Best verbal response (5)

1. No verbal response
2. Incomprehensible sounds.
3. Inappropriate words.
4. Confused
5. Orientated

Best motor response (6)

1. No motor response.
2. Extension to pain.
3. Abnormal flexion to pain.
4. Normal flexion to pain.
5. Localising pain.
6. Obeys commands.

Box 7.1 The Glasgow Coma Scale table for adults.[12]

painful stimulus is required then this must be recorded, a guide to undertaking eye response testing is seen in Table 7.1.

Best verbal response

The best verbal response assesses two aspects of cerebral function:

- Comprehension or understanding of what has been said.
- Ability to express thoughts into words or expression.

This can be achieved by speaking to the patient in a normal voice. It is best practice not to ask yes or no questions as they can lead to missed information. The best verbal response also assesses the patient's awareness of themselves in relation to time and space. An element of consideration is required when assessing a best verbal response, many authors suggest that the patient must be able to state the day and date to be considered orientated.[7] However thought must be given to the patient's status, as many patients who have been hospitalised for a long time for example will have little need to know the date. A guide to undertaking a best verbal response can be seen in Table 7.2.

Discrepancies can occur in the assessment of verbal response; therefore it is imperative that the practitioner uses language that the patient can understand to reduce the likelihood of misunderstanding.

Best eye response (4)

1. No eye opening.
2. Eye opening to pain.
3. Eye opening to verbal command.
4. Eyes open spontaneously.

Best verbal response (5)

1. No vocal response.
2. Occasionally whimpers and/or moans.
3. Cries inappropriately.
4. Less than usual ability and/or spontaneous irritable cry.
5. Alert, babbles, coos, words or sentences to usual ability.

Communication with the infant or child's caregivers is required to establish the best usual verbal response. A 'grimace' alternative to verbal responses should be used in pre-verbal or intubated patients.

Best grimace response (5)

1. No response to pain.
2. Mild grimace to pain.
3. Vigorous grimace to pain.
4. Less than usual spontaneous ability or only response to touch stimuli.
5. Spontaneous normal facial/oro-motor activity.

Best motor response (6)

1. No motor response to pain.
2. Abnormal extension to pain (decerebrate).
3. Abnormal flexion to pain (decorticate).
4. Withdrawal to painful stimuli.
5. Localises to painful stimuli or withdraws to touch.
6. Obeys commands or performs normal spontaneous movements.

Box 7.2 Paediatric version of the Glasgow Coma Scale.[14]

THINK

What difficulties can arise in assessing a verbal response? What can you do to improve or assist in these situations?

Table 7.1 Best eye response[18]

Observation	Score	Method
Eye response: If the patient is unable to open their eyes as a result of trauma or surgery the letter 'c' indicating closed should be recorded. This will ensure that false recordings are reduced.		
This score indicates the level of arousal/ consciousness	4 - Spontaneously	The patient's eyes should open as you approach. If the patient is asleep wake them first as the assessment is based upon best response.
	3 - To speech	The patient will respond to your voice. The simplest way is to use their name. If there is no response consider using a raised voice as the patient may be hearing impaired.
	2 - To pain	The patient should open their eyes to painful stimulus (discussed below)
	1 - No response	The patient's eyes remain closed despite painful stimuli.

Table 7.2 Best verbal response[19]

Observation	Score	Method
Verbal response: The patient may have difficulty in speaking (dysphasia). If this is the case 'D' should be indicated in the chart, if the patient is intubated then the letter 'T' should be used.		
This score indicates the level of orientation to time, place and self.	5 - Orientated	The patient must be able to state their name, who they are, where they are and what the month is (or time of day - morning, evening, night).
	4 - Confused	If the patient is able to hold a conversation but unable to answer the previous questions correctly they should be considered confused. Correct any wrongly answered questions and re-ask them later in the assessment using a different order to avoid copying.
	3 - Inappropriate words	The patient will use random words that make little sense or are out of context. This typically consists of swearing and shouting. A painful stimuli may be required to gain a response.
	2 - Incomprehensible sounds	The patient will only respond with moaning and groaning. Painful stimuli may be required to gain a response.
	1 - No response	There is no verbal response despite painful stimuli.

Best Motor Response

The best motor response is used to test how well the brain is functioning as a whole by testing the identification of sensory input and the subsequent motor response. The best possible motor response is the ability to understand simple commands and respond.[11] A guide to undertaking an assessment of best motor response can be seen below in Table 7.3.

It is not recommended to use the command of 'squeeze my fingers' as an obeyed command as this is a primitive reflex and may occur involuntarily.[16] It is recommended that a central response is used to test a response to pain as a peripheral stimulus may provoke a spinal reflex and therefore not assess cerebral functioning.[11] Spinal reflexes may cause limbs to flex briskly and can even be elicited in patients who have been certified as brainstem dead.[15] It can also be very difficult to differentiate flexion from pain and withdrawal from pain if using a peripheral pain stimuli.

Painful stimuli

A response to painful stimulus is a very contentious issue and should only be applied if the patient does not respond to other stimuli.[8] There are numerous legal and ethical issues that should be considered on each occasion, therefore it is recommended that explanation is given to any onlookers to save confusion and later complications.[11] There are two overarching approaches to painful response, both having inherent flaws and benefits that must be considered; these approaches are central and peripheral stimuli.[16]

Table 7.3 Best motor response[11,19]

Observation	Score	Method
Motor response: If the patient is receiving paralytic drugs as Glasgow coma scale cannot be assessed.		
This indicates brain function.	6 - Obeys commands	Ask the patient to perform a series of different movements such as sticking out their tongue or raising their arms.
	5 - Localises to pain	Apply a central painful stimulus (as described later in Table 7.4). The patient should purposefully move the arm towards the site of pain to remove the cause.
	4 - Withdraws from pain	The patient will flex their arms in response to a painful stimulus but will not move towards the source of the pain.
	3 - Flexion to pain	Also referred to as decorticate positioning. It occurs when there is a block in the motor pathway between the cerebral cortex and brain stem. It is a slower response to a painful stimulus. It is recognised by a flexion of the upper arm and rotation of the wrist. It may also result in the thumb flexing across the fingers.
	2 - Extension to pain	Also known as decerebrate positioning. This is the result of a blocked or damaged motor pathway within the brainstem. This is characterised by straightening of the elbow and internal rotation of the shoulder. The legs may also straighten with the toes pointing downwards.
	1 -	There is no physical response despite painful stimuli.

Table 7.4 Eliciting painful stimuli[18,19]

Stimulus	Procedure	Rationale
Trapezium squeeze	1. This is achieved by using the thumb and two fingers as 'pincers'. Feel for the large muscle mass of the trapezius (located at the angle where the neck and shoulders meet) and twist or squeeze.	A gentle pinch of approximately half an inch hurts but does not cause real pain.
Supraorbital pressure	2. Pain is achieved by applying pressure over a branch of the facial nerve. This can be found upon the inner aspect of the eyebrow in a small notch. Place the hand upon the patients head and the flat of the thumb or knuckle is placed over the notch. Pressure should gradually be applied for a maximum of thirty seconds.	Pressure applied here causes pain in the form of a headache. This method should not be used in facial trauma or glaucoma as it may further injury.[34] Caution is also required as orbital pressure may also cause bradycardia.
Jaw pressure	3. Apply pressure to the angle of the jaw just in front of the ear lobe using the thumb.	This method should not be used in cases of facial trauma.
Sternal rub	4. This involves grinding the knuckles or palm upon the centre of the sternum.	This method can cause bruising over time and is considered to be an outdated and should only be used with extreme caution.[16]

Central stimuli

There are four commonly used distinct methods of providing a central painful stimulus: trapezium squeeze, supraorbital pressure, jaw pressure and sternal rub as described in Table 7.4.

The use of the centralised pain response to elicit eye opening response can be difficult as it may cause grimacing or eye closure as a natural response therefore making it counter-productive when assessing for eye opening.[8] However central stimuli are perceived to be more reliable as they can produce an overall body response thus making a centralised stimulus more reliable when assessing motor function.[17] Whilst there are little data to suggest a recommended method of centralised painful stimuli, anecdotal evidence suggests that the sternal rub technique should be discontinued due to concerns over potential patient injury including bruising and skin breakdown.[11] In addition the use of supra-orbital pressure should only be undertaken by those who are competent in its' use due to concerns of potential injury or adverse reaction.

Peripheral stimuli

A peripheral stimulus is interpreted by the peripheral nervous system and communicated to the central nervous system via the spinal cord to the brain. However a peripheral response may also elicit a spinal reflex making the use of peripheral stimuli limited in terms of motor assessment. Due to reasons stated earlier a peripheral stimulus is more suited to best eye opening response.[2,8] Table 7.5 describes the common techniques in applying a peripheral pain stimulus.

Table 7.5 Peripheral pain stimulation

Stimulus	Procedure	Rationale
Lateral finger or toe pressure	Using a pen or similar object (consider infection control) apply pressure to the lateral aspect of a finger or toe, avoid the nail bed. Rotate the object around the finger/toes away from the nail. This should be performed for no longer than 10 seconds.	It is advisable to avoid the nail bed as beneath the bed are a number of structures such as tendons, nerves and blood vessels.[2] These can be damaged by the use of extreme pressure upon the nail.

By avoiding pressure over the nail short term pain can be applied with a reduced likelihood of longer term damage to underlying structures.

Pupillary assessment

Careful examination of the pupils is an important part of a neurological assessment and is often the only way to assess the neurological status of a sedated patient. Pupils should be assessed for size, shape, and response to a light stimulus. Any change of pupil response may be an indication of raised intracranial pressure or lesion.[19]

Pupil size and shape

Pupil size will vary for a variety of reasons such as light, anxiety, drug use and pain, as a result of sympathetic and parasympathetic responses to stimuli,[2] suggested causes of pupil size abnormality can be found in Table 7.6. Pupil size is measured in millimetres (diameter) with a normal pupil size ranging from 2–6 mm.[19] Each pupil should be assessed individually and documented, this should be undertaken prior to any light being shone in them – it is important to note that levels of ambient light

Table 7.6 Abnormal pupil sizes – Common causes. Adapted from Cox and Roper (2006).[21]

Pupil size	Common causes
Pin point pupils	Opiate overdose, brainstem CVA (pontine), miotic eye drops, Horner's syndrome.
Dilated pupils	Fear, anxiety, anti-cholinergic drug overdose, brainstem CVA (mid brain), pain, mydriatic eye drops.
Unequal dilated pupils (unreactive)	IIIrd nerve palsy, mydriatic eye drops.
Unequal constricted pupils (unreactive)	Miotic eye drops, Horner's syndrome.

may affect pupil size. Many forms of documentation and some pen torches have a guideline scale for the measurement of pupils, these should be used to ensure objectivity of measurement. In the average patient the pupils will be of equal size, however it is estimated that up to 20% of patients will have unexplained unequal pupils (anisocoria).[20] A difference of up to 1mm is acceptable and may be physiological, especially if this is maintained in both light and dark conditions.[21]

There are numerous causes of abnormal pupil size, these are just some of the common causes that may be found.

Pupils are generally round in shape and equal. However certain conditions such as glaucoma (oval pupil) and ocular trauma (grossly irregular pupil) can alter the shape of both or an individual pupil. It is therefore important in the presence of an abnormal pupil size or shape to ask the patient or relative whether this is new to the patient.

Pupil response

In the presence of a bright light the pupils should constrict to reduce the amount of light that enters the eye.[2] However in the presence of an insult the sensory (afferent) or motor (efferent) pathways may be damaged and reduce or eliminate pupil response. With a light stimulus to one eye there should be experienced a direct response (constriction of the pupil) and consensual light reflex (constriction of the other pupil).[2] For this to take place an intact sensory and motor pathway is required. This response should occur in both light and dark conditions, although the response may be more difficult to spot in very light conditions. Pupil response to a light source should be relatively swift, therefore sluggish or slow responses should be noted, as should exceptionally brisk response as they can suggest neurological injury.[21]

A guide for the examination of direct and consensual light reflex can be seen below.

Assessing light response[21]

Procedure	Rationale
1. Gain informed consent from the patient to undertake the procedure.	This will help to reduce anxiety and make the patient easier to examine. It is also a basic requirement for professional practice.
2. Reduce the light from ambient sources wherever possible.	This enables a better view of the pupil and makes any response easier to view.
3. Wash the hands thoroughly.	As manual opening of the eye may be required this can reduce cross infection.
4. With the eyes open review the size and shape of the pupil.	See section upon pupil size and shape.

Procedure	Rationale
5. Using a bright pen torch move a light source from the outer aspect of the eye toward the pupil. This should cause pupil constriction (direct light reflex). The light only needs to be shone into the pupil for a very brief period to elicit a response. Assess the level of constriction and the speed of response.	This will assess the sensory and motor pathways.
6. Repeat the process, this time watch the other eye to assess consensual light reflex.	This will assess the motor pathway for the opposing eye.
7. Repeat the previous two steps shining the light into the opposing eye.	This will assess the sensory and motor pathways of the opposing eye.

Assessing motor function

Damage to the nervous system may result in changes in the patient's ability to move. To assess patient motor function an evaluation of the following areas should be undertaken:

- Inspection and palpation of muscle mass
- Assessment of tone
- Assessment of reflexes
- Assessment of movement and power
- Assessment of co-ordination
- Assessment of abnormal movements.

Inspection and palpation of muscle mass

Long standing motor neurone lesions/damage may result in the loss of muscle bulk due to atrophy and lack of muscle use. Diseases such as motor neurone or stroke are common causes of such signs.[22]

Assessment of tone

This involves the assessment of the resistance to passive movement of the limbs. Increased resistance suggests increased tone whereas decreased resistance suggests decreased tone. These tests are not routinely undertaken in prehospital care.

Assessment of reflexes

There are a variety of reflexes that can be tested. Typically these require great skill and experience to undertake and are not commonly used in prehospital care, examples include the deep tendon reflexes such as the knee jerk. However there are some reflexes that may be assessed within the community environment. These include the blink, gag, swallow, oculocephalic and plantar reflexes.

- Blink reflex: This is a protective reflex that can be affected by damage to the trigeminal and facial cranial nerves. These may be noted by a lack of blinking to stimulation of the cornea.
- Gag and swallow reflex: These are not routinely tested however history and clinical examination may suggest a loss of gag or swallow function. For example aspiration of foodstuffs. Altered responses suggest damage to the glossopharyngeal or vagus cranial nerves.
- Oculocephalic: This reflex is an eye movement that occurs in patients with severely decreased level of consciousness. When the reflex is present if the head is moved to one side the eyes will move in the opposite direction. However in patients with absent brain stem reflexes the eyes will appear to remain stationary in the centre.
- Plantar reflexes: An abnormal plantar reflex is evident upon the stimulation upon the lateral border of the underside of the foot. A normal response is the flexion of the great toe and adduction of the other toes. An abnormal response is noted when the great toe extends (or dorsiflexes) and the other toes abduct. This is a sign of upper motor neurone damage, however may be normal in babies under the age of one year.[23]

Assessment of movement and power

This involves the assessment of the patients muscle power and movement against resistance. If the patient is unable to generate any power against resistance then gravity should be used. These tests are not commonly used in prehospital care.

Assessment of co-ordination

Any disease or injury that affects the cerebellum or basal ganglia can affect co-ordination. The ability to perform complex movement smoothly and efficiently requires intact sensory and motor pathways. This can be simply tested with tasks such as asking the patient to run their heel up and down the shin of the opposite leg or by asking the patient repeatedly and rapidly pat the palm of one hand with the palm of the other hand and then with the back of the hand. This should be performed as quickly and regularly as possible.

Assessment of abnormal movements

When carrying out a neurological examination the patient should be observed for any abnormal movements such as jerks, tremor, tics, seizures or fasciculation (ripples or twitches underlying the skin in muscles at rest). These are all suggestive of neurological deficiency.

Sensory function assessment

Sensory functions and input allows the individual to respond to input from the external environment. When injury or illness damages the sensory pathways the ability to respond is decreased. This occurs in conditions such as spinal injury and stroke.[22] Assessment of sensory function should include:

- Central and peripheral vision: this can be achieved briefly by asking the patient about their vision or the use of standardised visual acuity charts.
- Hearing and ability to understand verbal communication: This can be briefly achieved by asking the patient about their hearing or asking them respond to simple commands such as tested in the Glasgow Coma Scale.
- Superficial sensations: This can be tested by applying a light stimulus to the skin (light touch or pain). Areas that can be tested are linked to sensory areas known as dermatomes that relate to specific nerve routes as seen below.
- Deep sensations: This relates to sensations of muscle and joint pain and the ability to recognise joint position. This can be briefly assessed by asking the patient to identify the position a joint is placed in when the patient has their eyes shut.

FAST

The FAST test is the acronym for the face, arm, speech test. This procedure is the current recommended technique for pre-hospital care staff in the recognition of stroke to allow for prompt management and referral.[24] Limited studies have been undertaken upon this technique; however initial findings suggest that there is a high level of diagnostic accuracy in the use by pre-hospital care personnel.[24]

The FAST approach is a simplified approach to a rapid assessment of a suspected stroke patient. Through the assessment of three specific areas of neurological functioning a level of suspicion of stroke can be gained. The FAST approach is shown in Table 7.7.

Table 7.7 The FAST approach to stroke recognition.[24]

Test	Findings
Face - Does the patient have a symmetrical face or are there any signs of a facial droop?	The presence of a facial droop can be indicative of stroke or facial nerve palsy.
Arm - Does the patient have equal power in their arms? Place the patients arms straight out in front of them, does one arm drift downwards?	The presence of an arm drift suggests a weakness to that limb and potential for hemiparesis.
Speech - Is there evidence of slurred speech? Are they able to speak normally?	Slurring of speech may indicate stroke due to weakness of facial muscles.

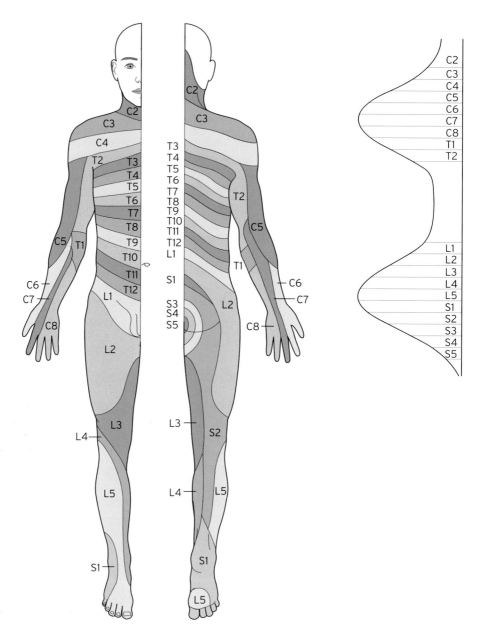

Figure 7.1 The dermatomes – sensory areas related to spinal nerves. Reproduced from Faiz, O. and Moffat, D., *Anatomy at a Glance*, copyright 2006, with permission of Blackwell Publishing.

Vital signs

There are a variety of vital signs that should be undertaken as a routine part of neurological assessment, these include:

- Respirations
- Temperature
- Pulse
- Blood pressure
- Blood sugar.

The assessment of these key areas can offer vital information into the functioning of the neurological system. See chapters upon Respiratory Observations and Assessment and Cardiovascular Observations and Assessment for further information. The assessment of blood sugar is often taken as a part of the neurological examination and will therefore be discussed in this chapter.

Blood glucose testing

The body regulates blood glucose levels through the production of insulin and glucagon by the pancreas. These hormones are responsible for the metabolism and release of glucose from body stores respectively, alongside other functions.[2] Blood glucose levels are normally maintained within relatively narrow limits of about 5-7 mmol/L (millimoles per litre).[25] However conditions such as diabetes affect the body's ability to produce insulin and subsequently control blood sugar. In the diabetic patient the normal blood sugar level may vary between individuals therefore trends over time and norm values for the individual are paramount in the identification of abnormal blood sugar values.[26]

Abnormal blood sugar values

There are two broad categories of abnormal blood sugar; hypoglycaemia (low blood sugar) and hyperglycaemia (high blood sugar). Hypoglycaemia occurs when the blood sugar falls below 4.0 mmol/L and causes subsequent changes in neurological functioning such as confusion.[27] This can be caused by issues such insulin overdose, insufficient food intake, exercise or alcohol. Hyperglycaemia is often caused by current illnesses such as infections that lead to a raise in blood sugar beyond normal limits (>7 mmol/L or relative value for the patient).

Capillary blood glucose testing

Within the prehospital setting the common technique for blood glucose testing involves the use of capillary blood glucose monitors (glucometer) with blood samples taken by pin prick from the finger. Whilst this is a simple measurement previous research suggests that serious errors have occurred that have led to inappropriate decisions being made,[28] this has led to recommendations for the training of staff and the use of testing devices as seen below:

- Staff must be aware of what results to expect in normal and abnormal situations.

- Staff must be aware of the correct use of equipment and the consequences of incorrect use.
- Staff must be educated in the collection of blood samples including the gaining of consent and health and safety issues.
- Staff must be aware of the standards of documentation of such results.
- Staff must understand the limitations of equipment and when use is contra-indicated.
- Staff must have an in-depth knowledge of the equipment including error codes and calibration.

What site should be used?

There is little evidence to support a specific location for capillary blood testing, typically the finger tip is used,[29] however sites such as the earlobe and heel may also be used[30]. Initial studies suggest that the earlobe may provide a less painful site for testing.[30] There have been no demonstrated differences in accuracy between these sites therefore no specific recommendations can be made.

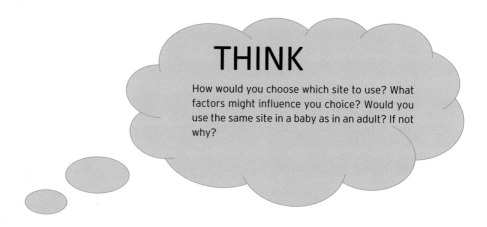

THINK

How would you choose which site to use? What factors might influence you choice? Would you use the same site in a baby as in an adult? If not why?

Skin preparation

Again there is little evidence to provide a recommendation for the use cessation or use of skin swabbing prior to capillary blood glucose testing. Some authors suggest that the use of alcohol skin swabs could cause erroneous results,[31] however small scale research suggests that no difference in readings are obtained following the use of an alcohol swab.[32] General advice provided by The National Library for Health[33] and the Royal College of Nursing[34] suggests that there is little need to clean healthy skin for routine injections outside of a hospital. The advice states that if chemical disinfection is used that it must be allowed to dry prior to injection. Manufacturers of glucometers suggest that the skin should be physically cleaned using soap and water.[32] This has the dual benefit of warming the digit to increase blood flow and subsequently make testing easier.

Which drop to test?

There has been anecdotal evidence to suggest that the initial drop of blood gained from a pin prick should be removed and a second drop tested to reduce the risk of inaccurate results. This is based upon the concept that the initial drop may contain excess tissue fluid and potentially alcohol from any swab that is used;[35] whilst there is little published evidence to dispute or support this notion, until proven otherwise it is suggested that the second drop be tested.

Capillary blood glucose testing: procedure

A step-by-step approach to capillary blood glucose testing is provided below.

Procedure	Rationale
1. Check and prepare the equipment for use-including functionality, use by date, calibration. Equipment required: glucometers, test strips, finger pricking device, cotton wool, sharps disposal container, gloves.	To ensure maximum efficiency, comfort and safety.
2. Prepare the patient – gain informed consent, if possible wash the digit (especially if physically dirty) and ensure the patient is comfortable.	This will reduce anxiety and make the testing process easier. Consent is also a legal requirement for practice.
3. Wash your hands and put on gloves.	Please refer to infection control chapter.
4. Take the blood sample – Using a single use retractable lancet take a sample from the side of the finger (or ear lobe or heel). If the site does not bleed then milk the site until enough blood is obtained.	A single use retractable lancet is recommended as this will reduce the risk of needle-stick injury and cross-infection. The side of the finger is generally less sensitive than the tip and sensitivity in tips of fingers may be lost if used regularly. Rotation of sites is advised to avoid over use of one site as the skin may become hard and painful.
5. Apply blood to the test strip.	Most strips are hydrophilic and draw blood up when applied. However some strips still require a drop of blood to be dropped onto them, this will vary between manufacturer and strip type.

Procedure	Rationale
6. Dispose of the lancet in a sharps disposal container and any contaminated non sharps material into a clinical waste container.	This conforms with infection control and sharps disposal policies and will reduce the risk of needlestick injury and/or contamination.
Document the findings appropriately.	To ensure accurate documentation of findings and to determine management.
7. Report or act upon any abnormal or unexpected findings.	It is important to recognise any abnormal or unexpected finding as this may influence care or priorities of management.

Scenario

You are called to a 25-year-old patient who suffers with diabetes (insulin controlled), he is suffering from acute confusion and is behaving irrationally. You test the blood sugar which is recorded as 6.8 mmol/L. What are your differential diagnoses? How could you further assess this patient to form a diagnosis?

Chapter Key Points

1. The assessment of neurological function is both complex and requires experience to gain competence.
2. The understanding of the concepts and interpretation of neurological assessments is a major facet in patient assessment and subsequent management.
3. Neurological assessment incorporates a number of potential examinations and vital signs therefore a thorough assessment may well be required to identify abnormal findings.

References and Further Reading

1   Teasdale G, Murray L. Revisiting the Glasgow coma scale and coma score. *Intens Care Med* 2000;26:153-154.

2   Marieb, E. & Hoehn, K. *Human Anatomy and Physiology*, 7th edn. San Francisco: Pearson International, 2007.

3   Joint Royal Colleges Ambulance Liaison Committee and Ambulance Service Association. *UK Ambulance Service Clinical Practice Guidelines*. London: JRCALC/ASA, 2006.

4   American College of Surgeons Committee on Trauma. *Advanced Life Support Course for Physicians*. Chicago, Illinois: American College of Surgeons, 1993.

5   McNarry A, Goldhill D. Simple bedside assessment of level of consciousness: comparison of two simple assessment scales with the Glasgow coma scale. *Anaesthesia* 2004;59:34-37.

6   Gill M, Martens K, Lynch E, Salih A, Green S. Interrater reliability of 3 simplified neurologic scales applied to adults presenting to the emergency department with altered level of consciousness. *Ann Emerg Med* 2007;49(4):403-407.

7   Teasdale G, Jennett B. Assessment of coma and impaired consciousness: a practical scale. *Lancet* 1974;2:81-84.

8   Palmer R, Knight J. Assessment of altered conscious level in clinical practice. *Br J Nurs* 2006;15(22):1255-1258.

9   Gill MR, Reiley DG, Green SM. Interratter reliability of Glasgow Coma Scales in the Emergency Department. *Ann Emerg Med* 2004;43:215-223.

10 Gill MR, Windemuth R, Steele R *et al.* A comparison of the Glasgow Coma Scale score to simplified alternative scores for the prediction of traumatic brain injury outcomes. *Ann Emerg Med* 2005;45:37-42.

11 Waterhouse, C. The Glasgow Coma Scale and other neurological observations. *Nurs Stand* 2005;19(33):56-64.

12 National Institute for Clinical Excellence. *Head Injury: Triage, assessment, investigation and early management of head injury in infants, children and adults*. London: NICE, 2007.

13 Fischer, J, Mathiesthon C. The history of the Glasgow Coma Scale: implications for practice. *Crit Care Nurs* 2001;23(4):52-58.

14 National Institute for Clinical Excellence. *Head Injury: Triage, assessment, investigation and early management of head injury in infants, children and adults*. London: NICE, 2007.

15 Stewart N. Neurological observations. *Profess Nurse* 1996;11(6):377-378.

16 Edwards S. Using the Glasgow Coma Scale. *Br J Nurs* 2001;10(2):92-101.

17 Barker E. *Neuroscience Nursing: A Spectrum of Care*, 2nd edn. St Louis: Mosby, 2002.

18 National Neuroscience Benchmarking Group. *Neurological Assessment*. London: NNBG, 2006.

19 Dawes E, Lloyd H, Durham L. Monitoring and recording patients' neurological observations. *Nurs Stand* 2007;22(10):40-45.

20 Littlejohns L. Ask the experts. *Crit Care Nurse* 2007;27(1);62-64.

21 Cox N, Roper T. *Clinical Skills*. Oxford: Oxford University Press, 2006.

22 McCance K, Heuther S. *Pathophysiology: The Biologic Basis for Disease in Adults and children*. St. Louis: Elsevier, 2006.

23 Dougherty L, Lister S. *The Royal Marsden Hospital Manual of Clinical Nursing Procedures*, 6th edn. Oxford: Blackwell Publishing, 2006.

24 National Institute for Clinical Excellence. Stroke: Diagnosis and initial management of acute stroke and transient ischaemic attack (TIA). *National Clinical Guideline for Chronic Conditions*. London: NICE, 2008.

25 Williams G, Pickup J (Eds) *Handbook of Diabetes*, 3rd edn. Oxford: Blackwell Publishing, 2004.

26 National Institute of Clinical Excellence. *Management of Type 2 Diabetes*. London: NICE, 2002.

27 Joint Royal Colleges Ambulance Liaison Committee. *UK Ambulance Service Clinical Practice Guidelines*. Warwick: JRCALC, 2006.

28 Medical Devices Agency. *Management and Use of IVD Point of Care Test Devices*. London: The Stationary Office, 2002.

29 Wallymahmed M. Capillary blood glucose monitoring. *Nurs Stand* 2007;21(38):35-38.

30 Toledo F, Taylor A. Alternative site testing at the earlobe tip. *Diabetes Care* 2004;27(2):616.

31 Burden M. Diabetes: Blood glucose monitoring. *Nurs Times* 2001;97(8):36-39.

32 Cave L. Effects of skin preparation on blood glucose monitoring results. *J Diabetes Nurs* 2002; March-April.

33 National Library for Health. *Primary Care Question Answering Service*, 2005. [on-line: www.clinical answers.nhs.uk/index.cfm?question=1386].

34 Royal College of Nursing. *Position Statement on Injection Technique*. London: RCN, 2002.

35 Albert Einstein College of Medicine. *Capillary Blood Glucose Testing*. Albert Einstein College of Medicine Research & Training Centre, 1997.

Chapter 8

History taking and communication

Content

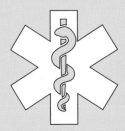

The taking of a medical history is a vast area that is acquired with both experience and knowledge. It is not the intention of this chapter to explain the full history taking requirements of all presentations of patients but to introduce key components and skills involved in the history taking process. There is little evidence to support specific approaches to history taking, however it is universally agreed that history taking is of paramount importance.

Definitions

History taking is the process of gaining a patient's account of their illness or injury and the eliciting of further information that is required to lead to a diagnosis, prioritise care and evaluate the impact of a patient's symptoms upon their lives. A medical history can be viewed as a conversation with a purpose, that of gaining information about a patient, their life and their condition. Taking a history is not a passive process; the practitioner needs to guide the patient so that a comprehensive history can be obtained. The importance of taking a history cannot be overestimated in the assessment and treatment of any patient.

To gain a comprehensive history the practitioner needs to understand the principles of communication with a wide variety of client groups and the importance of a structured yet flexible approach to history taking. There is an undoubted need for effective history taking and communication in the assessment of any patient group and professional role, therefore the underlying skills of gaining a medical history are a core competency for any health professional.[1,2,3]

Key communication skills

The patient–carer relationship should be based upon openness, trust and good communication.[1,2] It is therefore essential to have a good understanding of effective communication skills. Whilst there are no set rules for what is effective communication, there are some key skills that are of undoubted value:

- Be honest.
- Avoid medical jargon as it may confuse or mislead patients.
- Speak clearly and use unambiguous language.
- Actively listen to the patient, ask for and respect their views. This means encouraging the patient to talk by looking interested and consider encouraging comments such as, 'Tell me more about...'
- Try to develop a rapport, history taking requires honesty from both yourself and the patient, they must feel able to communicate any concerns they may have.
- Provide positive support and empathy, this may enhance health outcomes and the practitioner relationship.
- Consider verbal and non-verbal communication skills (see Table 8.1).

THINK

Are there any situations where communication can be especially difficult? Think of your own practice, what groups of patients are more difficult to communicate with and what can you do to improve this?

Table 8.1 Key examples of verbal and non-verbal communication skills. Adapted from Mehrabian (1981)[3]

Non-verbal skills	Verbal skills
• Eye contact • Interested posture • Hand gestures • Nodding of the head (provides a positive emphasis of listening) • Facial gestures	• Appropriate language • Avoid jargon and technical language • Consider the pitch and tone of your voice • Speak at a pace that can be easily understood • Speak at a volume that can be easily heard but not overpowering of lacking consideration for confidentiality

Communication models

There are a variety of communication models that are used and have been used in healthcare over many years. However the use of these models is a blend of personal preference and adaptation to specific situations. There are currently two main models that are commonly seen in practice. Each has inevitable benefits and flaws. The most commonly used models are:

• The biomedical model – This is a practitioner-led model, whereby the focus is upon the disease and subsequent management.
• The patient-centred model – This model seeks to holistically assess the patient and shares the decision making and power between the practitioner and the patient.

The biomedical model has recently fallen out of favour amongst the medical profession due to the rigid focus and lack of consideration for the patient experience and subjective effects of the disease process.[4] The patient-centred model seeks to understand the patient's experience of the disease whilst considering the whole person and agree a management plan in conjunction with the patient's wishes. There is no evidence to suggest that either model is more effective or desirable; however consensus of opinion suggests that the patient should be treated as a whole person as opposed to a disease or injury.[1-3]

The practitioner–patient relationship

This should not be mistaken for having a relationship with a patient! Any health or medical assessment and history should be considered as a partnership with the patient whereby the two parties work together toward a set goal (often a cure or appropriate treatment). The broad role of the practitioner in this relationship is to:

- Be polite, considerate and honest.
- To treat patients with dignity.
- Treat each patient as an individual.
- Respect patients' privacy and rights of confidentiality.
- To empower the patient in caring for themselves.

A standardised history framework

This is a structured approach to history taking that complements documentation skills as discussed within this book. It is generally accepted that it is important to have a logical and systematic approach to history taking to ensure quality and adequacy in a health history. As an element of this, consent must be sought prior to any assessment process including physical assessment and questioning. A standardised history taking structure can be seen below.

- Introductions
- The presenting complaint
- The history of the presenting complaint
- Past medical history
- Medication history
- Allergies
- Family history
- Social history
- Sexual history
- Mental health
- Occupational history
- Systematic enquiry
- Further information from a third party
- Summary.

Adapted from Thomas and Monaghan (2006)[4]; Douglas G, Nicol F, Robertson C. (2005).[5]

This outline above is just a guide as it will not always be appropriate or relevant to include all areas, for example in the critically ill patient such a history could detract from more pressing issues such as treatment. Each section of the history process will now be broken down and discussed individually.

Introductions

This is a key element in establishing a rapport with the patient and can provide information vital to the assessment of the patient. Greeting the patient with a simple hello is often an adequate verbal approach, as comments such as 'good morning' may not always be appropriate for a patient who may receive bad news. The shaking of hands can provide vital information about a patient such as their peripheral circulation (i.e. cold hands) and their neurological status (loss of power). However this may not always be appropriate. Take each consultation upon its own merits. It is vital to gain the name of the patient at the commencement of the history as reliance upon terms such as 'my dear' or 'sweetheart' may be misconstrued. The use of first names or surnames can also be problematic, as some patients may prefer to be called 'Mr or Mrs Smith'; however some patients would rather be called by their first name. It is simplest just to ask the patient what they would like to be called, as there are no strict rules. Don't forget to introduce yourself; this can be either just your name or may include your title (i.e. Paramedic/Technician/Emergency Care Assistant).

The presenting complaint

It is essential to define the problem that has caused the patient to seek medical assistance. This can often be a difficult to ask question as terms such as 'What are you complaining of?' or 'Why have you called for an ambulance?' may be misinterpreted as implying they should not have called or they are 'complainers'. As with many areas of history taking it is important to choose a technique suited to each individual. Open questions such as 'What would you say your main problem is?' or 'How can I help you today?' may be more appropriate.

The history of the presenting complaint

To evaluate the presenting complaint further, questions need to be asked that are aimed at working out the cause of the complaint. The required questions to achieve this can vary widely and are dependent upon experience and knowledge in terms of depth of questioning. Key components of the history of the presenting complaint are:

- Location of the symptom
- Duration of symptoms
- Onset of symptoms (i.e. provocation and worsening of symptoms)
- Aggravating and alleviating factors
- Any attributable causes
- Previous episodes
- Severity of symptoms (i.e. pain score)
- Nature of the symptoms (i.e. are the pains continuous)
- Any medication use to relieve symptoms.

Past medical history

The previous medical history of a patient is often key in understanding current medical conditions. There is often a strong probability that new symptoms may be caused by long-standing medical conditions. Also consideration of medical history is paramount for safety in treatment regimes as contra-indicated treatments must be avoided. It is important to remember that many patients may not consider conditions such as asthma or hypertension (amongst others) to be significant. It is therefore important to ask not only a generalised open question such as, 'Do you have any medical conditions?' but to consider asking about specific conditions such as, 'Do you have or have you had asthma, diabetes, heart attacks, epilepsy, strokes, high blood pressure?'. This list is not exhaustive so please consider ruling out any history that could relate to the presenting complaint. Do not forget to ask about any previous surgery as this may highlight further medical complications.

Medication history

This can be very important for a number of reasons that may relate to a current complaint, including:

- Contra-indication of treatments
- Side effects of current medications
- Identification of current medical conditions.

It is important to consider both prescribed and non-prescribed medications, alongside any herbal remedies as they often have a medicinal quality that may affect treatment. Therefore it is useful to ask, 'Do you take any medicines from your doctor/pharmacist/ or any herbal remedies?'. It may also be useful to expand this to enquire, 'Do you take any tablets, inhalers, or drops for anything?'. This may elicit further information. Ideally the patient will have their medication with them; this allows for you to review them thoroughly paying attention to dates, dosages, compliance with medications and frequency.

Allergies

Consideration of allergies is not only key to the safe administration of medications and treatments, but it may also provide clues to underlying causes of symptoms. Prior to any medication provision the checking of allergies is vital. Ask the patient if they 'have any allergies or medications that they cannot take?' this will allow for identification of not only allergies but often medications that they do not perceive as allergies but have been informed not to take by their GP or other healthcare professional. If any allergies or other medications are raised it is useful to clarify what reasons underlie the stated problem. This may give rise to further medical history not already stated.

Family history

With a prevalence of genetic inheritance in certain conditions such as heart disease or cancer among others, the consideration of family medical history may be important. Consider asking:

- Has anyone in your family had a similar problem?
- Do any diseases run in the family?
- Have any of your family members died at a young age? And if so how?

Social history

This can help to build a general picture of the patient and how the illness/injury is affecting their life. It is important to consider family commitments, occupation, where they live, quality of life at the present time and hand dominance (in the case of upper limb injury). All of these factors may influence either the establishment of a diagnosis or treatment regimen. For example it would be inappropriate to leave an elderly patient at home following a fall if they were unable to cope with the stairs to a flat. It may also be of relevance to enquire about smoking and alcohol consumption as it may relate to the current illness or treatment for the presenting complaint. Areas that should be considered as a part of a holistic social assessment include:

- The ability to cook or provide nutrition for self.
- The ability to undertake personal hygiene activities (i.e. washing).
- Social conditions such as heating and ability to maintain a healthy living environment.
- The ability to dress themselves.
- The availability of social support such as friends, family or carers.
- Access to healthcare should the need re-arise.

Sexual history

This is not commonly an area for enquiry in the prehospital field and if required should be undertaken sensitively. It may be of relevance in any patient however based upon presenting symptoms (such as vaginal discharge) or history provided.

Mental health

A mental health history is not commonly undertaken in the prehospital setting, however in cases such as deliberate self-harm it may be of utmost importance. It is important to recognise any mental health concerns. The patient should be assessed for issues such a low mood, anxiety, depression and risk of self-harm. Elements of the history that may indicate mental health concerns include; alcohol use, drug use (prescribed or illicit), previous use of mental health services or abnormal behaviour. Tools such as the SADPERSONS risk assessment chart may be of use when assessing the risk of deliberate self-harm as is now commonly in use in both nursing and pre-hospital environments (see Table 8.2). However it should be noted that there is limited evidence to support the use of such scales due to the complex nature of the assessment of suicide risk.[6,7]

Systematic enquiry

The purpose of the systematic enquiry is to uncover symptoms that the patient may have forgotten to mention or not have considered a symptom. The systematic enquiry involves questioning on a variety of body systems and symptoms to exclude or diagnose conditions. If positive answers are elicited then more focused examination of body systems and symptoms can be undertaken. Some key examples of systematic enquiry symptoms can be seen in Table 8.3.

Table 8.2 SADPERSONS risk assessment.[8]

SADPERSONS assessment		
Sex	Female	Male
Age	19-45	<19 >45
Depression or hopelessness	No	Yes
Previous attempts	No	Yes
Excessive alcohol or drugs	No	Yes
Rational thinking	Yes	No
Separated/divorced/widowed	No	Yes
Organised or serious attempts	No	Yes
Social support	Yes	No
Stated future suicide intent	No	Yes
Number of ticks in right hand column indicates score		
<3 low risk		
3-6 medium risk		
>6 high risk		

Table 8.3 Systematic Review: Key points. Adapted from Douglas G, Nicol F, Robertson C. (2005).[5]

General health	• Well-being: Energy
	• Appetite (loss or increased): Sleep patterns
	• Weight loss/gain: Mood
Cardiovascular system	• Chest pain: Breathlessness
	• Orthopnoea: Palpitations
	• Ankle/sacral oedema: Dizziness
Respiratory system	• Shortness of breath: Cough
	• Phlegm/sputum: Wheeze
	• Haemoptysis: Chest pain
	• Exercise tolerance
Gastrointestinal system	• Nausea and vomiting: Haematemesis
	• Indigestion: Heartburn
	• Abdominal pain: Change in colour of stools
	• Difficulty swallowing: Change in bowel habit
Genitourinary system	• Pain passing urine: Frequency passing urine
	• Discharge: Blood in urine
	• Last menstrual period: Unprotected sexual intercourse
Nervous system	• Headaches: Visual disturbances
	• Fits: Altered sensation
	• Weakness: Dizziness or faints
Musculoskeletal	• Joint pain or stiffness: Mobility
	• Falls: Joint swelling
Endocrine	• Excessive thirst: Heat or cold intolerance
	• Change in sweating
Other	
	• Bleeding or bruising: Skin rashes

THINK

Are these questions always needed? In what situations might you alter these questions and how? For example would all of these enquiries be useful in a patient with cardiac chest pain?

Further information from a third party

It may be pertinent to gain further information from a third party, especially in cases where the patient is unable to provide a valid or reliable history, for example young children or unconscious patients. If such information is used remember to document this and consider the reliability of third party data at all times, as it may not always be correct. Third party information can be a vital tool in assessing the effects of an illness or injury upon the life of a patient, or may provide sensitive information that the patient may not have mentioned.

Summary

Upon completing history taking it may be useful to clarify the main points with the patient to ensure that you have understood and recorded them correctly. This also allows the patient to add any further information that they may wish.

Questioning techniques

There are a variety of questioning techniques that can be utilised in the assessment and history taking process. These are commonly grouped into five main areas; open, closed, limiting, leading and comparative questions. Each style of question has its own benefits and flaws, therefore it is not recommended to use a single style but to adapt the questioning process to gain maximal information. Open questions are broad questions such as, 'Tell me about your health problems?' that allow for the recipient to respond with a wide array of information. It is important that if these questions are used that time is taken to listen to the responses. Whilst open questions can provide a great breadth of information, there is often little structure to the answers, therefore listening is essential. These questions can also be time-consuming and are not always suited to a time-critical environment.

Closed questions are narrowly focused and typically provide the option of yes or no answers. These questions are often used to clarify issues and can provide key information in a brief period of time. However these questions may limit answers to such a narrow field that key information may not be gained. Examples of closed questions are: 'Do you have any allergies?' or 'Does breathing affect your chest pain?'. It is important to note that if a closed question is asked, such as 'Are you allergic to aspirin?', that the patient will only provide the information requested despite the fact that they may be allergic to other medications or substances.

Limiting questions are often utilised to gain clarity and focus as they are designed to limit the answers to one key area or subject, for example 'Do you have any heart problems?'. This again can be useful in clarifying issues or gaining specific information, but can limit the amount of information provided in response. Leading questions are the use of questions that suggest the answer within the question. These questions should be avoided wherever possible as they do not provide the patient with the freedom to answer truthfully. A common example of such a question is, 'You don't want to go to hospital do you?'; whilst this provides the patient the opportunity to respond, it is clear from the question that the patient is being encouraged to say no.

Comparative questions can be useful in the assessment process. A comparative question allows the patient to compare two things, for example 'Is the pain worse than your normal pain?'. This can provide vital information into how the current situation is perceived against a prior experience. Whilst there is no evidence to suggest that one technique is superior to another, review of questioning skills suggests that the use of differing methods can be used dependant upon each individual situation.

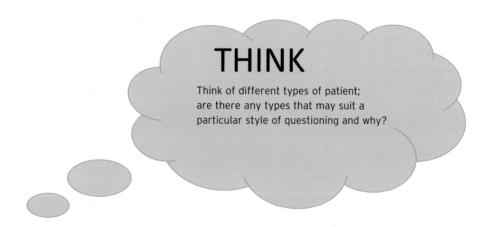

THINK

Think of different types of patient; are there any types that may suit a particular style of questioning and why?

Consent

Prior to undertaking any healthcare intervention or action including the collection of a history it is imperative that informed consent is gained.[9,10] Patients can only provide valid consent if they are able to act under their own free will, understand what they are agreeing to and have enough information upon which to base a decision. Consent can be verbal, written or implied. Often consent for history taking and assessment will be implied as the patient will willingly pass on information after seeking help. However it is best practice to enquire whether the patient is happy for you to ask pertinent questions.

Scenario

You are called to an 80-year-old patient who has fallen in her own home; she is complaining of hip pain and is unable to mobilise. She appears confused and is unable to recall the day, date and where she is. You decide that she has a potential neck of femur fracture and wish to convey her to the hospital for further assessment. Unfortunately the patient refuses to attend the hospital and her husband tells you that you must take her to hospital as he cannot cope with caring for her. What consent issues does this raise? What actions could you take to assist this patient?

Further useful information upon consent and capacity can be found in the Mental Capacity Act (2005).[11]

Chapter Key Points

1. There are a variety of formats for history taking and each individual practitioner should base their approach around each individual situation.
2. The importance of a thorough and objective history cannot be underestimated.
3. It is essential to consider both verbal and non-verbal communication techniques to ensure that a thorough history is gained.

References and Further reading

1 General Medical Council. *Good Medical Practice*. London: GMC, 2006.
2 Health Professions Council. *Standards of Proficiency: Paramedics*. London: HPC, 2007.
3 Mehrabian A. *Silent messages: Implicit Communication of Emotions and Attitudes*, 2nd edn. Belmont, CA: Wadsworth, 1981.
4 Thomas J, Monaghan T. *The Oxford Handbook of Clinical Examination and Practical Skills*. Oxford: Oxford University Press, 2006.
5 Douglas G, Nicol F, Robertson C. *MacLeod's Clinical Examination*. London: Elsevier, 2005.
6 Khan S. *SADPERSONS Scale in the Assessment of Self-harm Risk*. BestBets Review, 2008. Accessed on-line at: http://www.bestbets.org/cgi-bin/bets.pl?record=01556
7 Department of Health. *Best Practice in Managing Risk*. London: HMSO, 2007.
8 Patterson *et al*. Evaluation of suicidal patients: The SADPERSONS scale. *Psychosomatics* 1983;24(4):343-349.
9 Department of Health. *Good Practice in Consent Implementation Guide: Consent to Examination or Treatment*. London: The Stationary Office, 2001.
10 Health Professions Council. *Code of Conduct, Performance and Ethics*. London: HPC, 2007.
11 Her Majesty's Government. *Mental Capacity Act*. London: HMSO, 2005.

Chapter 9

Documentation and record keeping

Content

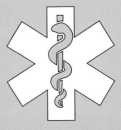

Record keeping is a professional duty of care for all healthcare practitioners; therefore failure to maintain reasonable standards can have both professional and legal implications. High quality record keeping and documentation is linked to quality patient care, as such this chapter will provide guidance upon standards of record keeping, identifying key legislative documents and professional requirements.

Definitions

The Data Protection Act 1998[1] defines a health record as:

> *'any information relating to the physical or mental health or condition of an individual that has been made by or on the behalf of a health professional in connection with the care of that individual. This includes a variety of materials including case report forms, printouts from electronic measuring devices, photographs and computerised records.'*[2,3]

In the year 2004–05, the ambulance services in England alone received more than 5.6 million emergency calls and undertook more than 12.8 million planned patient journeys[4] this resulting in a vast quantity of healthcare records.

Whilst there are a variety of forms that health records can take, the focus of this chapter will be upon note taking and manual/electronic patient case notes. It is important to note that each individual workplace will have a differing set of documentation requirements however adherence to these general principles is widely accepted.

Why keep healthcare records?

There is considered opinion that good record keeping is a mark of a skilled and safe practitioner.[2,3,5] However, beyond this opinion there are many functions served by healthcare records and these reasons can be split into primary and secondary functions (see Box 9.1).

The primary purpose of healthcare records is to support quality patient care and maximise safety for all parties.[6,9] The ability to utilise documentation as an aide memoire can assist in the provision of timely and effective patient care. Within a multidisciplinary healthcare system the ability to communicate is key, with both written and verbal communications commonplace. To ensure this continuity and quality of care, professional standards and expectations are set by the registering bodies of all healthcare professions.[5,7,8] Records are a valuable resource because of the information they can and should contain. High-quality information underpins the delivery of high-quality evidence based healthcare and other key service deliverables. Information has most value when it is accurate, up to date and accessible when it is needed.[8,11]

A secondary function of health records as a medico-legal document is a core function in an ever-increasing litigation aware society. With increased public awareness of litigation and complaints policies, accurate and comprehensive records are essential in safeguarding the healthcare practitioner.[10] This is perhaps best emphasised by the Nursing and Midwifery Council (2002)[5] who state that, 'If it is not

Primary functions: Supporting direct patient care

- Aide memoire
- Communication

Secondary functions: Medico-legal record
Source of information for:

- Clinical audit and research
- Resource allocation
- Epidemiology
- Service planning
- Performance monitoring
- Evidence based clinical care
- To meet legal requirements, including requests from patients under subject access provisions of the Data Protection Act or the Freedom of Information Act

Box 9.1 Primary and Secondary functions of healthcare records. Adapted from Mann and Williams (2003)[6] and Department of Health (2006)[11]

recorded, it has not been done'. The value of high quality accurate records is key in any complaint or claim that may arise; as such resources are a key piece of evidence.[12]

As well as enabling high quality care for patients, good medical and health records are of value in improving standards of care. The continued audit of records plays an important part of the clinical governance process. Clinical governance was introduced in 1998, at the centre of the NHS drive to create a modern, patient-led health service, with the fundamental aim being the provision of responsive, consistent, high-quality and safe patient care. Clinical governance was born out of the need for accountability for the safe delivery of health services. This was due partly to the public's and professionals' perception of systemic failings within the NHS. Clinical governance was defined in the 1998 consultation document 'A First Class Service: Quality in the New NHS' (p.33)[13] as 'A framework through which NHS organisations are accountable for continuously improving the quality of their services and safeguarding high standards of care by creating an environment in which excellence in clinical care will flourish'. Through high quality documentation and record keeping the health service is able to monitor a variety of areas such as epidemiology of disease and the effectiveness of current treatments. Within this culture high quality care is proposed to flourish.

What constitutes good medical records?

Whilst the need to keep accurate patient, client and user records is recognised by the bodies that govern healthcare practice including the Health Professions Council (HPC),[7] General Medical Council (GMC)[8] and the Nursing and Midwifery Council (NMC),[5] there is currently very little evidence to support a specific standard of record keeping. Current guidelines are based upon expert opinion of what should constitute good medical records and documentation.

Recommendations

- Records should be clear, accurate and legible, reporting the relevant clinical findings, the decisions made, the information given to patients, and any drugs prescribed or other investigation or treatment.[8]
- Record any important negative findings that occur. For example the absence of a non-blanching rash in a sick child.[2,3]
- Records should be made at the same time as the events you are recording or as soon as possible afterwards.[8]
- You must keep notes for any patient that is treated or who asks you for professional advice or services.[7]
- Any records should be objective – opinions should be based upon facts that you have recorded not speculation. Remember the patient has a right to view their records, therefore any unjustified statements may be disputed.[2,3]
- First hand – if the information has been passed to you by anyone other than the patient, record that person's name and position.[2,3] For example are they a friend or a relative?
- Records should be tamper proof – any attempt to amend records should be apparent. For example write in pen, not pencil.
- Records should be the original documentation; any alterations should be dated, timed and signed. This is to make it clear that it is not an attempt to tamper with the document but to make a correction or addition.[2,3,7]
- If you make a correction to any health record the data should not be erased or made difficult to read; instead it should be made clear that it has been superseded.[7] For example place a single line through it. Again any change must be signed, timed and dated.
- Involve the client and/or carers in the documentation process.[18]
- Ensure that records are kept confidential and secure.[18]
- Only use accepted terminology in health records.[19]

Models of record keeping

Whilst there is no evidence to support a single method of documenting clinical findings the principle of a consistent, organised and structured approach is vital. Below you will find a suggested model for the free text documentation of any patient (Box 9.2); this is by no means the only model available and each individual practitioner should consider what model is best suited to their own and organisational needs. The described format provides basis for documenting any clinical episode.

Whilst this model encourages a thorough and comprehensive examination, it may not always be the most suited to a critically ill patient, therefore it can be modified with irrelevant sections being minimised. The use of a single structure will allow for continued standards of documentation to be adhered to.

Demographic Details - Always ensure that there is a record of the patients name, age, date of birth, address, source of referral (i.e. 999 call), GP, source of the history and the date/time of the examination.

Presenting Complaint (PC) - State the major problem in the patients own words. Medical terminology is not required.

History of Presenting Complaint (HPC) - Describe the onset, nature and course of each symptom. You may have to paraphrase the patients' words. Consider highlighting key facts by underlining.

Past Medical History (PMH) - Provide all details of the patients' current and past medical problems including medical and surgical history. Include important negatives also, for example exclude previous myocardial infarction or angina in patients presenting with chest pain.

Drug History (DH) - Record all current prescribed and over the counter medications. Also consider herbal remedies that the patient may be taking.

Allergies - Document any allergies the patient states they have.

Family History (FH) - Consider any health issues within the patients close family, for example early death due to cardiac disease in a parent.

Social History (SH) - Consider and document any relevant social issues, for example occupation, family/social care support, smoking or illicit drug use, or even hand dominance (especially in hand or arm injury).

On examination (O/E) - Provide a general examination of the patient, for example are they alert? Orientated? Pale? What is their mental and physical status?

Respiratory System (RS) - Document all respiratory information, for example chest sounds, use of accessory muscles and percussion.

Cardiovascular System (CVS) - Document all relevant cardiovascular investigations and observations, for example pulse, blood pressure and electrocardiograph.

Central Nervous System (CNS) - Include all relevant neurological examinations, for example Glasgow Coma Score, pupil reaction and Face, arm speech test (FAST).

Abdominal System (AS) - Consider any relevant examination or observations, for example pulsatile masses, scars, guarding and bowel sounds.

Musculoskeletal System (MSS) - Document any relevant musculoskeletal examinations. Consider gait, pain swelling, deformities and ranges of movement for joints.

Clinical Diagnosis or Impression - Record any potential diagnoses.

Plan - Document treatments, investigations and any information given to the patient.

Box 9.2 Documenting the findings adapted from Douglas G, Nicol F, Robertson C. (2005) *Macleod's Clinical Examination*[22] and Bickley L. (2003) *Bates' Guide to Physical Examination and History Taking*[23]

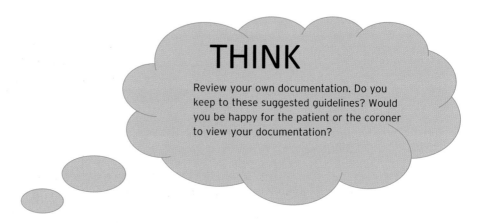

Abbreviations

The use of abbreviations in health records remains controversial, the use of abbreviations can save time however they can also lead to problems. Any abbreviation used should be unambiguous and be universally understandable,[3] for example the use of PID can mean pelvic inflammatory disease or prolapsed intervertebral disc. The use of humorous or sarcastic abbreviations are definitely not recommended and have no place in health records. Remember the patient has the right of access to their records.

Key documents in record keeping and documentation

There have been numerous key documents and legislation that have impacts upon standards of record keeping and documentation for the individual practitioner and organisation; these include:

Access to Health Records Act (1990) Department of Health[14]

The Access to Health Records Act (1990)[14] was published to establish a right of access to health records by the individuals to whom they relate and for others to allow for the correction of inaccuracies, the avoidance of contractual obligations and any related purposes. Whilst this act allows for access it does require written application for approval.

The Patient's Charter (1991) Department of Health[15]

In the following year the Patient's Charter (1991)[15] empowered patients and their relatives in the provision of their healthcare, allowing them access to standards of care and increased patient choice. This was replaced in 2001 by 'Your Guide to the NHS: getting the most from your National Health Service'[18] a guide to all standards and services within the National Health Service.

The Data Protection Act (1998) Department of Health[1]

In 1998 the Data Protection Act[1] was revised to encompass advances in healthcare records and technology, updating the previous act in 1984. This act sought to make new provision for the regulation of the processing of information relating to individuals, including the obtaining, holding, use or disclosure of such information.

Freedom of Information Act (2000) Department of Health[17]

The Freedom of Information Act (2000)[17] superseded previous legislation and was fully implemented in 2005. The Act gives a general right of access to all types of recorded information held by public authorities; the Act does however set out exemptions to this right. Any request that falls within the bounds of the exemptions must be considered using a 'public interest' test prior to access.

Essence of Care (2003) National Health Service[16]

This document was published as a toolkit for benchmarking of fundamental aspects of care including record keeping. Collaboratively written by patients, carers and professionals Essence of Care set out standards of care and best practice throughout the NHS. This document proposed seven key factors in record keeping that were considered best practice including:

- Access to current health care records.
- Integration - patient and professional partnership.
- Integration of records - across professional and organisational boundaries.
- Holding lifelong records.
- High quality practice - evidence based guidance.
- High quality practice - Records should demonstrate that care follows evidence based guidance.
- Security and confidentiality - Records should be safeguarded through explicit measures.

Records Management: NHS Code of Practice (2006)[11]

The Records Management: NHS Code of Practice was published by the Department of Health as a guide to the required standards of practice in the management of records for those who work within or under contract to NHS organisations in England. It is based on current legal requirements and professional best practice as agreed by a committee of professional representatives from all areas of the NHS. The Code provides a key component of information governance arrangements for the NHS; as such it is subject to continual review as best practice and records management evolve. This Code of Practice relates to all forms of record that may be required in practice, setting one key standard for the individual practitioner, stating 'Under the Public Records Act all NHS employees are responsible for any records that they create or use in the course of their duties. Thus any records created by an employee of the NHS are public records and may be subject to both legal and professional obligations'.

In addition a variety of professional standards have been introduced by the professional bodies that govern healthcare practitioners in the United Kingdom, these include:

- Guidelines for Records and Record Keeping (2005) Nursing and Midwifery Council.[5]
- Code of Conduct, Performance and Ethics (2007) Health Professions Council.[7]
- Standards of Proficiency – Paramedics (2007) Health Professions Council.[19]
- Good Medical Practice (2006) General Medical Council.[8]

These standards offer key overarching guidance upon record keeping in each specific profession, therefore paramedics will be governed by the standards of the Health Professions Council,[7,19] nurses by the Nursing and Midwifery Council[5] and doctors by the General Medical Council.[8] A review of these documents suggests that the expectations of each governing body differ very little, with only generic standards as set out earlier in this chapter.

The Caldicott Guardian

In 1997 a report on the review of patient identifiable information (The Caldicott Report) put forward a series of recommendations for the regulation of the use and transfer of patient identifiable information within the NHS and to non-NHS bodies.[20] The aim of these recommendations was to ensure that information was only shared for justified purposes and only the minimum information required was shared. Central to these requirements was the appointment of a 'Guardian' in each trust or organisation to oversee the sharing of information within these regulations (The Caldicott Guardian). The appointed guardian must ensure that any patient identifiable information released must meet a set of agreed principles.[20]

Electronic patient records

In recent years there have been moves to modernise the record keeping infrastructure within the NHS by the evolution of the electronic patient record.[21] The Governmental organisation Connecting for Health has sought to introduce a central electronic record spine within the NHS to allow for 24/7 access to patient records. This had had increasing influence upon the Ambulance Service and Acute Care Services with the intended introduction of an Electronic Patient Report Form (EPRF) in 2008. Whilst the final format of these care records are yet to be published an implemented the standards of record keeping required will undoubtedly remain.

Whilst this is a new initiative standards for documentation and record keeping will continue to be set by previous guidance.

> ## Scenario
>
> You have been called to a patient who has been assaulted in the street and suffered limb and facial injuries. You are not concerned that the patient has been knocked out, but feel the wounds need assessment and closure at the local hospital. The patient refuses to attend the emergency department. What details do you need to document upon this case? Consider both clinical and non-clinical issues.

Chapter Key Points

1. The recording of patient and clinical information is paramount in a quality healthcare system.
2. There is a wide range of guidance provided for documentation standards to ensure that any documentation and care is logical, well-structured and demonstrates adherence to key principles.
3. It is essential to review your own documentation and compare how you document episodes according to these standards. If you do not meet these standards you may place yourself or the patient at risk.

References and Further reading

1   Department of Health. *Data Protection Act*. London: HMSO, 1998.
2   Medical Protection Society. *Keeping Medical Records: A Guide for Medical Students*. London: Medical Protection Society, 2005.
3   Medical Protection Society. *Keeping Medical Records: A Complete Guide for GPs*. London: Medical Protection Society, 2005.
4   National Statistics Office – Health and Social Care Information Centre. *Ambulance Service Bulletin 2005/01/HSCIC*. London: HMSO, 2005.
5   Nursing and Midwifery Council. *Guidelines for Records and Record Keeping*. London: NMC, 2005.
6   Mann R, Williams J. Standards in medical record keeping. *Clin Med* 2003;3(4):329-332.
7   Health Professions Council. *Standards of Conduct, Performance and Ethics*. London: HPC, 2007.
8   General Medical Council. *Good Medical Practice*. London: GMC, 2006.
9   Royal College of Physicians. *Generic Medical Record Keeping Standards*. London: RCP, 2007.
10 Owen K. Documentation in nursing practice. *Nurs Stand* 2005;19(32):48-49.
11 Department of Health. *Records Management: NHS Codes of Practice*. London: HMSO, 2006.
12 National Health Service Litigation Authority. *Clinical Negligence Litigation: A Guide for Clinicians*. London: NHSLA, 2003.
13 National Health Service. *A First Class Service: Quality in the New NHS*. London: NHS, 1998.

14 Department of Health. *Access to Health Records Act 1990*. London: HMSO, 1990.

15 Department of Health. *The Patient's Charter*. London: HMSO, 1991.

16 Department of Health. *Essence of Care*. London: HMSO, 2003.

17 Department of Health. *Freedom of Information Act*. London: TSO, 2000.

18 Department of Health. *Your Guide to the NHS: Getting the Most from your National Health Service*, 2001.

19 Health Professions Council. *Paramedics – Standards of Proficiency*. London: HPC, 2007.

20 Department of Health. *The Caldicott Guardian Manual*. London: HMSO, 2006.

21 Department of Health. *Delivering 21st Century IT Support for the NHS: National Strategic Programme*. London: HMSO, 2002.

22 Douglas G, Nicol F, Robertson C (Eds) *Macleod's Clinical Examination*. London: Elsevier, 2005.

23 Bickley L. *Bates' Guide to Physical Examination and History Taking*. London: Lippincott Williams & Wilkins, 2003.

Chapter 10
Drug administration

Content

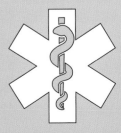

The paramedic has access to an increasing number of drugs and has a legal and ethical responsibility to deliver the correct dose of the correct drug to the correct patient at the correct time. An understanding of pharmacology and the associated subjects is essential if drugs are to be delivered safely and legally.

Definitions

The definition of a drug is complex and depends to a certain extent upon who is being asked to define the term. In medicine, the World Health Organization suggest that the term refers to a substance with the potential to prevent or cure disease or enhance physical or mental welfare, and in pharmacology to any chemical agent that alters the biochemical physiological processes of tissues or organisms.[1]

Legislation related to paramedic administration of drugs

Medicines approved for use in the UK are categorised in one of three ways:[2]

- General Sales List (GSL) medicines can be bought in places such as supermarkets and do not require the supervision of a pharmacist.
- Pharmacy (P) medicines can only be bought at a pharmacy and are sold under the supervision of a pharmacist.
- Prescription only medicines (POM) must be prescribed by a doctor, dentist, or exceptionally, another qualified health professional.

There is a range of exemptions from these restrictions which allow certain groups of health professionals, including paramedics, to sell, supply and administer particular medicines directly to patients. The exemptions are distinct from prescribing, which requires the involvement of a pharmacist in the sale or supply of the medicine. They also differ from the arrangements for Patient Group Directions (PGDs) as the latter must comply with specific legal criteria, be signed by a doctor or dentist and a pharmacist and authorised by an appropriate body. The exemptions that allow suitably trained ambulance paramedics to administer these drugs in specified circumstances exist under Part III of Schedule 5 to the Prescription Only Medicines (Human Use) Order 1997. For this purpose, a Paramedic is defined as being on the register of Paramedics maintained by the Health Professions Council pursuant to paragraph 11 of Schedule 2 to the Health Professions Order 2001.[3]

Diazepam and morphine are both controlled drugs regulated under the Misuse of Drugs Act 1971. This Act and its Regulations control the availability of drugs that are considered sufficiently 'dangerous or otherwise harmful', with the potential for diversion and misuse.[4] The drugs which are subject to the control of the Misuse of Drugs Act 1971 are listed in Schedule 2 of the Act and are termed CDs. The Act establishes a series of criminal offences for their unauthorised, and therefore unlawful, possession, possession with intent to supply, supply, importation and unlawful production.

As many CDs have legitimate medical purpose, the Regulations made under the Misuse of Drugs Act 1971, authorise and govern certain activities that would otherwise be illegal under the Act. The Regulations identify those health care professionals who may legitimately possess and supply CDs. They also establish a regime of control around prescribing, administrating, safe custody, dispensing, record keeping and destruction or disposal.[4]

Ambulance paramedics serving at any approved ambulance station are able to administer diazepam and/or morphine sulphate injection (to a maximum of 20 mg) for immediate necessary treatment of sick or injured persons. Currently there is wide variation in how CDs are obtained, stored and recorded by qualified paramedics working in the ambulance service.[4]

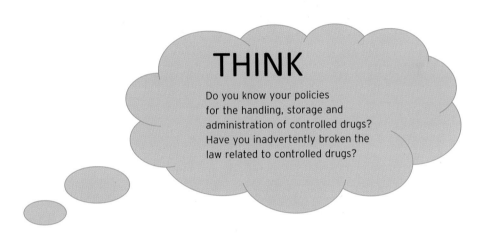

THINK

Do you know your policies for the handling, storage and administration of controlled drugs? Have you inadvertently broken the law related to controlled drugs?

A list of medicines which may only be administered by ambulance paramedics on their own initiative for immediate, necessary treatment of sick or injured persons can be found on the Medicines and Healthcare Products Regulatory Agency website at www.mhra.gov.uk.

Drug formulations

Drugs can be delivered in a variety of forms including tablets, capsules, solutions, inhalers, and by a variety of different routes – e.g. oral, rectal, intravenous, and intramuscular. A drug formulation may allow for selective targeting of specific tissues or may prevent systemic absorption. The formulation of the drug and the route administered determine the absorption and distribution of the drug.

Formulations for oral administration

Tablets

e.g. Aspirin.

Tablets are presented in a variety of different sizes, colours, shapes and types. The formulation of the tablet will be based upon the requirements of the drug, e.g. modified release tablets control the rate of release of a drug as it passes through the gastrointestinal tract. Tablets may be formulated to be chewed, held under the tongue (sublingual) or between the gum and the inside of the mouth (buccal), swallowed or to dissolve readily in liquid (soluble or effervescent).

Sprays

e.g. Glyceryl trinitrate (GTN).

Sprays such as GTN are designed to be taken sublingually because the first-pass mechanism destroys the majority of any drug that is swallowed.

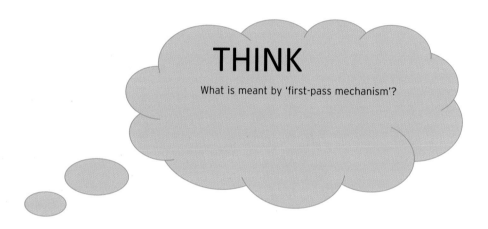

THINK

What is meant by 'first-pass mechanism'?

Liquids

Liquids, such as Calpol, are usually sweet, syrup-like solutions often designed to be taken by children where a tablet may be inappropriate.

Formulations for rectal administration

There are many different drug formulations that use the rectal route including enemas and suppositories; these are not commonly used in prehospital emergency care. Most commonly used is the rectal tube for delivery of diazepam. Rectal diazepam is formulated to be absorbed via the rectal mucosa and is highly effective.

Formulations for nebulisation

Nebulisation involves the passage of a gas (usually oxygen in paramedic care) through a solution of drug to create a fine mist to be inhaled by the patient. The drugs most commonly administered via this route in emergency prehospital care are bronchodilators. Studies have shown that only between 10% and 30% of an inhaled drug is actually deposited in the lungs, the rest is generally swallowed and passes into the gastrointestinal tract.[5]

Formulations for injection

Injections are sterile solutions, emulsions or suspensions where an active ingredient is either dissolved or requires to be dissolved in an appropriate solution. The injection may come in a pre-filled syringe, Mini-Jet, powder with solute to be mixed, an ampoule or a vial.

Most preparations are single-dose formulations that provide the correct volume to allow withdrawal and administration of the appropriate dose using standard techniques. However, initial doses of certain drugs may require the administration of less than is in the delivery system. An example is morphine, which has a typical presentation of 10 mg in 1mL, although the initial adult dose is usually between 2.5 and 5 mg.

Drug documentation

Documentation of drugs is a legal requirement and also essential for patient safety. Good practice related to documentation will minimise the risk of misunderstandings and ensure that there is some uniformity of practice across different health disciplines.

The following points should be noted:[6]

- Unnecessary use of decimal points should be avoided, e.g. 2 mg not 2.0 mg.
- Quantities of 1 gram or more should be written as 1g etc.
- Quantities less than 1 gram should be written in milligrams, e.g. 500 mg not 0.5 g.
- Quantities less than 1mg should be written in micrograms, e.g. 100 micrograms not 0.1mg.
- When decimals are unavoidable a zero should be written in front of the decimal point where there is no other figure, e.g. 0.5 mL not .5 mL.
- Use of the decimal point is acceptable to express a range, e.g. 0.5 to 1g.
- 'Micrograms' and 'nanograms' should not be abbreviated nor should 'units'.
- In medicine and pharmacy the term 'millilitre' (ml or mL) is used; cubic centimetre, (cc, or cm^3) should not be used.
- Unit abbreviations are not followed by a full stop (mL, not m.L. or mL.).
- A single space is left between the quantity and the symbol (24 kg not 24kg).
- Unit abbreviations are not pluralised (kg not kgs).
- As a rule, fractions are not used, only decimal notation (0.25 kg not ¼ kg).

Storage of drugs

General guidelines

Whilst in the possession of the ambulance service the responsibility for the safekeeping of the medicines rests with the Chief Executive. The security of medicines in specialist kits (e.g. paramedic bags) should be checked by pharmacy staff periodically, normally every 3 months, in accordance with locally agreed procedures. They should carry out inspections of medicines in specialist kits with reconciliation, where necessary. Prescription only medicines may only be issued by non-clinical staff for whom training and Standard Operational Procedures are agreed and in place.[7]

Security

Security should be of prime concern to the paramedic, especially when carrying and administering CDs. The Misuse of Drugs (Safe Custody) Regulations 1973 imposes controls on the storage of Schedule 1, 2 and Schedule 3 CDs.[8]

On station

Drugs should be kept in a locked storage area where general access is not possible; this helps to minimise the risk of unauthorised access and to deter abuse or misuse. Each service should have written procedures surrounding the signing in and out of medicines.

On vehicles

Where drugs are left on an unattended vehicle, the vehicle should be closed and locked – this alone is not adequate where CDs are involved.

'Doctor's bag'

A 'doctor's bag' is a locked bag, box or case for home visits, etc. which should be kept locked at all times, except when in immediate use. The person in lawful possession of this bag, or an individual authorised by them, must always retain the keys. Legal precedent holds that such a bag is regarded, once locked, as a suitable receptacle for storing CDs, but a locked vehicle is not.[4]

Stability

Medicines should be stored where they will not be subject to substantial variations in temperature. It is important that medicines are not stored close to heaters in ambulance vehicles as some may be damaged by heat.

Some medicines require storage under well-defined conditions, such as in a refrigerator. If ambulance services carry such medicines, provision should be made to meet these requirements.

Stock control

Stock rotation must be in operation to prevent the accumulation of 'old' stocks; this applies to vehicle or personal drug issue and drug supplies on station. It is the responsibility of the attending paramedic to ensure that all personal/vehicle drugs are checked and replenished, where necessary, on a day-to-day basis. Normally a supervisor will be responsible for monitoring the rotation of drugs held in station stores.

Routes of administration

Oral administration

Procedure	Additional information/rationale
1. Perform hand hygiene.	Minimises risk of infection.
2. Explain the reasons for administration of the drug to include potential side effects; gain consent from the patient.	Informed consent necessitates explanation of a procedure or medicine.
3. Prepare the medication for administration: • Confirm drug • Confirm dosage • Expiry date • Integrity of package.	To ensure that the patient receives the correct dose of the correct drug using the appropriate diluent and via the correct route. To protect the patient from harm.
4. Empty the required dose into a medicine container; avoid touching the medicine.	Reduces the risk of cross-infection.
5. Offer water if permitted.	Facilitate swallowing of medication.
6. Document administration of the drug as per Trust guidelines.	Legal requirement and patient safety. Other health professionals need documentation of interventions to guide further treatment.
7. Do not break a tablet unless it is scored.	Breaking may cause incorrect dosing.
8. Do not interfere with enteric coated or delayed release capsules; ensure that patients swallow them whole and do not chew them.	Changing the formulation of the medicine can affect rates of absorption and the amount of drug that is destroyed by the first pass mechanism.
9. Sublingual tablets should be placed under the tongue; buccal tablets should be placed between gum and cheek.	Allows for correct absorption.

Note – Chewing aspirin is not a pleasant experience and current prehospital guidance suggests that it may be swallowed with water or chewed.[9] The American Heart Association recommends that the tablet is chewed for speed of effect despite the unpleasant taste.[10]

Administration of Inhaled drugs (nebulised)

Procedure	Additional information/rationale
1. Perform hand hygiene.	Minimise risk of infection.
2. Explain the reasons for administration of the drug to include potential side effects; gain consent from the patient.	Informed consent necessitates explanation of a procedure or medicine.
3. Prepare the medication for administration: • Confirm drug • Confirm dosage • Expiry date • Integrity of package.	To ensure that the patient receives the correct dose of the correct drug using the appropriate diluent and via the correct route. To protect the patient from harm.
4. Administer only one drug at a time unless specifically indicated to the contrary.	Several drugs used together may produce adverse side-effects.
5. Empty contents of nebule into the nebuliser.	
6. If the prescribed dose does not require the entire contents of the nebule to be administered, measure the appropriate amount with a syringe.	Ensures the correct dose.
7. Connect nebuliser and mask to appropriate gas supply (oxygen or air) and turn to between 6 and 8 L/min. A fine mist should be apparent.	If the flow is too low there will be insufficient pressure to aerosolise the medication. If the pressure is too high, the oxygen tubing or nebuliser may become damaged at their weakest points.
8. Place the mask over the patient's face and pull the elastic to create a comfortable seal.	Ensures that the drug does not escape through a poorly fitted mask.
9. Coach the patient's breathing. Advise them to inhale slowly and as deeply as possible and to hold the medication for a short period before exhaling.	This maximises the deposition of the drug in the bronchial tree and improves absorption.
10. Document administration of the drug as per Trust guidelines.	Legal requirement and patient safety. Other health professionals need documentation of interventions to guide further treatment.

It is possible to nebulise bronchodilators in an intubated patient – the nebuliser should be connected to the oxygen supply as normal and then connected via a 'T' piece to the catheter mount immediately after the bag-valve ventilator or mechanical ventilator. It is essential that the nebuliser is maintained in an upright position to ensure that sufficient gas passes through the drug to aerosolise it.

Subcutaneous Injection

A subcutaneous (SC) injection is given beneath the skin into the connective tissue or fat immediately beneath the dermis. This route is generally used for small volumes of drugs (0.5 mL or less) that do not irritate tissue. The maximum volume that should be used for this route is 2 mL.[11] It is not commonly used in the emergency situation due to the slow absorption rates although there may be benefit from the prolonged effects when given via this route.

Traditionally, SC injections have been given at a 45° angle into a raised skin fold.[12] However, there is a recommendation that with the introduction of shorter needles (5, 6 or 8 mm), the injection is now administered at an angle of 90°.[13,14] The skin should be pinched up to lift the adipose tissue away from the underlying muscle, especially in thin patients. When injecting at 45° or into the buttock areas, which have the densest fat layer, lifting up of the skin fold is not required.[15] Traditional teaching has suggested that an attempt be made to aspirate once the needle is inserted in order to confirm that the needle is not in a blood vessel. This is no longer considered necessary as piercing of a blood vessel in a SC injection has been shown to be very rare.[16]

Suitable sites include the lateral aspects of the upper arm, lower abdomen (umbilical region), and the upper outer quadrant of the buttocks.[11] The lower back may also be used if necessary.

Procedure

Select the correct equipment:

- Appropriate sized syringe
- 25-gauge needle
- Filter needle
- Cleansing swab
- Drug to be administered.

Procedure	Additional information/rationale
1. Explain the procedure and gain consent from the patient.	Legal requirement
2. Perform hand hygiene and put on clean gloves.	Minimises risk of cross-infection.
3. Check and prepare all equipment.	Check that none is damaged, if so, discard.
4. Prepare the medication for injection: • Confirm drug • Confirm dosage/concentration • Expiry date • Diluent as appropriate • Integrity of package.	To ensure that the patient receives the correct dose of the correct drug using the appropriate diluent and via the correct route To protect the patient from harm.
5. Confirm with colleague.	Minimise risk of error.

Procedure	Additional information/rationale
6. Draw up the drug using a filter needle and then change for the appropriate administration needle.	This ensures that the needle used for administration is clean, sharp and the right length.
7. Use a two-finger 'pinch-up' technique to lift the skin fold away from the underlying muscle.	Helps to ensure SC administration.
8. Using a 90° angle of entry, pierce the skin and advance needle into the subcutaneous region.	
9. Administer the drug and withdraw the needle – the skin fold should be held until the needle has been removed.	
10. Dispose of sharps safely.	Drop sharps into container do not push. Colleagues should NOT hold the sharps container so as to avoid risk of accidental needlestick injury.
11. Document the administration and any untoward events at the site of injection.	Legal requirement and allows hospital staff to monitor any untoward occurrences.

Intramuscular Injection

Intramuscular injections deliver medication into well perfused muscle, providing rapid systemic action and absorbing relatively large doses – from 1mL in the deltoid site to 5mL elsewhere in adults (these values should be halved for children).[11] Administration of an IM injection is a complex psychomotor task that requires considerable dexterity and underpinning knowledge.[17] It is a two-handed procedure requiring the practitioner to use one hand to stabilise the injection site, and the other to administer the injection.

Site selection is of vital importance as the effect of the medication can be enhanced or diminished depending upon the selected site; complications are also associated with the chosen site.[17] The most common complications are muscle contracture and nerve injury.[18,19] Site selection should take into consideration the patient's general physical status and age, and the amount of drug to be given. The proposed site for injection should be inspected for signs of inflammation, swelling, and infection, and any skin lesions should be avoided.

Older and emaciated patients are likely to have less muscle than younger, more active patients. The proposed sites should be assessed for sufficient muscle mass and where there is reduced muscle mass it is helpful to 'bunch up' the muscle before injecting.[11]

There are five sites considered to be useful for IM injections although paramedics tend to use only two of these:

- The deltoid muscle of the upper arm.

- The dorsogluteal site using the gluteus maximus muscle, the traditional site in the UK.[20] Complications are associated with this site as there is a possibility of damaging the sciatic nerve or the superior gluteal artery if the needle is misplaced. Several studies show that even in mildly obese patients, injections into the dorsogluteal area are more likely to be into adipose tissue rather than muscle, and consequently slow the absorption rate of the drug.[21]
- The ventrogluteal site is a safer option which accesses the gluteus medius muscle. This site is recommended as the primary location for IM injections as it avoids all major nerves and blood vessels and there have been no reported complications.[21] In addition, the thickness of adipose tissue over the ventrogluteal site is relatively consistent at 3.75 cm as compared to 1-9 cm in the dorsogluteal site. This ensures that a standard size 21-gauge needle will usually penetrate the gluteus medius muscle area.[11]

Techniques

The angle of needle entry may contribute to the pain of the injection. For many years it has been stated that intramuscular injections should be given at a 90° angle to ensure the needle reaches the muscle and to reduce pain; most of the literature tends to support this contention.[22] One study seems to indicate that the 90° angle is less important in terms of the depth of injection as an angle of 72° penetrates to 95% of the depth of a needle angled at 90°.[23] Based on this, the practitioner should endeavour to give the injection with the needle perpendicular to the patient's body, which should ensure that it falls within the range of 72-90°.[17]

Fewer needlestick injuries and improved site accuracy have been reported when the hands are positioned near the intended entry site.[11] To ensure entry at the correct angle, the heel of the dominant palm should rest on the thumb of the non-dominant hand. It is suggested that by holding the syringe between the thumb and forefinger, a firm and accurate thrust of the needle at the correct angle can be achieved.[11]

The traditional method of giving an intramuscular injection has been to stretch the skin over the site to reduce the sensitivity of nerve endings and to insert the needle in a dart like action at 90° to the skin.[24] Two different techniques are also available, the Z track technique and the air bubble technique.

Z-track technique

The Z-track technique is believed to reduce pain, as well as the incidence of leakage.[25] It involves pulling the skin downwards or to one side at the intended site, which moves the cutaneous and subcutaneous tissues by 1-2 cm. The needle is inserted and the injection given. Ten seconds should be allowed before removing the needle to facilitate diffusion of the medication into the muscle. On removal, the retracted skin is released so that the tissues close over the deposit of medication thus preventing leakage from the site. Exercising the limb afterwards is believed to assist absorption of the drug by increasing blood flow to the area.[21]

Aspiration should be practised in IM injections. If a needle is mistakenly placed in a blood vessel, the drug may be given intravenously.

Air bubble technique

This technique arose historically from the use of glass syringes which required an added air bubble to ensure an accurate dose was given. It is no longer necessary to allow for the dead space in the syringe and needle, as plastic syringes are calibrated more accurately than glass ones, and it is no longer recommended by manufacturers.[21] Studies comparing this technique with the Z-track technique have been inconclusive with one suggesting that the air bubble technique is more successful at preventing leakage than the Z-track technique,[26] whilst the findings of the other were inconclusive.[27] There are issues related to the accuracy of the dose when using this technique – it may significantly increase the dose.[28] Further research needs to be undertaken on this method as it is relatively new to the UK; it is recommended that the Z-track technique be used in preference.[29]

Procedure (Z-track)[29]

Procedure	Additional information/rationale
1. Explain the procedure and gain consent from the patient.	Legal requirement
2. Perform hand hygiene and put on clean gloves.	Minimises risk of cross-infection.
3. Check and prepare all equipment.	Check that none is damaged, if so, discard.
4. Prepare the medication for injection: • Confirm drug • Confirm dosage/concentration • Expiry date • Diluent as appropriate • Integrity of package.	To ensure that the patient receives the correct dose of the correct drug using the appropriate diluent and via the correct route To protect the patient from harm.
5. Confirm with colleague.	Minimise risk of error.
6. Determine the appropriate injection site (see preceding information).	
7. Position the patient and identify the injection site by using body landmarks. Make sure the area is intact and free from abnormalities such as infection, bruising, or tenderness.	
8. Clean the skin as per guidelines.	Minimise risk of infection.
9. Using the subdominant hand, displace the skin and subcutaneous tissue by pulling the skin laterally or downward from the injection site. Holding it taut, quickly and smoothly insert the needle into the muscle at a 90-degree angle.	Displaces cutaneous and subcutaneous layers. Needle is inserted at 90° to ensure that the needle reaches muscle tissue, and it also reduces pain.

Procedure	Additional information/rationale
10. Continue to hold the skin taut with the subdominant hand. With the dominant hand, aspirate for approximately 5 seconds. If no blood returns with aspiration, slowly inject the medication (10 seconds/mL). If blood is seen in the syringe, withdraw the needle, discard both the medication and syringe properly, and prepare another dose for injection.	Prevents inadvertent intravenous administration.
11. Wait 10 seconds to withdraw the needle Withdraw it slowly and smoothly at a 90-degree angle.	Allows the medication to disperse evenly in the muscle tissue.
12. Release the skin to create a zigzag path.	Minimises seepage of the drug.
13. Apply gentle pressure at the injection site with a sterile pad but DO NOT massage the site as this can cause irritation.	
14. Discard all equipment properly, remove gloves, and perform hand hygiene.	Reduces risk of cross-infection.
15. Document the date and time of administration, the drug name and dose, the injection route and site, and the patient's response.	Legal requirement.

Rectal administration

The rectal route is not frequently used by paramedics, but it is suitable for patients who are having seizures where it may not be possible to cannulate. The drug is absorbed rapidly through the rectal mucosa.

Equipment required

- Clean, non-sterile gloves
- Lubricating jelly
- Rectal tube.

Procedure	Additional Information/rationale
1. Explain the procedure and gain consent from the patient (if possible).	Legal requirement.
2. Perform hand hygiene and put on clean gloves.	Minimises risk of cross-infection.
3. Check and prepare all equipment.	Check that none is damaged, if so, discard.

Procedure	Additional Information/rationale
4. Prepare the medication: • Confirm drug • Confirm dosage/concentration • Expiry date • Integrity of package.	To ensure that the patient receives the correct dose of the correct drug and via the correct route. To protect the patient from harm.
5. Confirm with colleague.	Minimises risk of error.
6. Remove the cap of the rectal tube and lubricate with lubricating jelly.	Reduces trauma on insertion.
7. Position the patient on the abdomen or side with a cushion under the hip. A small child can lie across the practitioner's knees.	Allows ease of passage of the tube into the rectum.
8. Insert the nozzle into the anus.	Most rectal tubes have a mark to indicate depth of insertion for young children.
9. Keep the tube with the nozzle pointing downwards during administration.	
10. Squeeze the tube between thumb and finger to deliver drug.	
11. Keep pressing the tube whilst withdrawing. Hold the buttocks together for a few moments.	Prevents aspiration of drug back into tube and prevents seepage.
12. A small amount of fluid left in the tube will not affect the dose administered.	
13. Discard all equipment properly, remove gloves, and perform hand hygiene.	Reduces risk of cross-infection.
14. Document the date and time of administration, the drug name and dose, the injection route and site, and the patient's response.	Legal requirement.

Chapter Key Points

1. Medicines approved for use in the UK are categorised as either General Sales List (GSL); Pharmacy (P) or Prescription Only Medicine (POM).
2. There are a range of exemptions from legal restrictions that allow paramedics to supply and administer particular medicines directly to patients.
3. Paramedics are responsible legally and ethically for the safe administration of drugs; the law is clear on how drugs should be stored and administered.
4. Clear, accurate documentation is essential.
5. Drugs can be delivered in a variety of forms including tablets, capsules, solutions, inhalers, and by a variety of different routes. They may be administered via a number of different routes.
6. The paramedic needs to know which drugs can be administered via which route and the procedures for using any given route.

References and Further reading

1 World Health Organization. *Lexicon of alcohol and drug terms published by the World Health Organization*. Available online at http://www.who.int/substance_abuse/terminology/who_lexicon/en/ [accessed 04 Dec 2008].
2 Medicines and Healthcare Products Regulatory Agency. Availability of Medicines. Available online at http://www.mhra.gov.uk/Howweregulate/Medicines/Availabilityprescribingsellingandsupplyingofmedicines/Availabilityofmedicines/index.htm [accessed 03 April 2008].
3 Statutory Instrument 2002 No. 880. The Health Professions Order 2001 (Consequential Amendments) Order 2002. London: HMSO, 2002.
4 National Prescribing Centre. *A Guide to Good Practice in the Management of Controlled Drugs in Primary Care (England)*, 2nd edn. Liverpool: The National Prescribing Centre, 2007.
5 New Zealand Medicines and Medical Devices Safety Authority *Ipratropium Steri-neb Data Sheet*. 2005. Available online at http://www.medsafe.govt.nz/Profs/Datasheet/i/Ipratropiuminh.htm [accessed 23 Nov 2008].
6 British Medical Association and Royal Pharmaceutical Society of Great Britain. *British National Formulary 53*. March 2007. available online at http://www.bnf.org.uk/bnf/ [accessed 03 April 2008].
7 Royal Pharmaceutical Society of Great Britain. The Safe and Secure Handling of Medicines: A Team Approach. London: Royal Pharmaceutical Society, 2005.
8 Home Office – Action Against Drugs Unit. Misuse of Drugs (Safe Custody) Regulations 1973. London, UK: Home Office.
9 Joint Royal Colleges Ambulance Liaison Committee. *UK Ambulance Service Clinical Practice Guidelines* v4. London: IHCD, 2006.
10 ACC/AHA Guidelines for the Management of Patients With ST-Elevation Myocardial Infarction - Executive Summary: A Report of the American College of Cardiology/American Heart Association Task Force on Practice Guidelines (Writing Committee to Revise the 1999 Guidelines for the Management of Patients With Acute Myocardial Infarction). *Circulation* 2004;110;588-636.
11 Workman B. Safe injection techniques. *Nurs Stand* 1999;13(39):47-52.
12 Thow J, Home P. Insulin injection technique. *Br Med J* 1990;301(7):3-4.

13 Burden M. A practical guide to insulin injections. *Nurs Stand* 1994;8(29):25-29.

14 Nicol M, Bavin C, Bedford-Turner S, Cronin P, Rawlings-Anderson K. *Essential Nursing Skills*, 2dn edn. Philadelphia: Mosby, 2004.

15 Wood L, Wilbourne J. Kyne-Grzebalski D. Administration of insulin by injection. *Pract Diabetes Internat* 2002;19(2)(Suppl):S1-S4.

16 Peragallo-Dittko V. Rethinking subcutaneous injection technique. *Am J Nurs* 1997;97(5): 71-72.

17 Nicoll LH, Hesby A. Intramuscular injection: an integrative research review and guideline for evidence-based practice. *Appl Nurs Res* 2002;16(2):149-162.

18 Beecroft PC, Redick SA. Possible complications of intramuscular injections on the pediatric unit. *Pediat Nurs* 1989;15(4):333-336,376.

19 Bergeson PS, Singer SA, Kaplan AM. Intramuscular injections in children. *Pediatrics* 1982;70(6):944-948.

20 Campbell J. Injections. *Profess Nurse* 1995;10(7):455-458.

21 Beyea SC, Nicholl LH. Administration of medications via the intramuscular route: an integrative review of the literature and research-based protocol for the procedure. *Appl Nurs Res* 1995;5(1):23-33.

22 Warren BL. Intramuscular injection angle: evidence for practice? *Nurs Prax NZ* 2002;18(2): 52-53.

23 Katsma DL, Katsma R. The myth of the 90 degrees-angle intramuscular injection. *Nurse Educ* 2000;25(1):34-37.

24 Stilwell B. *Skills Update*. London: MacMillan Magazines, 1992.

25 Keen MF. Comparison of Intramuscular injection techniques to reduce site discomfort and lesions. *Nurs Res* 1986;35(4):207-210.

26 Quartermaine S, Taylor R. A comparative study of depot injection techniques. *Nurs Times* 1995;91(30):36-39.

27 MacGabhann L. A comparison of two injection techniques. *Nurs Stand* 1998;12(37):39-41.

28 Chaplin G *et al*. How safe is the air bubble technique for IM injections? Not very say these experts. *Nursing* 1985;15(9):59.

29 Pullen R. Administering medication by the Z-track method. *Nursing* 2005;35(7):24.

Chapter 11

Medical gases

Content

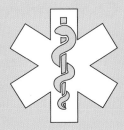

Entonox and oxygen have been available to ambulance personnel for many years and at one time were the only medicines available in the ambulance service. When given appropriately, both drugs have proven beneficial effects for patients; however, there is disquiet surrounding the amount of oxygen that is administered by ambulance staff in the prehospital environment.

Definition and indications for the use of Entonox

Entonox is an inhaled analgesic gas comprising of 50% nitrous oxide and 50% oxygen that is indicated in the management of moderate pain and also for labour pain.[1] Entonox is rapidly absorbed into the blood stream of the pulmonary vasculature, but does not combine with haemoglobin or with any other body tissues. Its low solubility in blood produces the rapid onset and offset of effect.[2] Nitrous oxide (the anaesthetic agent within Entonox) has very few side-effects and no incompatibility with other drugs has ever been demonstrated. [2] It has been noted that the nitrous oxide constituent of Entonox inactivates vitamin B_{12}.[3] The mixture of nitrous oxide and oxygen remains stable at temperatures above $-6\,^{\circ}$C.

There are different theories as to the exact mechanism of action of Entonox. It has been suggested that Entonox interacts with the endogenous opioid system,[4] and it has been shown to act preferentially on areas of the brain and spinal cord that are rich in morphine sensitive cells.[5] BOC suggest that it also has an effect on gamma aminobutyric acid (GABA), which increases inhibition of nerves cells, causing drowsiness and sleep.[6]

Advantages of Entonox

Entonox offers the practitioner and patient several advantages:

- Analgesic effect is rapid and side-effects are minimal.
- It confers no cardiac or respiratory depression.
- It can be self-administered.
- It has a very short half-life so the effects wear off rapidly once inhalation has ceased. This may be useful for short-term relief when carrying out painful procedures such as wound dressings or applying traction to fractures. In addition, Entonox may be administered as a temporary analgesic agent whilst preparing the patient for the administration of intravenous analgesia.
- The oxygen content may confer benefit to patients with certain medical or trauma conditions.

Contraindications to the use of Entonox

According to the Joint Royal Colleges Ambulance Liaison Committee (JRCALC), Entonox is contraindicated in the following circumstances:[1]

- Severe head injuries with impaired consciousness.
- Decompression sickness (anybody who has been diving in the previous 24 hours should be considered at risk).

- Violently disturbed psychiatric patients.

Caution should be applied when administering Entonox to a chest injured patient when a pneumothorax is suspected as it may expand the pneumothorax.

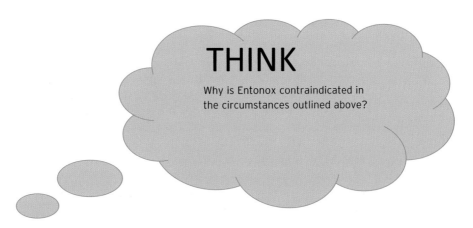

THINK

Why is Entonox contraindicated in the circumstances outlined above?

There appears to be some conflict between JRCALC and the contraindications listed by the BOC datasheet, which includes any patient:

- Where air is entrapped within a body and where its expansion might be dangerous.
- Artificial, traumatic or spontaneous pneumothorax.
- Air embolism.
- Gross abdominal distension.
- Intoxication.
- Maxillofacial injuries.

Essentially N_2O is contraindicated where there is trapped air, which covers the first four in the BOC list. Dr Tom Clarke of JRCALC states that intoxication is not defined by BOC but would appear to indicate a state where the 'balance of the mind is disturbed' due to alcohol, drugs or psychosis.[7] Maxillofacial injuries are contraindicated due to the possible access of Entonox to the sinuses and also due to the difficulty of administration.

It has been suggested that Entonox should not be given during the first trimester of pregnancy due to the risk of skeletal teratogenic complications; however no increased incidence of foetal malformation has been discovered in 8 epidemiological studies and case reports in human beings. There is no published material showing that nitrous oxide is toxic to the human foetus, therefore, there is no absolute contra-indication to its use in the first 16 weeks of pregnancy.[3]

Recommendations

- Entonox should be contraindicated to patients where air is entrapped within a body and where its expansion might be dangerous, those with severe head injuries with impaired consciousness, decompression sickness, and intoxication or psychiatric patients where the balance of the mind is disturbed.

Equipment

- Entonox cylinder
- Regulator
- Face mask or mouthpiece.

The neck on an Entonox cylinder is blue and white segmented, which is a UK norm; colours may vary in other Countries. The newer CD (440 L) and HX (2200 L) cylinders feature a valve with built in regulator, an Entonox Schrader outlet connection, and a permanently live contents gauge. The cylinders are 25% lighter than conventional steel, which makes them ideal for prehospital use. The traditional 500 L, D sized cylinder is still in use and requires the application of a pin-index pressure regulator.

Use of cylinders and general safety for both Entonox and Oxygen are covered at the end of this chapter.

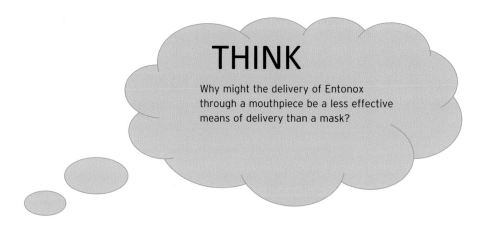

THINK

Why might the delivery of Entonox through a mouthpiece be a less effective means of delivery than a mask?

Principles of administration of Entonox

Entonox is self-administered by the use of a face mask or mouthpiece connected through a demand valve to the Entonox cylinder. Gas is drawn from the cylinder by the negative pressure created during the patient's inhalation; as soon as the face mask or mouthpiece is removed, delivery stops. For this reason, the face mask must be held firmly over the face or the mouthpiece to the lips to produce an airtight seal.

Doses are regulated by the patient and the risk of overdose is low. Since pain is usually relieved by a concentration of 25% nitrous oxide, continued inhalation does not occur. However, should inhalation continue, light anaesthesia supervenes and the mask drops away as the patient relaxes.[3]

Mouthpiece or face mask?

Searches revealed no studies investigating the relative effectiveness of delivering Entonox via a mouthpiece or mask. One study evaluated patient preferences and the efficacy of pre-oxygenation using face mask or mouthpiece with or without nose clip, which may provide some insight into the best method of administering Entonox.[8] Most conscious patients tolerated a mask well but a significant minority (12%) refused it. The mouthpiece on its own was insufficient to attain full preoxygenation owing to nose breathing of room air, which may explain why anecdotally, Entonox does not always provide analgesia. The mouthpiece with nose clip produced comparable results to the face mask but was less popular amongst patients.

Recommendation

Entonox should preferentially be delivered via face mask or mouthpiece with nose clip to maximise the effect of the drug.

Complications

Inappropriate, unwitting or deliberate inhalation of Entonox will ultimately result in unconsciousness, passing through stages of increasing light-headedness and intoxication. The treatment is removal to fresh air and resuscitation as appropriate.[3]

Procedure for administering Entonox

Procedure	Rationale/further information
1. Ensure that the patient is in a comfortable position prior to administration.	
2. Check the patient has no contraindications for the administration of Entonox.	Avoids exacerbating underlying conditions.
3. Explain the procedure and effects of the medication to the patient and gain informed consent.	Aids patient compliance and is a legal requirement.
4. Ensure that the cylinder is turned on; check the gauge to determine how much Entonox is in the cylinder.	Avoids risk of running out of medication.
5. Demonstrate how to obtain a seal with the face mask or mouthpiece. Explain that when the patient is breathing in and out regularly and deeply a hissing sound will be heard.	Maximises inhalation of the gas and indicates that the gas is being inhaled.
6. Encourage the patient to breathe deeply for at least two minutes before attempting any painful procedures.	Allows time for the analgesic effect to take place.
7. Coach the patient's respirations as necessary.	To ensure maximum inhalation of the gas.
8. Evaluate the effectiveness of Entonox by using verbal or visual pain scoring tools.	Identifies if further measures are required.

Procedure	Rationale/further information
9. Evaluate the effect during and after painful procedures, and throughout the duration of use.	
10. Turn off Entonox supply on completion.	Avoids inadvertent leakage..
11. Dispose of mask/mouthpiece as per Trust guidelines, or clean in accordance with guidelines if using reusable items.	
12. Record the administration, effects and side-effects of Entonox on the case report form. Any adverse effects should also be recorded.	A legal requirement and provides information for those caring for the patient afterwards

Troubleshooting

Procedure

Problem	Possible explanation	Suggestion
1. Patient not achieving adequate analgesia.	Cylinder empty.	Check prior to administration, change if necessary.
	Patient not inhaling deeply enough.	Coach respirations. Reassess suitability of Entonox for the patient and find alternative analgesia if necessary.
2. Patient refuses or can't tolerate a mask.	Feeling of claustrophobia or dislike of the smell of the mask.	Use mouthpiece with nose clip as an alternative.
3. Feelings of nausea, drowsiness or giddiness.	Effect of nitrous oxide accumulation.	Discontinue therapy and effects will wear of rapidly.
4. Patient afraid to use Entonox.	Possible associations with previous experiences.	Reassure patient about the benefits of receiving Entonox and the short-term effects. Reiterate the procedure for administration.

Definition of oxygen therapy

Oxygen (O_2) is a colourless, odourless gas that supports combustion and is essential to human life. It is provided in compressed form in a cylinder that is typically colour coded white. Modern cylinders are lightweight and feature a valve with built in regulator, an Oxygen Schrader outlet connection, and a permanently live contents gauge. The sizes most commonly used in prehospital care are the CD size (460L) and the HX size (2300L).

Oxygen is the most frequently used drug in prehospital emergency care and may be lifesaving when given correctly. However, it is often administered without careful consideration of its potential benefits and side-effects.[9]

Indications for use

JRCALC revised the oxygen guidelines in April 2009 to reflect concerns surrounding inappropriate administration of oxygen by practitioners in prehospital care.[1] The new guideline challenges many of the traditional practices, such as the routine administration of high concentration supplemental oxygen to all patients suffering a suspected or confirmed acute myocardial infarction. It also advocates the more widespread use of pulse oximetry to guide supplemental oxygen therapy and the use of alternative methods of delivery, such as nasal cannulae.

It is imperative that the practitioner is aware of the updated guidelines and also understands the physiology of respiration and tissue oxygenation. It is recommended that this be reviewed in a suitable physiology textbook.

> ## Scenario
>
> You are called to attend a case where a 65-year-old known COPD patient is suffering from cardiac related central chest pain. His 12-lead ECG is showing signs of a new inferior myocardial infarction whilst his oxygen saturations are 92%. Will you administer oxygen to the patient? If so, how much and why? If not, why not?

Cautions and contraindications to the use of oxygen

Paraquat poisoning

Paraquat is a bipyridyl herbicide which if ingested causes irreversible pulmonary fibrosis by generation of superoxide radicals. Treatment is by immediate gastric lavage and gastric decontamination. As high concentrations of oxygen worsen the lung damage, supplementary oxygen should be withheld for as long as practicable, then used at the lowest concentration that will maintain tissue oxygenation.[10]

Chronic obstructive pulmonary disease (COPD)

There remains much discussion surrounding what constitutes appropriate oxygen therapy in the emergency management of acute exacerbation of COPD. A number of studies[11] have concluded that oxygen therapy may lead to hypercapnia and acidosis, so it is imperative that patients with COPD do not receive excessive concentrations of oxygen.

Current guidelines recommend that:[11]

- The oxygen saturation should be measured in patients with an exacerbation of COPD, if there are no facilities to measure arterial blood gases.
- If necessary, oxygen should be given to keep the SaO_2 within range of 88-92% or pre-specified range detailed on patient's alert card.

During the transfer to hospital the following points should be considered:

- It is not desirable to exceed an oxygen saturation of 93%. Oxygen therapy should be commenced titrated upwards if saturation falls below 90% and downwards if the patient becomes drowsy or if the saturation exceeds 93-94%.
- Patients with known type II respiratory failure need special care, especially if they require a long ambulance journey or if they are given oxygen at home for a prolonged period before the ambulance arrives.

Oxygen should be given to all patients with an exacerbation of COPD who are breathless, if the oxygen saturations are not known.

JRCALC suggests that where the primary illness in a patient with COPD requires a high concentration of oxygen (e.g. serious trauma) then oxygen should not be withheld.[1] However, the patient should be continuously monitored and oxygen therapy amended if the patient deteriorates. For a further and fuller explanation of the most recent guidelines surrounding the indications and use of oxygen in emergency care, refer to the British Thoracic Society Guideline for emergency oxygen use in adult patients.[12]

NOTE - COPD is not a contraindication to the administration of oxygen.

Defibrillation and explosive environments

Oxygen supports combustion so should not be used during defibrillation or in an explosive environment.

Equipment

- Oxygen cylinder
- Regulator
- Flowmeter
- Disposable tubing
- Disposable oxygen mask or nasal cannula.

Oxygen cylinder

The neck on an oxygen cylinder is white, which is a UK norm; colours may vary in other Countries. Newer oxygen cylinders feature a valve with built in regulator, an oxygen Schrader outlet connection, and a permanently live contents gauge. Older cylinders have a black body with white neck and require the application of a pressure regulator to the valve. These cylinders will either have a 'bull-nose' valve or a pin-index valve.

Sizes typically used in prehospital care include the CD size (460 L) and the HX size (2300 L).

Regulator

The pressure contained within gas cylinders is initially very high and falls as the contents are used. The function of the regulator, or reducing valve, is to convert this variable, high-pressure gas supply to a constant, low-pressure gas supply. Ensure that only the appropriate regulator is fitted to the cylinder.

Flowmeter

The flowmeter allows the practitioner to select an appropriate flow of gas to the patient. The flow meter may be a glass tube with a ball that floats on the stream of gas or a twist-knob dial. The flow selected will depend up the requirements of the patient.

Oxygen tubing

Oxygen tubing may be packaged with the chosen mask or may be separate. Tubing is single-use and should be disposed of following patient treatment.

Oxygen masks and nasal cannulae

Nasal cannulae

See Figure 11.1.

Nasal cannulae are rarely used in prehospital care mainly because a constant oxygen concentration is not possible since the nasal catheter delivers a constant oxygen flow, and the resulting partial pressure received by the patient depends on the minute ventilation. In addition, the design is uncomfortable, there is a need for frequent replacement due to obstruction, and damage to the nasal mucosa.[13]

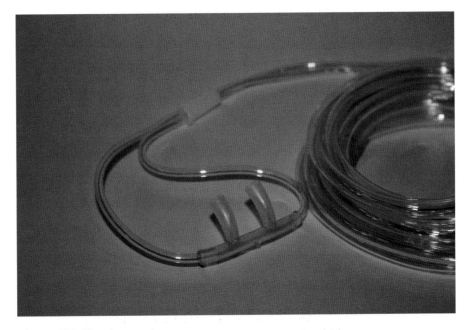

Figure 11.1 Nasal cannula.

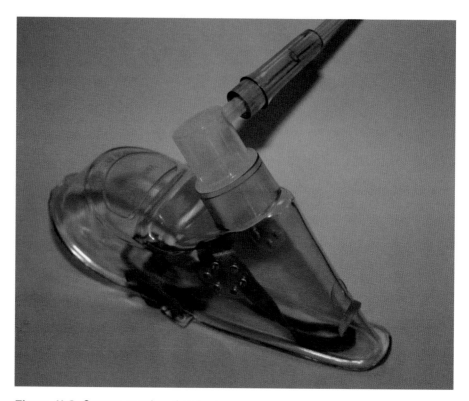

Figure 11.2 Oxygen mask - standard.

Simple face mask

See Figure 11.2.

The simple face mask has side-ports that allow the entrainment of ambient air, which dilutes the concentration of oxygen delivered to the patient and restricts oxygen concentrations. With flow rates of between 6 and 10 L/min, concentrations of between 40% and 60% can be attained. These masks are suitable for patients requiring moderate to high concentrations of oxygen.

Non-rebreather mask

See Figure 11.3.

These masks have one-way side ports that allow air to escape on exhalation but restrict entrainment of air during inspiration. The mask also has a reservoir bag to hold oxygen ready for inhalation. At a flow rate of 15 L/min, oxygen concentrations of 80%-95% can be achieved. These masks should be reserved for those patients who have adequate ventilation but who require high concentrations of supplementary oxygen.

Venturi mask

See Figure 11.4.

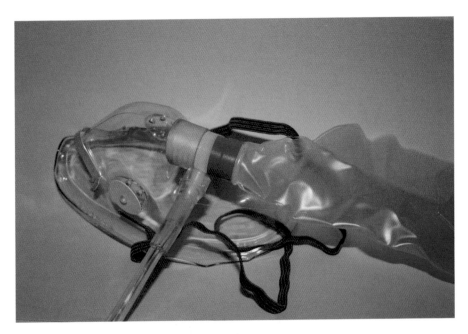

Figure 11.3 Non-rebreathe oxygen mask.

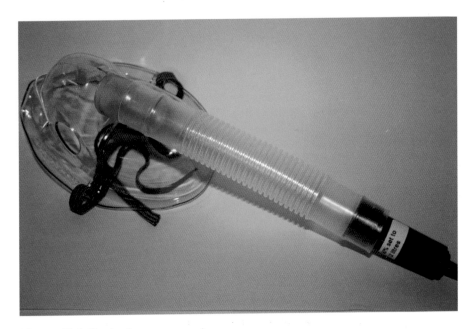

Figure 11.4 Venturi oxygen mask.

Venturi masks are not commonly used in UK prehospital practice even though they are capable of delivering a relatively constant concentration of oxygen irrespective of the patient's rate and depth of breathing. Masks generally deliver 24%, 28%, 35% or 40% oxygen, and may be particularly useful for COPD patients.

Oxygen passes into the mask through a jet orifice where it entrains room air. This mixture is then delivered to the patient. In order to change the concentration it may be necessary to change the cap on the mask.

Procedure for administering oxygen[14]

Procedure	Rationale/further information
1. Ensure that the patient is in a comfortable position prior to administration.	
2. Explain the procedure and effects of the medication to the patient and gain informed consent.	Aids patient compliance and is a legal requirement.
3. Ensure that the cylinder is turned on; check the gauge to determine how much oxygen is in the cylinder.	Avoids risk of running out of medication.
4. Select the most appropriate mask for the needs of the patient and remove from packaging.	Ensures appropriate concentration of oxygen is delivered. Do not remove oxygen masks from package until just before use to avoid contamination
5. Connect the oxygen tubing to the flowmeter and select the correct flow rate for the desired concentration	The flow required to attain a given concentration is normally provided with the mask.
6. Place the mask over the patient's nose and mouth and tighten the strap until the mask is firmly held in place.	
7. Coach the patient's respirations as necessary.	Maximises inhalation of the gas.
8. Evaluate the effectiveness of oxygen by reassessing observations; adjust flow rate as required.	Determines the need to amend concentration delivered.
9. Dispose of face mask and tubing on completion.	
10. Record the administration, effects and side-effects of oxygen on the case report form. Any adverse effects should also be recorded.	Legal requirement and provides information for those caring for the patient afterwards.

Use of cylinders and cylinder safety[14]

The following section is taken from BOC Medical guidelines and demonstrates best practice.

Storage of cylinders

Compressed medical oxygen cylinders should be:

- Stored under cover, preferably inside, kept dry and clean and not subjected to extremes of heat or cold, and away from stocks of combustible material.
- Stored separately from industrial and other non-medical cylinders.
- Stored to maintain separation between full and empty cylinders.
- Used in strict rotation so that cylinders with the earliest filling date are used first.
- Stored separately from other medical cylinders within the store.
- F size cylinders and larger should be stored vertically. E size cylinders and smaller should be stored horizontally.

Preparation for use[14]

- Remove the tamper evident seal and the valve outlet protection cap. Ensure the cap is retained so that it can be refitted after use.
- Do not remove and discard any batch labels fitted to the cylinder.
- Ensure that an appropriate compressed medical oxygen regulator is selected for connection to the cylinder.
- Ensure the connecting face on the regulator is clean and the sealing washer fitted is in good condition.
- Connect the regulator, using moderate force only and connect the tubing to the regulator/flowmeter outlet.
- Only the appropriate regulator should be used for the particular gas concerned.
- Open the cylinder valve slowly and check for any leak.
- Cylinder valves and any associated equipment must never be lubricated and must be kept free from oil and grease.

Leaks[14]

Cylinders used with a pressure regulator

- Having connected the regulator or manifold yoke to the cylinder check the connections for leaks.
- Should leaks occur this will usually be evident by a hissing noise.
- Should a leak occur between the valve outlet and the regulator or manifold yoke, depressurise and remove the fitting and fit an approved sealing washer.
- Reconnect the fitting to the valve with moderate force only, fitting a replacement regulator or manifold tailpipe as required.
- Sealing or jointing compounds must never be used to cure a leak.
- Never use excessive force when connecting equipment to cylinders.
- If leak persists, label cylinder and return to supplier.

Cylinders with an integral regulated valve

- Should leaks occur this will usually be evident by a hissing noise.
- Close valve, remove connection, check and refit.
- If leak persists, label cylinder and return to supplier.

Cylinder safety[14]

When compressed medical oxygen cylinders are in use, ensure that they are:

- Only used for medicinal purposes.
- Turned off, when not in use, using only moderate force to close the valve.
- Only moved with the appropriate size and type of trolley or handling device.
- Handled with care and not knocked violently or allowed to fall.
- Firmly secured to a suitable cylinder support when in use.
- Not allowed to have any markings, labels or batch labels obscured or removed.
- Not used in the vicinity of persons smoking or near naked lights.

When the compressed medical oxygen cylinder is empty ensure that the:

- Cylinder valve is closed using moderate force only and the pressure in the regulator or tailpipe released.
- Valve outlet cap, where fitted, is replaced.
- Empty cylinders are immediately returned to the empty cylinder store for return to supplier.

Chapter Key Points

1. Entonox is an inhaled analgesic gas comprising of 50% nitrous oxide and 50% oxygen that is indicated in the management of moderate pain and also for labour pain.
2. Entonox has a rapid onset of action and the side-effects are minimal; it confers no cardiac or respiratory depression, can be self-administered, and has a very short half-life so the effects wear off rapidly.
3. Contraindications to the use of Entonox and the difficulty of self-administration encountered by some patient groups may mean that an alternative analgesic is required.
4. Entonox should preferentially be delivered via face mask or mouthpiece with nose clip to maximise the effect of the drug.
5. Oxygen (O_2) is a colourless, odourless gas that supports combustion and is essential to human life.
6. Oxygen is the most commonly administered medicine in prehospital care, but caution should be exercised in its use. Oxygen should only be administered to those patients presenting with an indication for its use.
7. The most appropriate equipment should be used when administering oxygen. The choice between masks and nasal cannulae will be dependent upon patient needs.
8. It is essential that cylinders are stored and handled with care in order to minimise the risk of unwanted and dangerous occurrences.

References and Further reading

Tortora GJ, Derrickson B. *Principles of Anatomy and Physiology*, 11th edn. USA: Wiley, 2006.

National Institute for Health and Clinical Excellence. CG12, Chronic Obstructive Pulmonary Disease. 2004. available online at http://www.nice.org.uk/guidance/index.jsp?action=download&o=29303 [accessed 08-03-2008].

1   Joint Royal Colleges Ambulance Liaison Committee. *UK Ambulance Service Clinical Practice Guidelines version 4, Oxygen Update*. April 2009, available online at http://jrcalc.org.uk/newjrcalcguidance/oxygen guideline combined220409.pdf [29-08-2009]

2   O'Sullivan I. Benger J. Nitrous oxide in emergency medicine. *EMJ* 2003;20:214–217.

3   BOC Medical. *Data Sheet: Entonox*. Manchester: BOC Medical Gases, 1995.

4   Gillman MA. Analgesic (sub anaesthetic) nitrous oxide interacts with the endogenous opioid system. *Life Sci* 1986;39:1209–1211.

5   Haugen FP, Melzack R. The effects of nitrous oxide on responses evoked in the brain stem by tooth stimulation. *Anaesthesiology* 1957;18:183–195.

6   BOC Medical. Entonox. 1995 Available online at http://www.bocmedical.co.uk/product_information/entonox.asp [accessed 05-03-2008].

7   Clarke T. Entonox contraindications [Email to P. Gregory] [10 March 2008].

8   Everatt J, Ng WS. Pre-oxygenation using face mask or mouthpiece with and without nose clip: patient preferences and efficacy. *Anaesthesia* 1998;53:387–389.

9   Bateman NT, Leach RM. ABC of oxygen: acute oxygen therapy. *BMJ* 1998;317:798–801.

10 Haddad LM. Acute poisoning. In: Bennett JC, Plum F (Eds) *Cecil Textbook of Medicine*. Philadelphia: WB Saunders, 1996, pp. 509–510.

11 The National Collaborating Centre for Chronic Conditions. Chronic obstructive pulmonary disease; National Clinical Guideline on Management of Chronic Obstructive Pulmonary Disease In Adults in Primary and Secondary Care. 8, Management of Exacerbations of COPD. *Thorax* 2004;59:131–156.

12 British Thoracic Society. Guideline for emergency oxygen use in adult patients. *Thorax* 2008;63(Suppl VI):vi69–vi73 available online at: http://www.brit-thoracic.org.uk/

13 Domingo C. Home oxygen therapy for the 21st century. *Curr Resp Med Rev* 2006;2:237–251.

14 BOC Medical. *Medical Gas Data Sheet: Medical Oxygen*. Manchester: BOC Medical, 2006.

Chapter 12

Infection control

Content

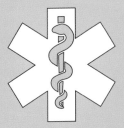

Infection control and aseptic techniques are vital tools in the battle to reduce infection acquired as a direct result of health care provision. Paramedics often work in environments that are unclean and unhygienic, and the risk of infection is unsurprisingly high. It is imperative that the paramedic optimises infection control techniques to minimise the risk of infection.

Definitions

Infection control is the application of standard principles to prevent health-care associated infections (HCAI) and is essential in the reduction of HCAI. Asepsis is described as the state of being free from living pathogenic organisms[1] and aseptic technique as the effort taken to keep a patient as free from micro-organisms as possible.[2] The incidence of HCAI in the United Kingdom is estimated to be 9%;[3] statistics specific to the ambulance service are not readily available.

Aseptic technique is used to minimise the risk of infection when managing wounds, or when carrying out invasive procedures such as intravenous cannulation. Asepsis in the out-of-hospital environment is classed as medical asepsis and aims to reduce the number and spread of organisms during patient contact with the ambulance service; this differs from surgical asepsis, which is undertaken in operating theatres.

The National Institute for Health and Clinical Excellence (NICE) divides the standard principles into three broad categories: [4]

- Hand hygiene
- Use of personal protective equipment (PPE)
- Safe use and disposal of sharps
- Education of patients, their carers, and healthcare personnel.

> ## Scenario
>
> You are called to transport a patient with diarrhoea and vomiting. What extra precautions need to be taken and what cleaning actions should be taken on completion of the case?

Indications for infection control

Patients have a right to clean and safe treatment wherever and whenever they are treated by the National Health Service (NHS).[5] Around 320,000 healthcare-associated infections occur every year (almost 3 million during the decade from 1993). These infections add an average of 11 days of hospitalisation for each person infected and cost the NHS an estimated £1 billion annually. Around a third of these infections could probably have been prevented.[6] The application of evidence-based infection prevention and control into every day practice is believed to be important in reducing preventable infections and could reduce the human and financial costs.[7] Healthcare professionals should routinely apply the principles of infection control to the management of every patient/client.

Hand hygiene

Several studies have demonstrated a clear link between handwashing and a reduction in infection[8-11] and, although these studies are hospital based, it is useful and reasonable to extrapolate the findings and apply them to the community setting. Expert opinion is consistent in asserting that effective handwashing reduces the number of pathogens carried on the hands and that this will logically decrease the incidence of preventable HCAI.[12-14]

Currently there is no compelling evidence to favour the general use of antimicrobial handwashing agents over soap, or one antimicrobial agent over another.[4] The acceptability of any preparation used in the community setting will need to be based upon ease of use and their dermatological effect; in most cases this will be determined by the employing Trust.

The latest recommendations from NICE[4] state that hands that are visibly soiled or potentially grossly contaminated with dirt or organic material must be washed with liquid soap and water. Hands must be decontaminated, preferably with an alcohol-based hand rub unless hands are visibly soiled, between caring for different patients or between different care activities for the same patient.

There is little high level evidence to support any given handwashing technique in terms of duration of washing and hand drying. Current guidelines are based on expert opinion that suggest that the time taken to decontaminate the hands, the exposure of all aspects of the hands and wrists to the decontaminant, the use of vigorous rubbing, thorough rinsing (in the case of handwashing), and drying are all key factors in the process of effective hand hygiene.[12,15]

Recommendations[4]

1. All wrist and hand jewellery should be removed prior to hand-cleansing. Cuts and abrasions must be covered with waterproof dressings. Finger nails should be kept short and free from nail polish.
2. Handwashing techniques involve three phases – preparation, washing and rinsing, and drying:
    a. Wet the hands under running tepid water BEFORE applying cleaning preparations.
    b. Hand wash solution MUST come into contact with ALL of the surfaces of the hand.
    c. The hands must be RUBBED together for between 10 and 15 seconds paying particular attention to the tips of the fingers, the thumbs and the areas between the fingers.
    d. Hands should be rinsed thoroughly before drying.
3. When decontaminating hands using an alcohol hand-rub, hands should be free of dirt and organic material. The hand-rub solution must come into contact with all surfaces of the hand. The hands must be rubbed together vigorously, paying particular attention to the tips of the fingers, the thumbs and the areas between the fingers, until the solution has evaporated and the hands are dry.

Areas that are commonly missed in handwashing are shown in Figure 12.1.

The handwashing technique that remains in vogue within the health service was first described by Ayliffe, Babb and Quoraishi in 1978[16] and is still the procedure recommended by the Ambulance Service Association (Figure 12.2).[17]

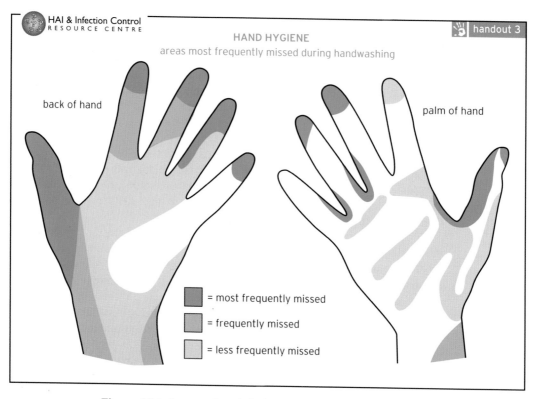

Figure 12.1 Areas missed during handwashing. Based on work by Taylor L (1978) An Evaluation of Handwashing Techniques, *Nursing Times* Jan 12, 1978 pp 54-55. Original material supplied by Health Protection Scotland. Responsibility for the editing and use of these materials lies with the individual and not Health Protection Scotland or Healthcare A2Z. Copyright 2006, original content developed by Healthcare A2Z, www.healthcareA2Z.org. Reproduced with permission.

Personal protective equipment

Most expert opinion regarding the use of personal protective equipment (PPE) has been based on studies in the hospital environment; however, it is safe to extrapolate the general findings and apply them to the community setting. This section discusses gloves, aprons, visors/eye protection, and face masks. The purpose of PPE is to protect both patients and staff, and to reduce the risk of transmission of microorganisms.[18,19] The decision to use PPE and the level of PPE is based upon an assessment of the anticipated risk of transmission of micro-organisms to the patient, and the risk of exposure to body fluid during patient management.

The guidelines in Figure 12.3 may be helpful in determining the level of PPE required.

Gloves

The use of gloves as a primary defence against infection has become common practice for health professionals in the hospital and community settings. There is expert agreement that gloves play a role in protecting the hands from contamination, and

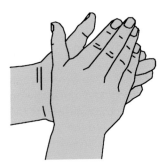

1. Palm to palm

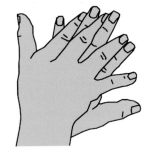

2. Right palm over left dorsum and left palm over right dorsum

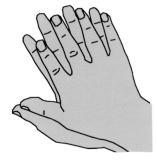

3. Palm to palm finger interlaced

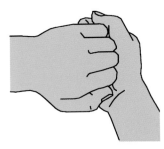

4. Backs of fingers to opposing palms with fingers interlocked

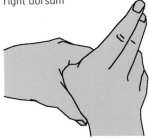

5. Rotational rubbing of right thumb clasped in left palm and vice versa

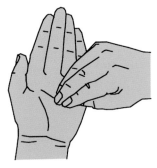

6. Rotational rubbing, backwards and forwards with clasped finger of right hand in left palm and vice versa

Figure 12.2 Hand-washing technique.

No exposure to blood/body fluids anticipated	→	No protective clothing
Exposure to blood/body fluid anticipated but low risk of splashing	→	Wear gloves and plastic apron
Exposure to blood/body fluid anticipated with high risk of splashing	→	Wear gloves, plastic apron and eye/mouth/nose protection

Figure 12.3 Adapted from ASA, 2004.[17]

reducing the risk of transmission of micro-organisms to both patient and practitioner,[20-22] but they should not be worn unnecessarily as prolonged and indiscriminate use may cause skin sensitivity and adverse reactions.[23] The guidance given above should be used to decide when it is appropriate to wear gloves.

Gloves must be discarded after every care activity for which they were worn in order to minimise the potential transmission of microorganisms to another site on the patient, or to a different patient.[4] The practicalities of this may be difficult in the emergency situation but every effort should be made to adhere to the guidelines where possible. Washing gloves rather than changing them is not safe so therefore, not recommended.[23,24]

It is also worth noting that the integrity of gloves cannot be taken for granted and there is evidence that hand contamination may occur when the gloves are removed.[20,23,24] The use of gloves reduces the risk of contamination but does not eliminate it and it cannot be presumed that hands are clean just because gloves have been worn. The practitioner should always wash hands in accordance with standard procedures after gloves have been removed.

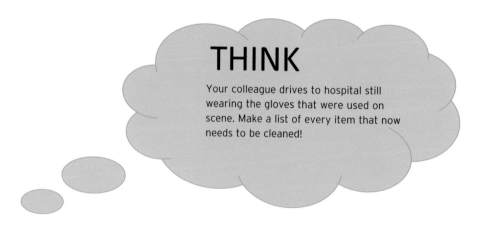

THINK

Your colleague drives to hospital still wearing the gloves that were used on scene. Make a list of every item that now needs to be cleaned!

Recommendations[4]

- Gloves must be worn for:
  - Invasive procedures (e.g. intravenous cannulation).
  - Contact with sterile sites and non-intact skin or mucous membranes.
  - All activities that have been assessed as carrying a risk of exposure to blood, body fluids, secretions or excretions, or sharp or contaminated instruments.
- Gloves must be worn as single-use items. They must be put on immediately before an episode of patient contact or treatment and removed as soon as the activity is completed. Gloves must be changed between caring for different patients, and between different care or treatment activities for the same patient.
- Gloves must be disposed of as clinical waste and hands decontaminated after the gloves have been removed.

Disposable aprons

Several studies show the potential for uniforms to become contaminated.[25-27] None of these studies were undertaken in the community setting but it is reasonable to suggest that the risk of contamination in the out-of-hospital setting is likely to be no lower than the in-hospital setting. Two of these studies[25,26] suggest the need for a clean uniform to be worn each shift, which may not be achievable in the community setting given that jackets and fleeces are frequently worn in cooler weather.

The routine use of aprons is not advocated,[15] but plastic aprons are recommended for use when there is a likelihood of contamination with blood, body fluids, excretions or secretions (excluding sweat), or when close contact with the patient, equipment or materials may lead to contamination of clothing.[23,24] Care should be taken to store disposable aprons away from potential sources of contamination prior to use and should be used once only. Full body gowns need only be worn where there is a risk of extensive splashing of body fluids, blood, secretions and excretions; e.g. serious trauma.[23,24]

Recommendations[4]

- Disposable plastic aprons should be worn when there is a risk that clothing may become exposed to blood, body fluids, excretions or secretions, with the exception of sweat.
- Plastic aprons should be worn for only one procedure or episode of patient care; they should then be disposed of as clinical waste.
- Full-body, fluid-repellent gowns should be worn where there is a risk of extensive splashing of body fluids, blood, secretions or excretions onto the skin or clothing of a healthcare practitioner.

Eye, mouth and nose protection

There is no robust evidence to support the use of surgical face-masks to protect the patient during routine procedures such as wound dressings.[15,23] In situations where protection is required, e.g., HIV-related or multiple drug-resistant tuberculosis, standard surgical masks do not provide effective protection and specialised equipment such as a particulate filter respiratory mask should be worn.[15,23,28]

Recommendations[4]

- Face masks and eye protection must be worn where there is a risk of splashing of body fluids, blood, secretions or excretions into the face and eyes.
- When clinically indicated, respiratory protective equipment must be used.

Environmental cleanliness

Maintaining a clean ambulance and equipment is essential, not only for reducing the risk of exposing patients to healthcare acquired infections, but also because it engenders confidence in the patients being conveyed by the ambulance service. In

2006 the Department of Health introduced the Standards for Better Health,[30] which states the following:

Healthcare organisations keep patients, staff and visitors safe by having systems to ensure that:

- The risk of health care acquired infection to patients is reduced, with particular emphasis on high standards of hygiene and cleanliness, achieving year-on-year reductions in MRSA.
- All risks associated with the acquisition and use of medical devices are minimised.
- All reusable medical devices are properly decontaminated prior to use and that the risks associated with decontamination facilities and processes are well managed.
- Medicines are handled safely and securely.
- The prevention, segregation, handling, transport and disposal of waste is properly managed so as to minimise the risks to the health and safety of staff, patients, the public and the safety of the environment.

Keeping the vehicle clean is everybody's responsibility.

This section does not endeavour to set policies for Ambulance Trusts, as these policies should be developed by managers utilising the National Patient Safety Agency Framework for setting and measuring performance outcomes in ambulance trusts.[29] Written local policies should be available for cleaning, decontamination, disinfection and sterilisation of all equipment and vehicles,[31] and should be followed rigorously by ambulance crews.

Recommendations[31]

- Ambulance interiors should be thoroughly cleaned on a weekly basis.
- All equipment used for patient treatment should be cleaned using detergent wipes or soap and water then either air dried or wiped with clean paper towels after EVERY patient.
- Extra attention must be given to items soiled with blood and/or body fluids; these should be decontaminated with detergent after cleaning.
- Additional cleaning is required following transportation of a patient suffering from diarrhoea as the infection status may be unknown. The vehicle interior, including walls and floors, and all equipment used to treat the patient must first be cleaned with soap and water and then disinfected with a chlorine-based fluid. *Clostridium difficile* is only removed when both soap and water and disinfectant are used in the above order.
- Ambulance stretcher beds should have linen changed after EVERY patient and the stretcher should be wiped down with detergent wipes or soap and water then air-dried or wiped dry with clean paper towels after EVERY patient.
- Where contaminated with blood and/or body fluids, a chlorine-based detergent should be used after it has been cleaned with soap and water or detergent wipes.
- Pillows should have a plastic cover, which should be wiped with a detergent wipe before a clean pillowcase is fitted. Pillowcases must be changed after EVERY patient.

Chapter Key Points

1. Effective handwashing reduces the number of pathogens present on the hands.
2. There is no compelling evidence to favour one handwashing agent over another – in the prehospital environment ease of use may be the over-riding factor.
3. The thumbs and finger tips are the most commonly missed areas during handwashing.
4. There is expert agreement that gloves play a role in protecting the hands from contamination, and reducing the risk of transmission of micro-organisms to both patient and practitioner.
5. The decision to use PPE and the level of PPE is based upon an assessment of the anticipated risk of transmission of micro-organisms to the patient, and the risk of exposure to body fluid during patient management.
6. Vehicle cleaning is the responsibility of everybody, not just of cleaning staff.
7. Written local policies should be available for cleaning, decontamination, disinfection and sterilisation of all equipment and vehicles.

References and Further reading

See Chapter 13 for management of sharps and needlestick injuries, and for swabbing prior to injection or intravenous cannulation.

Perry C. *Infection Prevention and Control*. Oxford: Blackwell, 2007.

Ambulance Service Association. *National Guidance and Procedures for Infection Prevention and Control*. London: Ambulance Service Association, 2004.

National Patient Safety Agency. *The national specifications for cleanliness in the NHS: A framework for setting and measuring performance outcomes in ambulance trusts*. London: NPSA, 2008.

1 Hart S. Using an aseptic technique to reduce the risk of infection. *Nurs Stand* 2007;21(47):43-48.
2 Crow S. Asepsis: an indispensible part of the patient's care plan. *Crit Care Nurse Quest* 1989;11(4):11-15.
3 Department of Health. *Saving Lives: the Delivery Programme to Reduce Healthcare Associated Infections (HCAI) Including MRSA*. London: The Stationery Office, 2005.
4 National Institute for Health and Clinical Excellence (NICE). *Infection control Prevention of healthcare-associated infection in primary and community care*. London: NICE, 2003.
5 Department of Health. *Clean, Safe Care: Reducing Infections and Saving Lives*. London: Department of Health Publications, 2008.
6 Sutcliffe A. Press release: *NICE launches new clinical guideline on prevention of healthcare associated infections in primary and community care*. London: NICE, 2003.
7 Haley RW, Culver DH, White JW, Morgan WM, Grace TG, Munn VP, Hooton TM. The Efficacy of Infection Surveillance and Control Programs in Preventing Nosocomial Infections in US Hospitals. *Am J Epidemiol* 1985;121(2):182-205.
8 Ryan MAK, Christian RS, Wohlrabe J. Handwashing and respiratory illness among young adults in military training. *Am J Prevent Med* 2001;21(2):79-83.

9 Fendler EJ, Ali Y, Hammond BS, Lyons MK, Kelley MB, Vowell NA. The impact of alcohol hand sanitizer use on infection rates in an extended care facility. *Am J Infect Control* 2002;30(4):226-233.

10 Gould D, Gammon J, Donnelly M, Batiste L, Ball E, De Melo AMSC *et al.* Improving hand hygiene in community healthcare settings: the impact of research and clinical collaboration. *J Clin Nurs* 2000;9(1):95-102.

11 Pittet D, Dharan S, Touveneau S, Sauvan V, Perneger T. Bacterial contamination of the hands of hospital staff during routine patient care. *Arch Intern Med* 1999;159(8):821-826.

12 Boyce JM, Pittet D. *Guideline for Hand Hygiene in Healthcare Settings: Recommendations of the Healthcare Infection Control Practice Advisory Committee and the HICPAC/SHEA/ APIC/IDSA Hygiene Task Force*, 2002, 58 pp.

13 Canada Communicable Disease Report Supplement. *Infection Control Guidelines: Hand washing, cleaning, disinfection and sterilization in health care. December* 1998;24(S8).

14 Infection Control Nurses Association. *Guidelines for Hand Hygiene*, 2002.

15 Pratt RJ, Pellowe C, Loveday HP, Robinson N, Smith GW, and the guideline development team. The epic project: Developing national evidence based guidelines for preventing healthcare-associated infections. Phase 1: Guidelines for preventing hospital-acquired infections. *J Hosp Infect* 2001;47(Supplement):S1-S82.

16 Ayliffe GA, Babb JR, Quoraishi AH. A test for 'hygienic' hand disinfection. *J Clin Pathol* 1978;31:923-928.

17 Ambulance Service Association. *National Guidance and Procedures for Infection Prevention and Control*. London: Ambulance Service Association, 2004.

18 Garner JS. The Hospital Infection Control Practices Advisory Committee: Guidelines for Isolation Precautions in Hospitals. *Infect Control Hosp Epidemiol* 1996;17(1):53-80.

19 Wilson J. *Infection Control in Clinical Practice*. London: Baillière Tindall, 1995:161-162.

20 Expert Advisory Group on AIDS and the Advisory Group on Hepatitis. *Guidance for Clinical Health Care Workers: Protection Against Infection with Blood-Borne Viruses*. London: Department of Health, 1998, 46 pp.

21 Centers for Disease Control Update. Recommendations for prevention of HIV transmission in health care settings. *Morb Mort Week Rep* 1987;37:24.

22 Garner JS. The Hospital Infection Control Practices Advisory Committee: Guidelines for Isolation Precautions in *Hospitals. Infect Cont Hosp Epidemiol* 1996;17(1): 53-80.

23 Pratt RJ, Pellowe C, Loveday HP, Robinson N, Smith GW, and the guideline development team. The epic project: Developing national evidence based guidelines for preventing healthcare-associated infections. Phase 1: Guidelines for preventing hospital-acquired infections. *J Hosp Infect* 2001;47(Supplement):S1-S82.

24 Clark L, Smith W, Young L. Protective Clothing; *Principles and Guidance*. London: ICNA, 2002.

25 Callaghan I. Bacterial contamination of nurses' uniforms: a study. *Nurs Stand* 2002;13(1):37-42.

26 Perry C, Marshall R, Jones E. Bacterial contamination of uniforms. *J Hosp Infect* 2001;48:238-241.

27 Huntley DE, Campbell J. Bacterial contamination of scrub jackets during dental hygiene procedures. *J Dent Hyg* 1998;72(3):19-23.

28 Health and Safety Commission. *Control of Substances Hazardous to Health Regulations 1999. Approved Codes of Practice*. London: HSE Books, 1999.

29 National Patient Safety Agency. *The National Specifications for Cleanliness in The NHS: A Framework for Setting and Measuring Performance Outcomes in Ambulance Trusts*. London: NPSA.

30 Department of Health. Standards for Better Health. London: Department of Health, 2006.

31 Department of Health. *Ambulance Guidelines: Reducing Infection Through Effective Practice in the Pre-Hospital Environment*. London: Department of Health, 2008.

Chapter 13

Vascular access devices

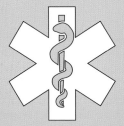

Vascular access and injections are tasks that are carried out quite commonly by ambulance paramedics. Intravenous cannulation is perhaps the most frequently used route of vascular access with the intraosseous route normally reserved for young children. The development of new devices may lead to an increase in the use of the intraosseous route in the emergency management of adults where intravenous access is unattainable.

The skills are fundamental for the administration of many drugs and fluids but have inherent risks attached to them; the paramedic should be aware of the options available and select the most appropriate for the circumstances.

Definition of a vascular access device

For the purposes of prehospital care, a vascular access device is a device that is inserted into a peripheral or central vein (intravenous), or into the marrow cavity of selected bones (intraosseous). The devices may be used to administer drugs or fluids, or as a prophylactic measure. They may be used for sampling blood for diagnostic tests although this is not currently within the remit of UK paramedics.

There is a variety of vascular access devices available and each has its own requirements; however, there are certain principles that are applicable to all devices.

Anatomy of veins

The superficial veins of the upper limbs are normally selected for siting a peripheral cannula in prehospital care. Use of the lower limbs may be indicated in very small children and where injury prevents the use of the upper limbs but cannulation of the lower limbs is associated with an increased risk of venous thromboembolism.[1]

Veins consist of three layers:[2]

- Tunica adventitia - the outer layer of fibrous connective tissue.
- Tunica media - the middle layer comprising of smooth muscle and elastic fibres.
- Tunica intima - the thin inner layer of endothelium.

The skin consists of two layers:[2]

- Epidermis - the superficial thinner layer of the skin composed of keratinised stratified squamous epithelium.
- Dermis - a layer of dense, irregular connective tissue lying deep to the epidermis. Blood vessels, nerves, glands and hair follicles are embedded in dermal tissue.

The structure and appearance of the skin alters with age as the dermal layers become thinner and elasticity is lost. The number of cells producing collagen and elastic fibres decrease leading to the development of wrinkles. The veins of older people may be easier to see as a result of these changes but they are more mobile, more fragile, and often tortuous and thrombosed.[3] It is perhaps best to avoid the dorsum of the hand in older people due to their fragile nature.[5]

Peripheral cannulas

There are two commonly used peripheral cannulas; a peripheral cannula, and a hollow-needle infusion device, often called a 'butterfly' (see Figures 13.1 and 13.2). The peripheral cannula is usually a catheter-over-needle design; the needle is withdrawn after the venepuncture whilst the flexible plastic catheter remains in the vascular compartment. The needle of the butterfly remains in the vein thereby causing increased risk of damage to the vein.[4]

Peripheral cannulas are available to paramedics in various sizes ranging from 22 gauge (smallest) through to 14 gauge (largest). Each device is colour-coded and information regarding flow rates and catheter diameters can be found on the device packaging. Modern catheters tend to be made from polyurethane, which is more flexible, less traumatic and less irritating on the intimal layer of the vein than earlier polyvinyl chloride (PVC) models.[5,6]

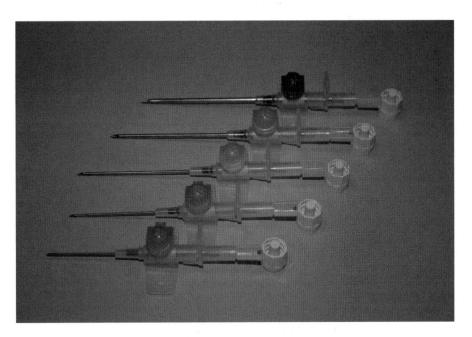

Figure 13.1 Intravenous cannulas.

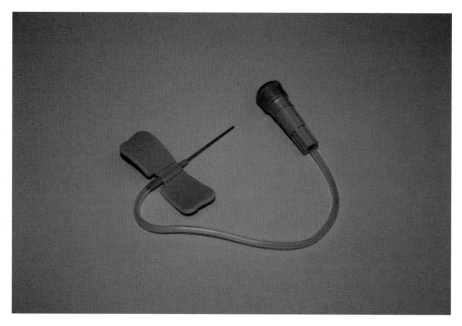

Figure 13.2 Butterfly cannula.

Indications for peripheral cannulation

Peripheral cannulas are indicated for:

- Drug therapy
- Fluid therapy
- Prophylaxis.

There are potential complications associated with intravenous cannulation so care should be taken to perform cannulation only on patients who are likely to benefit from the procedure. The risks associated with prophylactic cannulation probably outweigh the benefits so cannulation for this purpose is to be discouraged.

Selection of device for peripheral cannulation

The choice of cannula will be dependent upon several factors:

- **Purpose of cannulation.** A larger bore cannula will be required for rapid infusion of fluids whilst a smaller gauge will be adequate for drugs or for prophylactic purposes.
- **Size of veins.** Smaller veins will only tolerate a small cannula so irrespective of the purpose of cannulation, a small cannula may be required.
- **Shocked patients.** Shock leads to peripheral shutdown and may restrict the size of cannula that can be inserted.
- **Practitioner skill and confidence.** A newly qualified practitioner may be less confident at placing a large bore cannula so may take a pragmatic view that something is better than nothing.

Selection of vein

An advantage of peripheral venous cannulation is that the veins are normally visible; however, there may be occasions where this is not the case so palpation and familiarity with venous topography are useful. Figures 13.3 and 13.4 illustrate venous anatomy in the hand and forearm.

The vein should be selected before the device so that only an appropriate device is selected. The vein should be straight, free of valves and should feel 'bouncy' when palpated. It is best to avoid joints as there is increased risk of mechanical phlebitis and intermittent flow of fluids or drugs created by the patient's movements.

Vein selection will be dependent upon a number of factors including the reason for the cannulation, accessibility of the veins, injuries to the patient, and previous cannulation attempts. The initial attempt should be undertaken at the distal end of the limb as an unsuccessful attempt hinders the use of veins distal to the original site. A cannula should not be placed in areas of localised oedema, dermatitis, cellulitis, arteriovenous fistulae, wounds, skin grafts, fractures, stroke, planned limb surgery and previous cannulation.[5] It may also be beneficial to patient independence if the cannula is placed in the non-dominant limb.

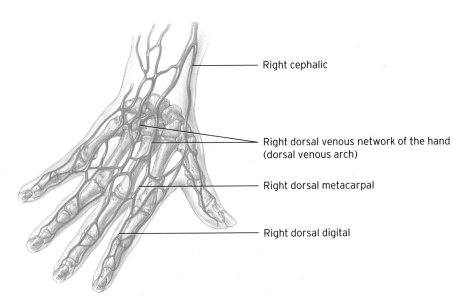

Right cephalic

Right dorsal venous network of the hand (dorsal venous arch)

Right dorsal metacarpal

Right dorsal digital

Posterior view of superficial veins of the hand

Figure 13.3 Veins of the hand. Reprinted from Jenkins, Kemnitz and Totora, *Anatomy and Physiology; From Science to Life*, copyright 2006, with permission of John Wiley & Sons Inc.

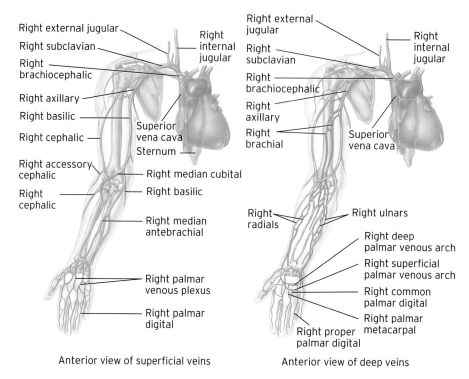

Figure 13.4 Veins of arm. Reprinted from Jenkins, Kemnitz and Totora, *Anatomy and Physiology; From Science to Life*, copyright 2006, with permission of John Wiley & Sons Inc.

Techniques of venodilatation

Tourniquet and Gravity

Apply venous tourniquet to limb and tightened to between the patient's systolic and diastolic pressures. If veins are not readily apparent or appear small in calibre, place the limb below the level of the heart.[8] Gravity serves to slow venous return, leading to increased venous volume and distention of veins of the upper extremity.[11]

Fist clenching

Opening and closing of the fist augments venous return by virtue of muscular compressive forces exerted on vessels to enhance arterial blood flow,[7] which results in local venous distention.[8] Increased blood velocity from fist clenching also increases venous flow to the basilic and cephalic veins.[9] Research has shown that this form of isometric activity also results in vasodilatation.[10]

Vein 'tap' and 'milking'

Tapping a superficial vein once or twice augments vein distention[11] although the mechanism by which this occurs is unclear.[8] Applying a mild, sliding pressure ('milking') along a short length of vein, from proximal to distal, displaces blood distally resulting in vein distention.[8] Care must be taken not to apply overly vigorous stimuli, especially to those with fragile superficial veins (e.g., elderly, those chronically on steroids) so as not to injure the veins or to result in pain related reflex vasoconstriction.[8] 'Slapping' the vein is painful and causes the release of histamine – this technique should not be used.

Local warmth

Blood flow in human skin increases greatly in response to direct heating [12] although care has to be taken not to induce thermal damage to the extremity. Applying local warmth in the prehospital environment may be difficult but consideration may be made to immersing the upper extremity in warm water for a few minutes, or applying a warm, moist compress.[13]

Dilatation of the external jugular vein (EJV)

The Valsalva manoeuvre (forced expiration through a closed glottis) for 30 sec (at a pressure of 40 mmHg) has been shown to result in an 86% increase in the area and 41% increase in the circumference of the right EJV.[14] Similarly, use of the Trendelenburg position augments venous return towards the right atrium and can result in EJV distention.[15,16]

Complications of peripheral venous cannulation

No clinical intervention is risk free but the benefits of appropriate intravenous cannulation are normally considered to outweigh the complications. One of the key concerns in prehospital care is the time delay for undertaking the task. Studies suggest that intravenous cannulation with no therapeutic treatment can increase on-scene times by an average of between 8 and 13 minutes,[17,18] this needs to be considered when making the clinical decision to cannulate as should the number of attempts that should be made.

Intravenous cannulation provides a direct portal of entry for infectious pathogens and is a considerable source of morbidity and mortality in hospital.[19,20] The incidence of infection secondary to intravenous cannulation by paramedics is not known but the nature of the work and the practice environment mean that it could be even higher. An increased risk of infection during emergency insertion has been noted as strict adherence to aseptic techniques may be less rigorous.[21] Places, people and equipment can all serve as reservoirs for infection.[22] For this reason infection prevention and control should consider not only patients, but also staff and bystanders as well as the environment and any equipment in use.[23] Whilst the paramedic may have limited control over the environment, they can minimise the risk of infection from equipment by ensuring that any packaging is intact and in date. When opening packaging, aseptic techniques should be employed. Compliance with hand hygiene and personal protective equipment policies is imperative in order to minimise the risks of contamination through this portal and, although there is debate regarding the efficacy of skin cleansing prior to insertion, current recommendations advocate the use of 2% chlorhexidine gluconate in 70% isopropyl alcohol, which should be allowed to dry.[24]

The incidence of vascular complications increases as the ratio of the external diameter of the cannula to vessel lumen increases;[25] therefore the smallest cannula for the prescribed therapy should be used.[5,26,27] Phlebitis related to intravenous cannulation has three underlying factors; mechanical (caused by friction and movement of the device within the vein), chemical (relating to infusates), and physical (related to the properties of the cannula).[28]

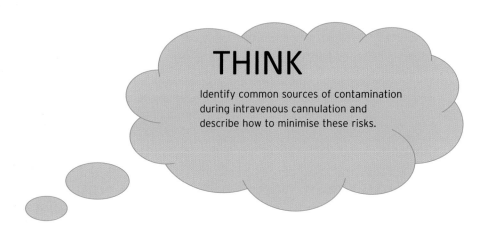

THINK

Identify common sources of contamination during intravenous cannulation and describe how to minimise these risks.

Other potential complications and their solutions are presented in Table 13.1.

Management in situ

Once sited, the peripheral cannula should be flushed with 0.9% sodium chloride or a heparin solution. The exact volume of fluid required to maintain patency is unclear but between 2 and 5 mL is adequate providing correct technique is used; i.e. a pulsatile flush ending with positive pressure.[25]

Once the cannula is in situ it should be taped into place for security. Non-sterile tape should not cover the site; it should be treated as an open wound. Specific cannula dressings are supplied and should be used as they are sterile and allow vision of the site during fluid/medication administration.

Table 13.1 Insertion and devices: complications and solutions

Risks with insertion of devices	Impact	Management
Failed technique	Delay in treatment and unable to use vein	Review technique, vein and equipment selection. Attempt again only if necessary and chances of success are high
Poor technique	Pain, nerve hit, overshot vein, bruising, increased risk of infection, patient anxiety, failed attempt	Refer to more experienced colleague; work to improve technique under supervision
Patient anxiety	Vein may be constricted, muscles may be tense so risk of pain	Reassure patient, select smallest suitable device, consider local anaesthetic, consider necessity of procedure in prehospital environment
Incorrect device	Device performs poorly, flow rate inadequate or fluid overload, causes mechanical phlebitis	Remove device and perform full assessment
Sharps disposal	Needlestick injury for staff or patient	Wash wound in running water and follow local policy
Plastic/air embolus	Risk of pulmonary embolism	Remove device and treat any symptoms, report on arrival at hospital and document incident
Patient compliance	Device removed or tampered with	Assess patient, ensure appropriate site selection and secure device
Haematoma	Bruising, pain, reduced access to vein	Remove device and apply pressure
Occluded cannula	Fails to allow fluid or medication delivery	Remove device and re-site

Adapted from Lavery and Smith 2007.[6]

Procedure for peripheral intravenous cannulation

Equipment required

- Gloves
- Selection of peripheral venous cannulas (select smallest for the intended purpose)
- Venous tourniquet
- 2% chlorhexidine gluconate in 70% isopropyl alcohol
- Sterile occlusive transparent semi-permeable membrane (e.g. Vecafix, Niko-Gard)
- Intravenous administration set or 0.9% sodium chloride flush
- Sharps box.

Procedure (Figures 13.5–13.13)	Additional information/rationale
Preparation	
1. Explain the procedure and gain consent.	Legal requirement.
2. Select site for cannula placement.	Straight, wide veins; 'bouncy' on palpation; avoid joints and valves.
3. Prepare equipment.	Check date and integrity of package. Check all component parts are present.
Technique	
1. Use a non-touch insertion technique[29]	Minimises risk of infection.
2. Apply tourniquet.	To engorge veins the tourniquet should be tightened to between the patient's systolic and diastolic pressures.
3. Perform hand hygiene and, wearing gloves, disinfect the selected venepuncture site, allowing at least 30 seconds for the site to dry.[27]	Minimises the risk of infection.
4. Inspect the chosen cannula to ensure product integrity. To avoid contamination do not touch the cannula shaft.	Ensure the package is intact and the expiry date has not been exceeded.
5. Hold the cannula in line with the vein at a 10–30° angle to the skin and insert the cannula through the skin.	
6. As the cannula enters the vein, blood will be seen in the flashback chamber.	Return of blood into the cannula is required to confirm correct placement of cannula in the vein.[30]
7. Lower the angle of the cannula slightly to ensure it enters the lumen of the vein and does not puncture the posterior wall of the vessel; advance the needle a little further.	The needle sits ahead of the catheter so the cannula may need to be advanced a little further to ensure that the catheter is in the vein.
8. Withdraw the stylet slightly and blood should be seen to enter the cannula. Slowly advance the cannula into the vein, ensuring that the vein remains anchored throughout the procedure. NB: The stylet must not be re-inserted as this can damage the cannula, resulting in plastic embolus.	Confirms the position in the vein.

Procedure (Figures 13.5–13.13)	Additional information/rationale
9. Release the tourniquet	Allows free flow of fluids/drugs and relieves pressure from patient's arm. Prevents flow of blood out of the distal end of the cannula as the needle is removed.
10. Place pressure distal to the end of the catheter and remove needle; immediately place needle into sharps bin then replace bung onto the end of the cannula or connect giving set.	Drop sharps into container; do not push. Colleagues should NOT hold the sharps container so as to avoid risk of accidental needlestick injury.
11. Connect cannula to pre-prepared infusion giving set or flush with 0.9% sodium chloride (or heparin solution).	Confirms patency and ensures easy administration without pain, resistance or localised swelling.
12. Apply a sterile dressing.	
13. Secure administration set tubing if an infusion is started.	
14. Remove gloves and perform hand hygiene.	

Post-procedure

1. Note the date and time of insertion on the case report form. Some cannula dressings may also have facility for documenting this information.	It is recommended that cannulas inserted in emergency conditions are replaced within 24 hours of insertion[21,32]
2. Document the number of attempts and any other complications.	Allows hospital staff to monitor any untoward occurrences.
3. Splints should only be used when the cannula is placed in an area of flexion or is at risk of dislodgment.[31]	If a splint is used, removal to allow assessment of the circulatory status of the limb is required at established intervals.[31]

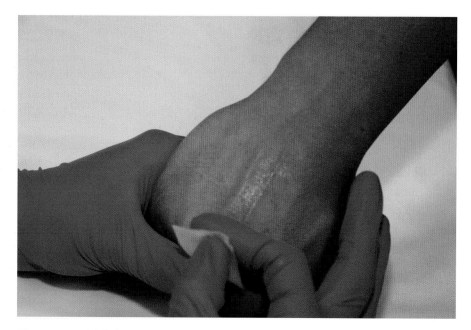

Figure 13.5 Disinfect chosen site.

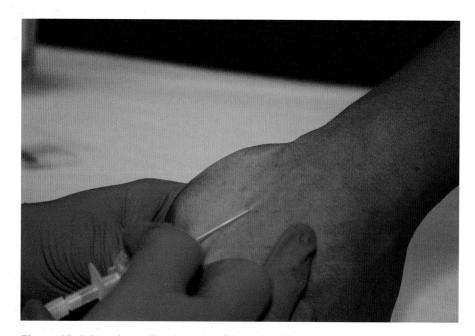

Figure 13.6 Insert needle at angle of between 10 and 30 degrees.

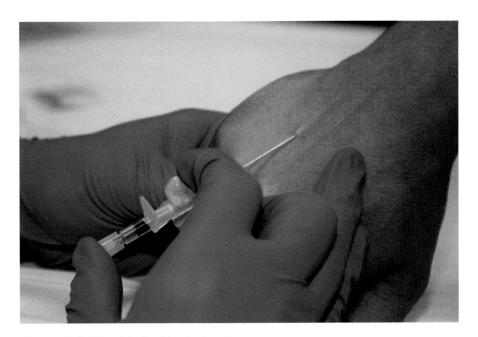

Figure 13.7 Blood in flashback chamber.

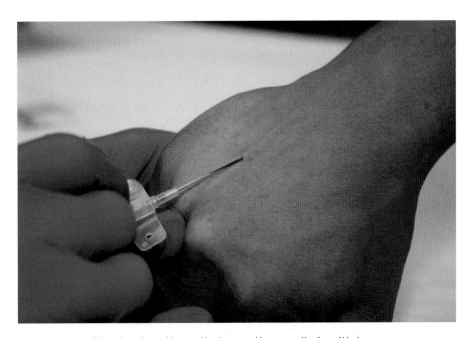

Figure 13.8 Blood enters the catheter as the needle is withdrawn.

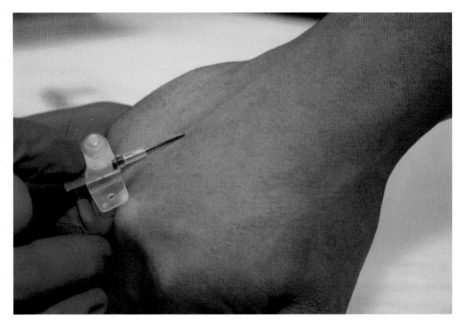

Figure 13.9 Advance cannula whilst anchoring the vein.

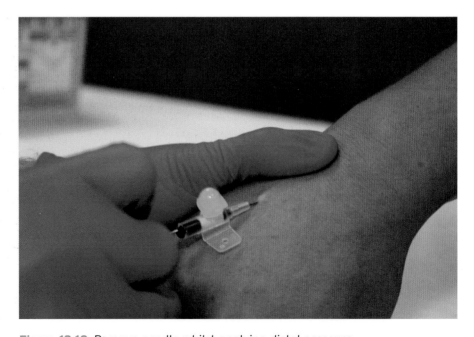

Figure 13.10 Remove needle whilst applying distal pressure

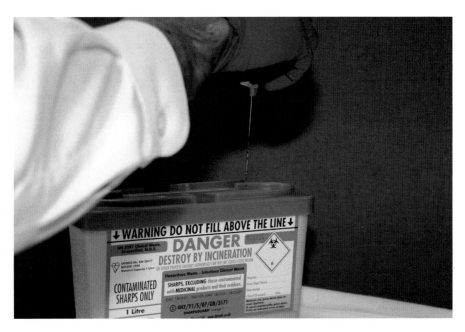

Figure 13.11 Safe disposal of sharps.

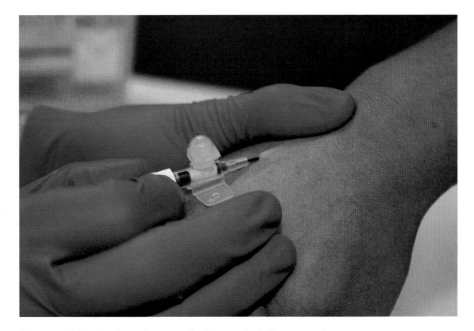

Figure 13.12 Replace bung onto the end of the cannula.

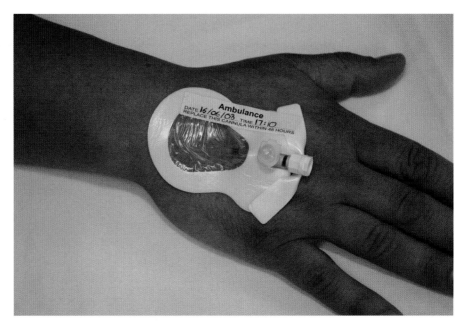

Figure 13.13 Secure cannula and document time.

Hollow needle device (butterfly)

These devices are suited for use on children or other patients with small, delicate veins. They do not have a polyurethane catheter; rather, the metal stylet is inserted into the vein and secured there. There is a risk of damage to the vein with the metal needle so care is needed when inserting and securing the device. A similar technique to standard peripheral cannulation is used except that there will be no flashback of blood and the needle remains in situ.

External jugular cannulation

The external jugular vein (EJV) crosses the sternomastoid muscle and then traverses the posterior triangle of the neck superficially. It is easily distended by a simple Valsalva manoeuvre. The EJV is superficial when it crosses the posterior triangle so it is safe for venepuncture. No important structures lie so superficially in the neck and therefore inadvertent muscle, arterial or nerve injury is avoided.[33]

The close proximity of the external jugular vein to the central venous system offers many of the benefits conferred by central venous cannulation; fluids and medications rapidly reach the core of the body from the EJV. Access to the EJV should only be considered where other means of peripheral access have been exhausted, so it will most likely be reserved for the cardiac arrest situation.

Cannulation of the EJV requires largely the same equipment as for cannulation at other peripheral sites although a 10 mL syringe is also required to aspirate blood to help confirm entry; a venous tourniquet is not required.

Complications

There are several complications in addition to those of other sites of peripheral intravenous cannulation:

- Puncture of the airway
- Damage to nearby arterial vessels
- The technique should not be used in suspected cervical spine injury
- Only one attempt may be used in prehospital care.

Procedure for external jugular cannulation

Procedure	Additional information/rationale
Preparation	
1. Explain the procedure and gain consent (where applicable).	
2. Prepare equipment.	Check date and integrity of package. Check all component parts are present. Draw 3-5 mL of saline into the 10 mL syringe and connect the syringe to the flashback chamber of a large-bore catheter over needle cannula.
3. Position the patient supine with feet elevated or use Trendelenburg position.	Increases blood flow to the chest and neck and decreases the chance of air entering the circulatory system during cannulation.[34]
4. Turn the patient's head in the direction away from the site to be cannulated.	Helps to expose the vein to be cannulated.
Technique	
1. Perform hand hygiene and, wearing gloves, disinfect the selected venepuncture site, allowing at least 30 seconds for the site to dry.[27] Start swabbing at the site of intended puncture and work outward 2.5-5 cm in increasing circles.	Minimises the risk of infection.
2. Engorge vein: Occlude venous return by placing a finger on the EJV just above the clavicle; this also anchors the vein.	Engorges vein prior to cannulation. *Never apply a tourniquet around the patient's neck.*

Procedure	Additional information/rationale
3. Point the cannula at the medial third of the clavicle and insert it at an angle of between 10° and 30°. The bevel of the needle should be up.	
4. As the cannula enters the vein, gently ease back on the plunger; if blood enters the syringe, proceed with insertion. Advance the entire cannula a further 0.5 cm so that the catheter has entered the vein; slide the catheter into the vein and remove the needle as previously described.	Return of blood into the syringe is required to confirm correct placement of cannula in the vein.[35]
5. Dispose of needle safely.	Drop sharps into container do not push. Colleagues should NOT hold the sharps container so as to avoid risk of accidental needlestick injury.
6. Connect cannula to pre-prepared infusion giving set and allow to run free for several seconds.	Ensures correct insertion.
7. Once position confirmed, set flow to appropriate rate.	
8. Apply a sterile dressing.	
9. Secure administration set tubing if an infusion is started.	
10. Remove gloves and perform hand hygiene.	

Post-procedure

1. Note the date and time of insertion on the case report form.	It is recommended that cannulas inserted in emergency conditions are replaced within 24 hours of insertion.[21,36]
2. Document the number of attempts and any other complications on case report form. Some cannula dressings may also have facility for documenting this information.	Legal requirement and allows hospital staff to monitor any untoward occurrences.

Intraosseous infusion

Intraosseous infusion (IOI) is an excellent alternative route for providing vascular access to administer fluids, blood products, and medications where alternative methods are not available or attempts have failed. IOI is particularly useful in children and studies have demonstrated that the use of IOI can decrease the time needed to obtain vascular access in paediatric patients in cardiac arrest.[37,38]

In addition, the rate of vascular access in paediatric cardiac arrest patients is higher for IOI (83%) than for all other forms of IV access,[39] and a recent study suggests that the IO route provides vascular access and fluid more quickly under HazMat conditions.[40] IO has been widely used in the United States for a number of years[41] and there is evidence that IO devices can be easily placed compared with intravenous access by combat medics.[42]

Anatomy of bones

Bone is made up of a dense outer layer surrounding a spongy inner layer that forms a meshwork occupied by bone marrow, blood vessels, nerves, and fat tissue.[43] Bone marrow consists of developing blood cells and a network of fibres that support the vascular complex in the medulla. The purposes of the medullary complex include production of red blood cells and provision of a blood supply to the bone itself. The medullary cavity of long bones provides a 'non-collapsible vein' for intraosseous access.

Indications for intraosseous access

The basic indication for IOI is the need for emergent vascular access when conventional methods have failed.[44] The Resuscitation Council state that the IO route should be considered for both adults and children where intravenous access is difficult or impossible.[45] IOI has also been recommended for conditions such as cardiopulmonary arrest, profound shock, status epilepticus, overwhelming sepsis, and major burns.[46,47]

THINK

You are about to administer an IOI to a young child – consider how you will gain consent from the parents and how you will reassure them during the procedure

Contraindications to intraosseous access

The only universally accepted absolute contraindication to IOI is a fracture of the bone near the access site.[48] Relative contraindications to IOI include cellulitis over the insertion site and inferior vena caval injury.[48]

Equipment for intraosseous access

Several devices are now available for use although most ambulance Trusts in the UK retain the traditional 'Cook' style device. The EZ-IO (a drill device), the Bone Injection Gun (BIG) (an automatic intraosseous device) and the FAST IO introducer are available and have met with varying reviews. The new devices will be discussed along with the traditional device in order to cover all of those used in UK practice.

Complications of intraosseous access

Very few complications have been reported in association with IO access.[49] In more than 4200 cases of IO access in children, osteomyelitis occurred in only 0.6%, and usually only if the infusion continued for a prolonged period or if the patient had bacteraemia at the time of insertion.[50] In a prospective, 250-patient, multi-centre study of the powered drill device, no observed cases of osteomyelitis, fat embolism, fracture, infection, extravasation, or compartment syndrome were found.[51]

Pain during insertion and infusion under pressure are likely to be of concern. One study showed average pain ratings of 5 on a 1-10 severity scale during IO infusion in conscious patients.[51] A separate study using the drill device in 125 conscious patients, recorded an average pain score of 1.2 on a five-point scale, 1 being lowest and 5 being greatest.[52] The use of 1% lidocaine injected into the marrow space over 60 seconds has been shown to be effective in reducing pain during infusion.[53]

Location sites for intraosseous access

The conventional site for IOI is the proximal tibia.[54] The tibial tuberosity can be located by palpation just below the patella. The usual insertion site is the relatively flat area 2 cm distal and 2 cm medial to the tibial tuberosity. Although this site is usually distal to the growth plate, it is still recommended that the needle be angled 10-15 degrees caudally to avoid injury to the growth plate.[44]

There are several alternative sites including the distal tibia in children. To avoid the saphenous vein, the distal tibia may be entered 1-2 cm superior to the medial malleolus. It is recommended that the needle be angled (10-15 degrees) away from the growth plate (i.e., cephalad in this instance).[44]

The sternum carries a number of problems: it may interfere with chest compressions and carries a risk of mediastinal injury, pneumothorax, great vessel injury, and death.[55] However, new devices such as the FAST have improved the safety of sternal access, and may now provide an option for prehospital providers.

Procedures for intraosseous access

Traditional IO device

Procedure	Additional information/rationale
1. Explain the procedure and gain consent of patient or relative.	Legal requirement.
2. Restrain the patient's leg and place padding under the knee.	Brings leg into best position for insertion and prevents accidental misplacement if patient moves during insertion.
3. Identify the chosen site – usually the tibia. The landmark on the tibia for all age groups can be found by: • Identifying the tibial tuberosity. • Find a point 2 cm inferior to the tibial tuberosity and then 2 cm medial to that point.	
4. Clean the skin.	There is no set method for doing this but the risk of infection and the problems associated with managing bone infections suggest that a rigorous technique be used.
5. If approved for use, administer local anaesthetic to the conscious patient (1% lidocaine injected subcutaneously and over the periosteum).	Reduces pain during procedure.
6. Insert IO needle through the skin and subcutaneous tissues until bone is felt. Using a twisting motion, insert the trocar into the bone until a loss of resistance or 'pop' is felt, do not insert any further.	Indicates entry into the marrow.
7. Remove the trocar from the needle dispose of safely.	Health and safety of sharps.
8. Attach a saline filled syringe; pull back on the plunger to attempt aspiration into the syringe.	Confirms correct placement.
9. If marrow is not aspirated, push a 5 to 10 mL bolus of isotonic sodium chloride solution through the syringe.	Correct medullary placement can be confirmed when bone marrow and blood can be easily aspirated.

Procedure	Additional information/rationale
10. If flow is good and extravasation is not evident, connect an intravenous line with a 3-way stopcock, and secure the needle with gauze pads and tape.	Resistance to flow should be minimal, and extravasation should not be evident. Observing the calf area for acute swelling or discoloration is important.
11. Fluids may infuse by gravity but the unpredictability of bone marrow blood flow by this method alone has been demonstrated [56] so it is usually necessary to use pressure to augment flow in IOI.	Flow rates can be dramatically increased by the use of pressure bags and infusion pumps. Flow rates of 10 mL/min by gravity can be increased to 41 mL/min by using pressurized bags.[58] An alternative method for rapid infusion is to manually infuse 30–60 mL boluses via a stopcock.
12. Only one IO attempt should be made in each bone. However, if the needle becomes plugged with soft tissue, it may be removed, and a new needle may be inserted through the same cannulation site.[57]	Multiple punctures in the periosteum may result in extravasation of fluid into the soft tissues.
13. Complete documentation.	

Virtually all drugs that can be administered via the IV route can be administered by IOI.[59] There is no need to adjust drug dosages when using the IO route because it has been demonstrated that different IOI sites (humerus, femur, malleolar, and tibia) are pharmacokinetically equivalent with regard to transit times and serum concentrations.[60]

EZ-IO

The EZ-IO® Intraosseous Infusion system is a system that allows for immediate vascular access in all patients larger than 3 kg. It comprises of a power driver that provides a minimum of 1000 insertions and has a shelf life of up to 10 years, and needle sets of varying sizes to match the needs of the patient. There is little research available at the moment, but the small scale studies that have been completed suggest that it is a useful tool. One study has shown that vascular access using the EZ-IO is achieved significantly more frequently at first attempt than a manual IO system (Cook),[61] whilst there has also been successful use by the military.[62] However, pain has been observed in conscious patients and in one study, insertion of the EZ-IO proved to be more painful than the original injury.[63] A small study investigated the use of the EZ-IO for humeral and tibial insertion and found that both sites had high-insertion success rates and there was no significant difference in tibial or humeral flow rates.[63] This may open up an alternative site for when tibial insertion is not an option.

Procedure EZ-IO[64]

See Figure 13.14.

- Follow first 5 steps above.
- Prepare infusion system.
- Ensure that the driver and needle set are securely seated.
- Remove and discard the needle set safety cap from the IO needle set installed on the EZ-IO power driver.
- Position driver at insertion site with needle set at a 90-degree angle to the bone. Gently power or press needle set until needle set tip touches bone.
- Ensure at least 5 mm of the catheter is visible.
- Penetrate bone cortex by squeezing the driver's trigger and applying gentle, steady downward pressure.
- Release driver's trigger and stop insertion process when:
  - A sudden 'give' or 'pop' is felt upon entry into the medullary space.
  - A desired depth is obtained.
- Remove power driver and stylet.
- Confirm catheter stability.
- Attach primed EZ-Connect® extension set to catheter hub's Luer lock and confirm position; proceed as before.

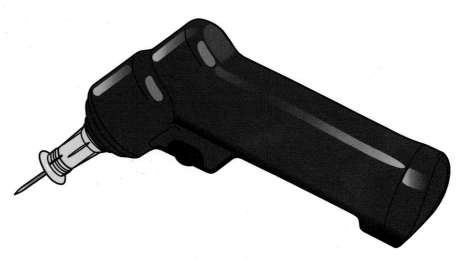

Figure 13.14 EZ-IO. Reproduced with permission of Vidacare (UK) Ltd.

FAST

The FAST™ is a sternal intraosseous infusion device that delivers life-saving drugs and fluids to the heart in under a minute. It is specifically designed for safe and effective use of IO under emergency conditions and features speedy access, a protected infusion site, and a depth-control mechanism. The tool allows IO infusion to be used as a standard protocol in adults. The FAST is only designed to be used in patients aged 12 years or older and is intended to be inserted only in the midline of the manubrium 1.5 cm inferior to the suprasternal notch. A second generation device, the 'FAST X', is being developed but was not available at time of writing; the information given here relates specifically to the FAST 1 (Figure 13.15).

Studies suggest that the FAST has considerable potential in prehospital care[65-67] although more work is probably required.

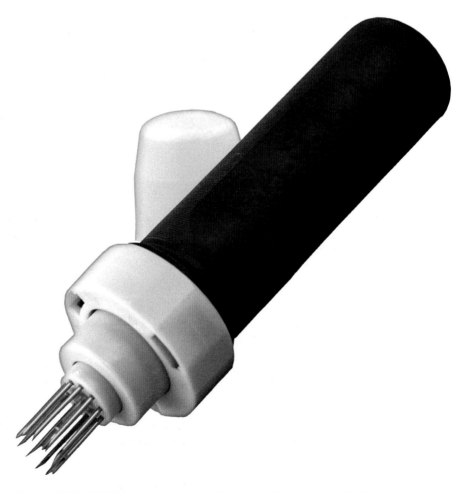

Figure 13.15 FAST 1. Reproduced with permission of Pyng Medical Corporation.

Procedure for FAST

Procedure	Additional information/rationale
1. Explain the procedure and gain consent of patient or relative.	Legal requirement.
2. Expose the sternum and clean the infusion site. Clean the skin.	There is no set method for cleaning the site but the risk of infection and the problems associated with managing bone infections suggest that a rigorous technique be used.
3. Remove top half of patch backing (labelled 'Remove 1'). Locate sternal notch with index finger held perpendicular to manubrium.	This point is needed to correctly place the 'target zone' of the patch.
4. Using index finger, align notch in patch with the patient's sternal notch ensuring that the target zone (circular hole in Patch) is over the patient's midline.	Ensures that the correct point on the manubrium will be entered by the device.
5. Remove the bottom half of the Patch backing (labelled 'Remove 2') and press Patch firmly to secure it to the patient.	
6. Verify that the target zone is over the patient's midline; adjust the Patch if the error is greater than about 1cm.	Errors of greater than 1cm may cause misplacement of the device and may cause injury.
7. Remove the sharps cap from the introducer.	
8. Place bone probe cluster (series of needles) in the target zone ensuring that the introducer axis is perpendicular (90°) to the skin at the insertion site. Ensure that the entire bone probe cluster is within the target zone.	The introducer must remain perpendicular in order that the insertion tube is correctly sited.
9. Pressing straight along the introducer axis, with hand and elbow in line, push with firm increasing pressure until a distinct release is heard and felt. The introducer must remain perpendicular to the skin during insertion.	
10. After release, pull straight back on the introducer to expose the infusion tube.	
11. Push the used bone probe cluster into the foam-filled sharps plug. Replace the original sharps cap over the sharps cover if desired.	Enables safe disposal of sharps.
12. Attach the elbow female connector (blue cap) on the patch to the infusion tube male Luer.	

Procedure	Additional information/rationale
13. Attach a syringe with 2–3 mL of sodium chloride to the infusion tube and push through quickly – NOTE: this will be very painful if the patient is conscious.	Required to create a clear passageway for fluid administration.
14. Attach the straight female connector on the patch to the IV set.	
15. If fluid does not flow or extravasation occurs, the infusion should be discontinued and an alternative vascular access method should be used.	
16. Complete documentation.	

Bone injection gun (BIG)

See Figure 13.16.

The bone injection gun was perhaps the first automatic IO device and was introduced into emergency medicine in 2000. There have been mixed reviews when compared with standard IO techniques or alternative powered/automatic devices. A Best Evidence Topic report from 2005[68] concluded that the bone injection gun appears to be equivalent in terms of success and possibly (but not clinically significantly) faster to use than standard IO needles at achieving IO access, whilst a prospective study suggested that the bone injection gun provides an effective alternative IV access for critical patients in whom a peripheral IV line cannot be

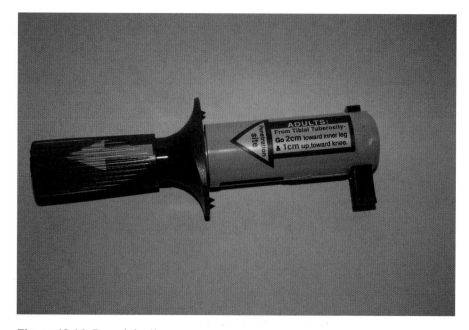

Figure 13.16 Bone injection gun.

readily obtained in the prehospital setting.[69] There have also been case reports of high failure rates when using the BIG device caused mainly by the inability to control the path of the catheter.[70] As with other recent automatic IO devices it is likely that more work needs to be done with the B.I.G before its effectiveness can be fully established.

Procedure for bone injection gun

Procedure	Additional information/rationale
1. Explain the procedure and gain consent of patient or relative.	Legal requirement.
2. Locate a suitable penetration site.	Primary site in adults is the proximal tibia, secondary sites include the medial malleolus, distal radius and anterior head of the humerus.
3. Clean the infusion site.	There is no set method for cleaning the site but the risk of infection and the problems associated with managing bone infections suggest that a rigorous technique be used.
4. Choose BIG with desired depth of penetration.	
5. With one hand holding firmly, position the BIG at a 90 degree angle to the surface of the skin.	Ensures that the correct point will be entered by the device.
6. With one hand holding the BIG firmly, pull out the safety latch by squeezing its two sides together.	Do not dispose of safety latch, it will be used later.
7. While continuing to hold the bottom part firmly against the leg, place 2 fingers of the other hand under the 'winged portion' and the palm of that hand on the top. Leaning on the device with straight elbows will activate the BIG.	No extra force is required.
8. Trigger the BIG by gently pressing down.	
9. Pull out the stylet trocar to leave the cannula in the bone.	
10. The safety latch can now be used to provide extra stability to the cannula.	Helps to prevent instability in the cannula and reduces the risk of displacement.
11. Proceed as for conventional IOI.	

Chapter Key Points

1. A vascular access device is a device that is inserted into a peripheral or central vein (intravenous), or into the marrow cavity of selected bones (intraosseous).
2. The structure and appearance of the skin alters with age as the dermal layers become thinner and elasticity is lost. The veins of older people may be easier to see as a result of these changes but they are more mobile, more fragile, and often tortuous and thrombosed.
3. There are two commonly used peripheral cannulas; a peripheral cannula, and a hollow-needle infusion device, often called a 'butterfly'.
4. The choice of cannula will be dependent upon several factors such as the purpose of cannulation, the size of veins, peripheral shutdown in shocked patients, and the practitioner's skill and confidence.
5. Appropriate techniques should be used to encourage venodilatation.
6. The benefits of appropriate venous cannulation normally outweigh the risks but the practitioner needs to be aware of the risks and minimise any dangers.
7. Intraosseous infusion is an excellent alternative route for providing vascular access to administer fluids, blood products, and medications where alternative methods are not available or attempts have failed.
8. New devices for obtaining intraosseous access mean that this route may become more widely used in the future.
9. The only universally accepted absolute contraindication to intraosseous infusion is a fracture of the bone near the access site.
10. Virtually all drugs that can be administered via the IV route can be administered by intraosseous infusion. There is no need to adjust drug dosages when using the IO route.

References and Further reading

1 Scales K. Vascular access in the acute care setting, in Dougherty L, Lamb J (Eds) *Intravenous Therapy in Nursing Practice*. London: Churchill Livingstone, 1999, pp. 261-299.
2 Tortora GJ, Derrikson B. *Principles of Anatomy and Physiology*, 11th edn. New Jersey: Wiley, 2006.
3 Dougherty L. Obtaining peripheral venous access. In: Dougherty L, Lamb J. (Eds) *Intravenous Therapy in Nursing Practice*. London: Churchill Livingstone, 1999.
4 Dougherty L. Obtaining peripheral venous access. In: Dougherty L, Lamb J. (Eds) *Intravenous Therapy in Nursing Practice*. London: Harcourt, 1999.
5 Scales K. Vascular access: a guide to peripheral venous cannulation. *Nurs Stand* 2005;19(49):48-52.
6 Lavery I, Smith E. Peripheral vascular access devices: risk prevention and management. *Br J Nurs* 2007;16(22):1378-1383.
7 Campbell J. Making sense of the technique of venepuncture. *Nurs Times* 1995;91:29-31.
8 Mbamalu D, Banerjee A. Methods of obtaining peripheral venous access in difficult situations. *Postgrad Med J* 1999;75:459-462.
9 Simons P, Coleridge Smith P, Lees WR, McGrouther DA. Venous pumps of the hand. Their clinical importance. *J Hand Surg* [Br] 1996;21:595-599.

10 Torok T, Bari F, Kardos A, Paprika D, Rudas L. Isometric handgrip exercise-induced musca-rinic vasodilation in the human skin microvasculature. *Acta Physiol Hung* 1997-98;85:193-198.

11 Millam DA. Tips for improving your venipuncture techniques. *Nursing* 1987;17:46-49.

12 Savage MV, Brengelmann GL. Reproducibility of the vascular response to heating in human skin. *J Appl Physiol* 1994;76:1759-1763.

13 Lenhardt R, Seybold T, Kimberger O, Stoiser B, Sessler DI. Local warming and insertion of peripheral venous cannulas: single blinded prospective randomized controlled trial and single blinded randomised crossover trial. *BMJ* 2002;325:409-410.

14 Attubato MJ, Katz ES, Feit F, Bernstein N, Schwartzman D, Kronzon I. Venous changes occurring during the Valsalva maneuver: evaluation by intravascular ultrasound. *Am J Cardiol* 1994;74:408-410.

15 Verghese ST, Nath A, Zenger D, Patel RI, Kaplan RF, Patel KM. The effects of the simulated Valsalva maneuver, liver compression, and/or Trendelenberg position on the cross-sec-tional area of the internal jugular vein in infants and young children. *Anesth Analg* 2002;94:250-254.

16 Lobato EB, Florete OG Jr, Paige GB, Morey TE. Cross-sectional area and intravascular pres-sure of the right internal jugular vein during anesthesia: effects of Trendelenburg position, positive intrathoracic pressure, and hepatic compression. *J Clin Anesth* 1998;10:1-5.

17 Sukumaran S, Henry JM, Beard D, Lawrenson R, Gordon MWG, O'Donnell JJ, Gray AJ. Pre-hospital trauma management: a national study of paramedic activities *Emerg Med J* 2005;22:60-63.

18 Johnson GS, Guly H. The effect of pre-hospital administration of intravenous nalbuphine on on-scene times. *Emerg Med J* 12(1):20-22.

19 Parker I. Management of intravascular devices to prevent infection. *Br J Nurs* 11(4):240-246.

20 Pinkowish M. Bloodstream infections and intravascular devices. *Am J Nurs* 106(12):72CC-72DD.

21 Tagalakis V, Kahn SR, Libman M, Blostein M. The epidemiology of peripheral vein infusion thrombophlebitis: a critical review. *Am J Med* 2002;113(2):146-151.

22 Chalmers C, Straub M. Standard principles for preventing and controlling infection. *Nurs Stand* 2006;20(23):57-65.

23 Damani NN. *Manual of Infection Control Procedures*, 2nd edn. London: Greenwich Medical Media, 2003.

24 Department of Health. High Impact Intervention No 2. Peripheral intravenous cannula care bundle. 2007 available online at www.clean-safe-care.nhs.uk [accessed 24-04-2008].

25 Mallet J, Dougherty L. *Manual of Clinical Nursing Procedures*, 5th edn. Oxford: Blackwell Science, 2000.

26 Fuller A, Winn C. Selecting equipment for peripheral intravenous cannulation. *Profess Nurse* 1999;14(4):233-236.

27 Royal College of Nursing. Infusion equipment. In: *Standards for Infusion Therapy*, 2nd edn. London: RCN; 2006, pp. 18-24.

28 Workman B. Peripheral intravenous therapy management. *Nurs Stand* 14(4):53-60.

29 Centre for Disease Control. Guidelines for the Prevention of Intravascular Catheter-Related Infections. *Morb Mort Week Rep* 2002;51(RR10).

30 Royal College of Nursing. Site selection and placement. In: *Standards for Infusion Therapy*, 2nd edn. London: RCN, 2005, pp. 25-32.

31 Royal College of Nursing. Infusion equipment. In: *Standards for Infusion Therapy*, 2nd edn. London: RCN, 2006, pp. 18-24.

32 NHS Lothian University Hospitals Division. *Venepuncture and/or Peripheral IV Cannulation Clinical Skills Education Pack*. Edinburgh: NHS LUHD, 2005.

33 Mason S, Watts A, Shiels S, Koorey D. Improving access to HCV treatment: external jugular venepuncture can overcome problems with difficult venous access. *Internat J Drug Policy* 2007;18(5):433-436.

34 Bledsoe B, Porter RS, Cherry RA. *Essentials of Paramedic Care*. New Jersey: Prentice Hall, 2003.

35 Royal College of Nursing. Site selection and placement. In: *Standards for Infusion Therapy*, 2nd edn. London: RCN, 2005, pp. 25-32.

36 NHS Lothian University Hospitals Division. *Venepuncture and/or Peripheral IV Cannulation Clinical Skills Education Pack*. Edinburgh: NHS LUHD, 2005.

37 Glaeser PW, Losek JD, Nelson DB *et al.* Pediatric intraosseous infusions: impact on vascular access time. *Am J Emerg Med* 1988;6:330-332.

38 Kanter RK, Zimmerman JJ, Strauss RH, Stoeckel KA. Pediatric emergency intravenous access: evaluation of a protocol. *Am J Dis Child* 1986;140:132-134.

39 Brunette DD, Fischer R. Intravenous access in pediatric cardiac arrest. *Am J Emerg Med* 1988;6:577-579.

40 Suyama J, Knutsen CC, Northington WE, Hahn M, Hostler D. IO versus IV access while wearing personal protective equipment in a HazMat scenario. *Prehosp Emerg Care* 2007;11:467-472.

41 Miner WF, Corneli HM, Bolte RG, Lehnhof D, Clawson JJ. Prehospital use of intraosseous infusion by paramedics. *Pediatr Emerg Care* 1989;5(1):5-7.

42 Calkins MD, Fitzgerald G, Bentley TB, Burris D. Intraosseous infusion devices: a comparison for potential use in special operations. *J Trauma* 2000;48(6):1068-1074.

43 Ross MH, Romrell LJ, Kaye GI. *Histology: A Text and Atlas*, 3rd edn. Baltimore, MD: Williams & Wilkins, 1995, pp. 150-153.

44 LaRocco BG, Wang HE. Intraosseous Infusion. *Prehosp Emerg Care* 2003;7:280-285.

45 Resuscitation Council UK. Adult advanced life support. 2005 available online at http://www.resus.org.uk/pages/als.pdf [accessed 04-05-2008].

46 Hurren JS, Dunn KW. Intraosseous infusion for burn resuscitation. *Burns* 1995;21:285-287.

47 Goldstein B, Doody D, Briggs S. Emergency intraosseous infusion in severely burned children. *Pediatr Emerg Care*. 1990;6:1995-1997.

48 Miner WF, Corneli HM, Bolte RG, Lehnhof D, Clawson JJ. Prehospital use of intraosseous infusion by paramedics. *Pediatr Emerg Care* 1989;5(1):5-7 .

49 Fowler R, Gallagher JV, Isaacs SM, Ossman E, Pepe P, Wayne M. The role of intraosseous vascular access in the out-of-hospital environment (resource document to NAEMSP position statement). *Prehosp Emerg Care* 2007;11:63-66.

50 Rosetti VA, Thompson BM, Miller J, Mateer JR, Aprahamian C. Intraosseous infusion: an alternative route of pediatric intravascular access. *Ann Emerg Med* 1985;14(9):885-888.

51 Davidoff J, Fowler R, Gordon D, Klein G, Kovar J *et al.* Clinical evaluation of a novel intraosseous device for adults: prospective, 250-patient, multi-center trial. *JEMS* 2005;30(10)(suppl):20-23.

52 Gillum L, Kovar J. Powered intraosseous access in the out-of-hospital setting. *JEMS* 2005;30(10)(suppl):24-26.

53 Waisman M, Waisman D. Bone marrow infusion in adults. *J Trauma* 1997;(2):288-293.

54 American College of Surgeons (Eds) ATLS, *Advanced Trauma Life Support for Doctors, Student Manual*. Chicago IL: American College of Surgeons, 1997, pp. 12, 97.

55 Fiser DH. Intraosseous infusion. *N Engl J Med* 1990;322:1579-1581.

56 Voelckel WG, Lurie KG, McKnite S *et al.* Comparison of epinephrine with vasopressin on bone marrow blood flow in an animal model of hypovolemic shock and subsequent cardiac arrest. *Crit Care Med* 2001;29:1587-1592.

57 Neal CJ, McKinley DF. Intraosseous infusion in pediatric patients. *J Am Osteopath Assoc* 1994;94(1):63-66.

58 Shoor PM, Berryhill RE, Benumof JL. Intraosseous infusion: pressure-flow relationships and pharmacokinetics. *J Trauma* 1979;19:772-774 .

59 Hazinski MF, Cummins RO, Field JM. (Eds) Basic life support for health care providers. In: *Handbook of Emergency Cardiovascular Care for Healthcare Providers*. Dallas TX: American Heart Association, 2002, pp. 1-2, 96.

60 Warren DW, Kissoon N, Mattar A, Morrissey G, Gravelle D, Rieder MJ. Pharmacokinetics from multiple intraosseous and peripheral intravenous site injections in normovolemic and hypovolemic pigs. *Crit Care Med* 1994;22:838-843.

61 Brennera T, Bernharda M, Helmb M, Doll S, Völkl A, Ganiona N, Friedmanna C, Sikingera M, Knappa J, Martina E, Gries A. Comparison of two intraosseous infusion systems for adult emergency medical use. *Resuscitation* 2008;78:314-319.

62 Cooper BR. Intra-osseous access EZ-IO for resuscitation: UK military combat experience. *J Royal Army Med Corps* 2007;153(4):314-316.

63 Ong ME, Chan YH, Oh JJ, Su-Yin Ngo N. An observational, prospective study comparing tibial and humeral intraosseous access using the EZ-IO. *Am J Emerg Med* 2009;27(1):8-15.

64 Vidacare. EZ-IO intraosseous infusion system directions for use. 2006 available online at http://www.vidacare.com/reports/VDAA168EZ-IODFU051707.pdf [accessed 06-05-2008].

65 Tiffany BR, Horwood BT, Pollack CV et al. Sternal intraosseous infusion: flow rates and utility. *Ann Emerg Med* 1999;34(4).

66 Tiffany BR, Adams J, Pollack CV et al. Prehospital use of a sternal intraosseous infusion device. *Ann Emerg Med* 1999;34(4).

67 Johnson DL, Findlay LM, Stair TO, Robinson DJ. Device for fast field intraosseous infusion via the adult manubrium. *Ann Emerg Med* 1998;32(3).

68 Curran A, Sen A. Bone injection gun placement of intraosseous needles. *Emerg Med J* 2005;22:366.

69 Schwartz D, Amir L, Dichter R, Figenberg Z. The use of a powered device for intraosseous drug and fluid administration in a national EMS: A 4-year experience. *J Trauma Injury Infect Critic Care* 2008;64(3);650-655.

70 David J-S, Dubien P-Y, Capel O, Peguet O, Gueugniaud P-Y. Intraosseous infusion using the bone injection gun in the prehospital setting. *Resuscitation* 2009;80:384.

Chapter 14
Needle thoracocentesis

Content

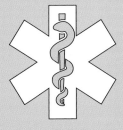

Needle thoracocentesis is a life-saving procedure that will rarely be used in prehospital care, but it may prove of significant value when it is indicated. The technique is only a temporary measure but it may 'buy' extra time to convey the patient to more definitive care or bring the definitive care to the patient.

Definitions

Needle thoracocentesis involves placing a wide-bore cannula into the mid-clavicular line of the second intercostal space, just above the third rib, in order to decompress a tension pneumothorax.[1] Normally, the pleural cavity is a potential space that is free from air and contains only a thin layer of fluid. When air enters the pleural cavity it is termed a pneumothorax.[2] Tension pneumothorax is a life-threatening condition that occurs when the intrapleural pressure exceeds atmospheric pressure. It is created when injury to the chest or respiratory structures allows air to enter but not to leave the pleural space, resulting in a rapid increase in pressure on the affected side. This causes collapse of the affected lung, compression atelactasis of the unaffected lung, mediastinal shift towards the opposite side of the chest, and compression of the vena cava.[2]

Resuscitation and trauma usually illustrate a patient in extremis and suggest that the clinical diagnosis is straightforward and that needle chest decompression always produces a rapid and reliable response.[3,4] This may be far removed from the real life situation, where the classically taught signs are not often present. Table 14.1 summarises the symptoms and signs that may be useful for diagnosing tension pneumothorax in awake and ventilated patients.[5]

THINK

You are at the scene of a Road Traffic Collision along with the police and fire service. How will you manage the noise at the scene to maximise your chances of identifying a life-threatening thoracic injury?

Table 14.1 Symptoms and signs of tension pneumothorax, adapted from Leigh-Smith and Harris (2005)[5]

Diagnosis of tension pneumothorax in awake patients	Diagnosis of tension pneumothorax in ventilated patients
Reliable and early	**Rapid disease progression**
• Pleuritic chest pain	**Reliable and early**
• Air hunger	• Decrease in SpO_2 - immediate
• Respiratory distress	• Decrease in BP
• Tachypnoea	• Tachycardia
• Tachycardia	
• Falling SpO_2	**Others**
• Agitation	• Increased ventilation pressure
Disease lateralisation - ipsilateral	• Surgical emphysema
• Hyper-expansion	Disease lateralisation
• Hypo-mobility	• Ipsilateral
• Hyper-resonance	• Hyper-resonance
• Decreased breath sounds	• Decreased breath sounds
• Added sounds–crackles/wheeze	• Chest hyper-expansion
Disease lateralisation - contralateral	• Chest hypo-mobility
• Hyper-mobility	• Added sounds
Pre-terminal	**Inconsistent**
• Decreasing respiratory rate	• Cyanosis
• Hypotension	• Distended neck veins
• Decreasing SpO_2	• Tracheal deviation
• Decreasing level consciousness	
Inconsistent	
• Tracheal deviation	
• Distended neck veins	

The literature surrounding needle thoracocentesis

The actual incidence of tension pneumothorax is not known, but it is more common in ventilated than awake patients and possibly most common in ventilated patients with visceral pleural injury from chest trauma.[4] Emergency needle decompression is widely advocated for use in the emergency management of tension pneumothorax[6,7,8] but there needs to be an appreciation of the potential problems associated with the technique; these will be discussed later.

Needle thoracocentesis is often ineffective on its own and requires subsequent tube thoracostomy,[9-14] hence why it should be seen as a temporary measure at best. There are also a number of factors that could cause needle decompression to fail; these include:

Needle too short[15,16,17]

The recommended point for insertion of a needle is between the 2nd and 3rd inter-costal space in the mid-clavicular line. Whilst this is easy to access, it does entail penetration of pectoral muscles and a variable quantity of subcutaneous tissue, which may be increased by oedema and subcutaneous emphysema. It has previously been recommended that the minimum length should be 4.5 cm (standard length 14-gauge cannula);[17] although up to one third of trauma patients have a chest wall thickness greater than 5 cm at the normal insertion point.[18,19]

A potential option is to use the 4th or 5th intercostal space in the midaxillary line and this has been recommended by ATLS as it contains less fat and avoids large muscles.[4] Unfortunately this site may have an increased risk of lung damage in the supine patient, as gas collects at the highest point and adhesions are most likely in more dependent parts of the lung.[20]

Obstruction[5,11]

- Kinking of the catheter
- Blood
- Pleural fluid
- Tissue.

Malposition

- Incorrect identification of landmarks; could lead to cardiac tamponade
- Inadvertent removal by patient
- Catheter too small to drain a large area[5]
- Missing a localised tension pneumothorax.

Despite these problems, needle decompression is a technique that has proved safe and therapeutic in the prehospital environment,[12,21-23] and leads to shorter on-scene times compared with tube thoracostomy.[23]

Equipment

- 14-gauge cannula
- 10 mL syringe (consider filling with sterile saline)
- Alcohol swab
- Asherman seal or other method of stabilising and securing the cannula.

Indications for use

When there are convincing signs of a tension pneumothorax (Table 14.1).

Contraindications for use

None in the emergency management of tension pneumothorax.

Potential problems of use

Problem	Solution
1. Obstruction of catheter: blood, fluid or tissue, or kinked catheter.	Try to aspirate, if unsuccessful, insert second needle close to original site.
2. Needle too short.	Consider using 4th or 5th intercostal space in the midaxillary line if authorised to do so.
3. Malposition	Leave in situ and secure. A small pneumothorax may be created by incorrect thoracocentesis, but this is unlikely to be a significant problem. However, if surgery and ventilation are required under anaesthesia, this can be expanded to a tension pneumothorax. If cannula has been removed, cover wound with sterile dressing and notify receiving hospital.
4. Displaced cannula	Insert a second cannula and secure well.

Box 14.1 Potential problems of needle thoracocentesis

There are a number of other potential problems associated with needle thoracocentesis, most of which the paramedic can do little about in the field (Box 14.2).

Unnecessary pain/discomfort for the patient if procedure was not required
Pneumothorax with potential to tension later - especially if ventilated
Cardiac tamponade
Life threatening haemorrhage
Intrapleural haematoma
Atelectasis
Pneumonia

Box 14.2 Morbidity associated with needle decompression[5]

Procedures for needle thoracocentesis

Procedure	Additional information/rationale
1. Ensure a patent airway and adequate oxygenation.	Maintains oxygenation
2. Ensure adequate ventilation	Ensures adequacy of ventilation.
3. Expose the chest.	Necessary to identify landmarks and perform technique.

Procedure	Additional information/rationale
4. Identify landmarks (Figure 14.1): • Locate suprasternal notch and move fingers down manubrium to the angle of Louis (this sits level with the second rib).	
• From angle of Louis, identify second intercostal space in the mid-clavicular line on the affected side. • Insertion should be on the superior border of the third rib.	The mid-clavicular line avoids the internal mammary arteries. Nerves, arteries and veins pass just below each rib so insertion point should be the superior margin of the third rib.
5. Clean the skin using alcohol wipe.	Reduces the risk of infection.
6. Remove the flashback chamber from a 10-16 g cannula and attach a 10-20 mL syringe.	
7. Insert needle fully at 90° to the skin. Withdraw on the plunger of the syringe until a free flow of air enters the syringe.	Free flow of air demonstrates that lung tissue has been reached.
8. Advance cannula and remove needle and syringe to allow a rush of air out of the syringe.	A rush of air signifies that the diagnosis was correct.
9. Secure cannula in place to prevent dislodgement.	Improper placement or movement may cause damage to other organs or structures.
10. There is no need to re-fit the cannula cap and time should not be wasted in applying a one-way valve.	
11. Complete documentation	

Chapter Key Points

1. Needle thoracocentesis is a potentially life-saving technique.
2. Diagnosis of tension pneumothorax may be difficult in the prehospital environment.
3. Many of the commonly taught signs and symptoms may not be present or may be unreliable indicators.
4. There are a number of potential problems related to needle thoracocentesis, some of which the paramedic may be able to manage, some may not be manageable in the field.

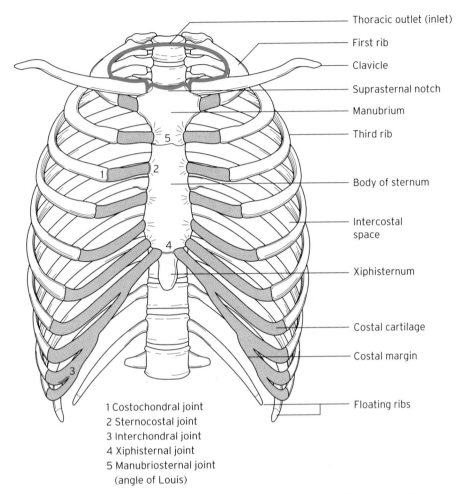

- Thoracic outlet (inlet)
- First rib
- Clavicle
- Suprasternal notch
- Manubrium
- Third rib
- Body of sternum
- Intercostal space
- Xiphisternum
- Costal cartilage
- Costal margin
- Floating ribs

1 Costochondral joint
2 Sternocostal joint
3 Interchondral joint
4 Xiphisternal joint
5 Manubriosternal joint
 (angle of Louis)

Figure 14.1 Sternal landmarks for needle thoracocentesis. Reproduced from Faiz O, Moffat D. *Anatomy at a Glance*, 2nd edn, copyright 2006, with permission of Blackwell Publishing.

References and Further reading

1 Ferrie EP, Collum N, McGovern S. The right place in the right space? Awareness of site for needle thoracocentesis. *Emerg Med J* 2005;22:788-789.

2 Porth CM. *Pathophysiology, Concepts of Altered Health States*, 7th edn. Philadelphia: LWW, 2005.

3 ALSG. *Advanced Life Support Manual*, 4th edn. London: Resuscitation Council (UK), 2001.

4 ATLS. *Advanced Trauma Life Support*. 6th edn. Chicago: American College of Surgeons, 1997.

5 Leigh-Smith S, Harris T. Tension pneumothorax - time for a re-think? *Emerg Med J* 2005;22;8-16.

6 Joint Royal Colleges Ambulance Liaison Committee. *UK Ambulance Service Clinical Practice Guidelines version 4*. London: IHCD, 2006.

7 National Association of Emergency Medical Technicians in Co-operation with the Committee on Trauma of the American College of Surgeons. *PHTLS Prehospital Trauma Life Support*, 6th edn. Missouri: Mosby/JEMS, 2006.

8 Sanders M. *Mosby's Paramedic Textbook*. Missouri: Mosby, 2006.

9 Britten S, Palmer SH. Chest wall thickness may limit adequate drainage of tension pneumo-thorax by needle thoracocentesis. *J Accid Emerg Med* 1996;13:426-427.

10 Britten S, Palmer SH, Snow TM. Needle thoracocentesis in tension pneumothorax: insufficient cannula length and potential failure. *Injury* 1996;27:321-322.

11 Conces DJ Jr, Tarver RD, Gray WC *et al.* Treatment of pneumothoraces utilizing small caliber chest tubes. *Chest* 1988;94:55-57.

12 Cullinane DC, Morris JA Jr, Bass JG *et al.* Needle thoracostomy may not be indicated in the trauma patient. *Injury* 2001;32:749-752.

13 Jenkins C, Sudheer PS. Needle thoracocentesis fails to diagnose a large pneumothorax. *Anaesthesia* 2000;55:925-926.

14 Jones R, Hollingsworth J. Tension pneumothoraces not responding to needle thoracocentesis. *Emerg Med J* 2002;19:176-177.

15 American College of Surgeons, Committee on Trauma. *Advanced Trauma Life Support Course Manual*. Washington DC: ACS, 1997.

16 Britten S, Palmer SH. Chest wall thickness may limit adequate drainage of a tension pneumothorax by needle thoracocentesis. *J Accid Emerg Med* 1996;13:426-427.

17 Britten S, Palmer SH, Snow TM. Needle thoracocentesis in tension pneumothorax: insufficient cannula length and potential failure. *Injury* 1996;27(5):321-322.

18 Marinaro J, Kenny C, Smith S *et al.* Needle thoracostomy in trauma patients: what catheter length is adequate? *Acad Emerg Med* 2003;10:495.

19 Zengerink I, Brink P, Laupland K. Needle thoracostomy in the treatment of a tension pneumothorax in trauma patients: what size needle? *J Trauma* 2008;64:111-114.

20 Goodman L, Putman C. *Intensive Care Radiology Imaging of the Critically Ill*, 2nd edn. Philadephia: W B Saunders, 1982:99-100.

21 Coats TJ, Wilson AW, Xeropotamous N. Pre-hospital management of patients with severe thoracic injury. *Injury* 1995;2:581-585.

22 Cameron PA, Flett K, Kaan E *et al.* Helicopter retrieval of primary trauma patients by a paramedic helicopter service. *Aust NZ J Surg* 1993;63:790-797.

23 Barton ED, Epperson M, Hoyt DB *et al.* Prehospital needle aspiration and tube thoracostomy in trauma victims: a six-year experience with aeromedical crews. *J Emerg Med* 1995;13:155-163.

Chapter 15

Pain assessment and management

Content

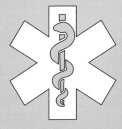

Pain is one of the most frequent symptoms presented by patients in the emergency care setting,[1-3] with a 2004 patient survey suggesting that 80% of patients experienced pain whilst in the ambulance.[4]

The ability to manage pain in emergency care is a key skill that provides comfort, minimises the stress associated with sudden illness or injury, and reduces the detrimental psychological and physiological effects associated with pain. Despite this, numerous studies have shown that pain is managed sub-optimally in emergency care.[5-9] A UK survey found that 1 in 5 patients were not satisfied with the way their pain was managed in the prehospital environment;[4] this is likely to be an underestimation as patients often report high levels of satisfaction even though their pain level has actually increased.[10]

Definitions

A widely used definition of pain is:

> *'... an unpleasant sensory and emotional experience associated with actual or potential tissue damage or described in terms of such damage'.*[11]

This definition does not address the autonomic responses associated with obnoxious stimuli, which is a key feature of pain in the emergency setting. A second definition proposed by Margo McCaffery as long ago as 1968 has become widely used by healthcare professionals. She states that pain is:

> *'... whatever the experiencing person says it is, existing whenever the experiencing person says it does'.*[12]

Pain is a complex phenomenon that comprises both physical and emotional elements; it is a subjective experience and should rely heavily on the patient's self-report whenever possible. A significant problem for the practitioner is related to this subjectivity. Paramedics interviewed by researchers expressed doubts as to the validity of some patients' pain descriptions, suggesting that patients may feel they need to increase their explanation of pain to be believed and to be taken seriously by the paramedics. Others felt that pain descriptions were exaggerated by patients with minor ailments so that they can justify calling an ambulance, also thinking that they will be seen more promptly at hospital.[13] The paramedics also believed that the cultural background of the patient had a major impact on their pain experience. They recognised a cultural difference to exist in the way that pain was expressed, with some cultures thought to be more vocal and emotional in expressing their pain. It was also held that older people may perceive pain differently to younger people and would be less likely to ask for help.[13] All of this indicates just how difficult assessment of pain can be, especially acute pain in the emergency setting.

Acute pain v chronic pain

Acute pain

Acute pain has been defined in a number of different ways but a common feature in definitions is that is a symptom with a discernible cause and usually subsides when injured tissues heal. Acute pain has a protective function.

Chronic pain

Chronic pain is, by definition, pain that has persisted beyond the time of healing; a classification based purely on causal agent is not achievable. Some patients become extremely disabled and suffer intractable pain even though their identifiable pathology appears to be relatively mild; other individuals with similar pathologies may report pain but do not present with the same level of disability.[14] Good evidence exists to show that quality of life for patients with chronic pain is more associated with beliefs about pain than the severity itself.[15] Although emergency care is often associated with acute pain, it is likely that those suffering from chronic pain (e.g., cancer, lower back pain, multiple pain localisations) will also access the emergency services.

The cornerstone of pain management is the assessment of the pain. A variety of pain assessment tools are available to assist in determining the level of pain and evaluating the effectiveness of interventions. These tools should be used in conjunction with a thorough history of the pain to help diagnose the most likely cause of the pain as well as the severity.

Assessing pain

- Look at the patient
- Taking the history of the pain
- Pain assessment tools.

Initial observations

It is worth noting the patient's position, any guarding of the site of pain and how well they mobilise. Significant information can also be obtained by watching the patient's face, especially during mobilisation. This is covered later in the chapter as a checklist of non-verbal indicators.

History of the pain

The history is vital to help make a differential diagnosis and several mnemonics have been suggested to help practitioners. Whether or not to use a mnemonic is for the individual practitioner to decide; two different ones will be presented here. It is important to remember that questions are only relevant if the practitioner understands the answers, so it is essential to have a sound understanding of the pathophysiology behind the clinical manifestations.

OPQRST mnemonic

This is probably one of the most commonly taught mnemonics in emergency care although some texts do not mention the 'O' element.

O Onset

P Provocation/palliation

Q Quality

R Region/radiation

S Severity

T Timing

O Onset

Did the problem develop suddenly or more gradually?
What was the patient doing when the pain came on?
Was the patient exercising or exerting themselves?
Was the patient eating or drinking, if so, what?

P Provocation/palliation

What provokes the pain (makes it worse)?
What palliates the pain (makes it better?)
Were there any precipitating factors e.g., did this come on after exercise?

Q Quality

What does it feel like, e.g., sharp, dull, stabbing, burning or crushing? Allow the patient to describe their pain otherwise they may say what they think you want them to say. Use their descriptors on the case report form.

R Region/radiation

Where is the pain?
Does the pain stay in one place?
Does it go anywhere else?
Ask the patient to point to the pain – can it be localised or is it diffuse?
If the pain radiates, where does it go?
Did the pain start elsewhere but become localised in one place?

S Severity/associated symptoms

How bad is the pain? (See section below on pain assessment tools)
Are there any associated symptoms – e.g., nausea, vomiting, dizziness?

T Time/temporal relations

When did the pain start?
How long did it last?
Is it constant or intermittent?
How long has it been affecting your patient for? (It may have been going on for some time)

Table 15.1 CHESTPAIN mnemonic

C	Commenced when?	When did the pain start? Was onset associated with anything specific? Exertion? Activity? Emotional upset?
H	History/risk factors	Do you have a history of heart disease? Is there a primary relative (parent/sibling) with early onset and/or early death related to heart disease? Do you have other risk factors, e.g., diabetes, smoking, hypertension, or obesity?
E	Extra symptoms	What else are you feeling with the pain? Are you nervous? Sweating? Is your heart racing? Are you short of breath? Do you feel nauseous? Dizzy? Weak?
S	Stays/radiates	Does the pain stay in one place? Does it radiate or go anywhere else in the body? Where?
T	Timing	How long does the pain last? How long has this episode lasted? How many minutes? Is the pain continuous or does it come and go? When did it become continuous?
P	Place	Where is your pain? Check for point tenderness with palpation.
A	Alleviates	What makes the pain better? Rest? Changing position? Deep breathing?
	Aggravates	What makes the pain worse? Exercise? Deep breathing? Changing positions?
I	Intensity	How intense is the pain?
N	Nature	Describe the pain (do not suggest descriptors)

Adapted from Newberry, Barnett and Ballard (2003).[16]

A recent mnemonic has been proposed specifically for the evaluation of chest pain (Table 15.1) and incorporates risk factors for cardiac problems. The mnemonic is CHESTPAIN.

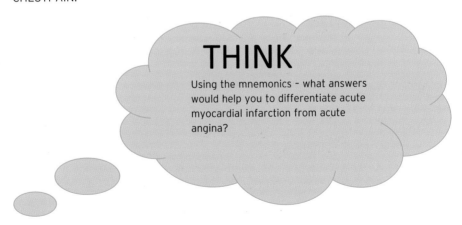

THINK

Using the mnemonics – what answers would help you to differentiate acute myocardial infarction from acute angina?

Pain assessment tools

The tools that will be covered in this section include:

- Numerical Rating Scale
- Visual Analogue Scale
- Verbal Rating Scale
- Wong-Baker FACES Pain Scale
- Checklist of non-verbal indicators.

Numerical Rating Scale (NRS)

The numerical rating scale is probably the most commonly used tool in prehospital emergency care and generally encompasses an 11 point scale ranging from 0 (no pain) to 10 (worst pain). It is simple to administer and requires no specific equipment. The NRS is often administered verbally in the prehospital setting but it could easily be completed as a paper exercise (see Figure 15.1), which may be helpful to those patients who have difficulty in allocating a pain score verbally. A study showed the NRS to have poor reproducibility[17] and highlighted the importance of consistency of terminology to ensure that confusion does not arise. A study in the emergency department has shown a verbally administered NRS to be a suitable substitute for the VAS, see below in the assessment of acute pain.[18]

Procedure	Additional information/rationale
1. Establish that the patient is able to use numbers to quantify their pain.	Improves likelihood of answers being accurate.
2. Explain the parameters of the scale and use descriptors at each end of the scale.	Patient needs to know which end of the scale represents severe pain for accuracy of measurement.
3. Ask the patient one of the following questions: • What number would you give your pain right now? • What number on a 0 to 10 scale would you give your pain when it is the worst that it gets and when it is the best that it gets? • At what number is the pain at an acceptable level for you?	
4. Record pain score and repeat at frequent intervals.	Allows evaluation of effectiveness of pain management strategies and whether more needs to be done.
5. For written NRS, follow the above but ask patient to circle the number that describes how much pain they are having.	

No pain   Worst Imaginable pain

0	1	2	3	4	5	6	7	8	9	10

Figure 15.1 Numerical Rating Scale.

Visual Analogue Scale (VAS)

The VAS is presented as a 10 cm line, anchored by verbal descriptors, usually 'no pain' and 'worst imaginable pain' (Figure 15.2). The patient is asked to mark a 100 mm line to indicate pain intensity and the score is measured from the zero anchor to the patient's mark. A millimetre scale can be used to measure the patient's score and will provide 101 levels of pain intensity.

One of the limitations of the VAS is that it must be administered on paper or electronically.[19] Caution is required when photocopying the scale as this can lead to significant changes in its length.[20]

THINK

You ask your patient to score their pain on a scale of 0-10, they reply 11. How would you feel and how would this impact on your management of their pain?

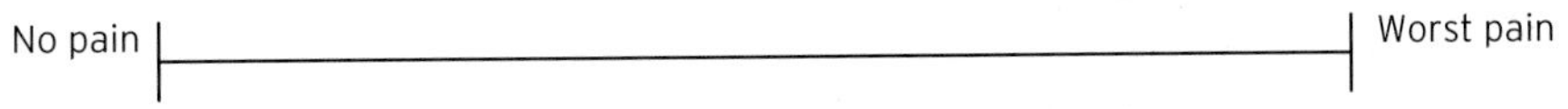

No pain |————————————————————————————————————| Worst pain

Figure 15.2 Visual Analogue Scale (VAS).

Procedure	Additional information/rationale
1. Explain procedure to patient.	
2. Ask patient to mark on the line how bad they feel their pain is.	
3. Measure pain score and repeat at frequent intervals using new VAS.	Allows evaluation of effectiveness of pain management strategies and whether more needs to be done.

Verbal Rating Scale (VRS)

The verbal rating scale employs a list of adjectives to denote increasing pain intensities. The most common words used being: no pain; mild pain; moderate pain; and severe or intense pain. For ease of recording these adjectives are assigned numbers.

0   no pain
1   mild pain
2   moderate pain
3   severe or intense pain

Sensitivity of pain scales

The sensitivity of a pain rating scale is the ability of that scale to detect change. The more levels a tool has the more sensitive it will be. A small change in pain is noticeable using a VAS but the small number of categories in the VRS demands that a much larger change in pain is required before the change shows up on the scale.[21] This lack of sensitivity can lead to over or under-estimation of pain changes.[22] Both the VAS and the NRS have increased sensitivity to change compared with the VRS [23,24] and should be used in preference.

There is compelling evidence that 11 or 21 point scales are more than adequate for the assessment of pain. 101 point scales (such as the VAS and 101 point NRS) have more levels of discrimination than most patients use.[22]

Wong–Baker FACES Pain Scale

The Wong-Baker smiley faces were originally designed for use in children although they have also been used with varied success with older people.[25,26] Stuppy[27] used an adapted version depicting older faces, and subsequently suggested that whenever practitioners suspect accuracy of pain measurement to be affected by fatigue, depleted physical or mental state, literacy or command of English, they should consider the use of this scale. A limitation of this system is that it cannot be administered verbally so is of limited use if patients have visual impairment.

Instructions

Explain to the person that each face is for a person who feels happy because he has no pain (hurt) or sad because he has some or a lot of pain. Face 0 is very happy because he doesn't hurt at all. Face 1 hurts just a little bit. Face 2 hurts a little more. Face 3 hurts even more. Face 4 hurts a whole lot. Face 5 hurts as much as you can imagine, although you don't have to be crying to feel this bad. Ask the person to choose the face that best describes how s/he is feeling.

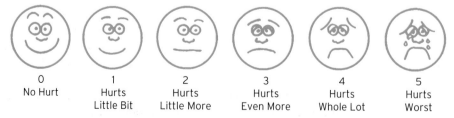

0	1	2	3	4	5
No Hurt	Hurts Little Bit	Hurts Little More	Hurts Even More	Hurts Whole Lot	Hurts Worst

Figure 15.3 Wong-Baker FACES Pain Scale. From Hockenberry MJ, Wilson D, Winkelstein ML. *Wong's Essentials of Pediatric Nursing*, 7th edn. St. Louis: Mosby, 2005, p. 1259. Used with permission. Copyright, Mosby.

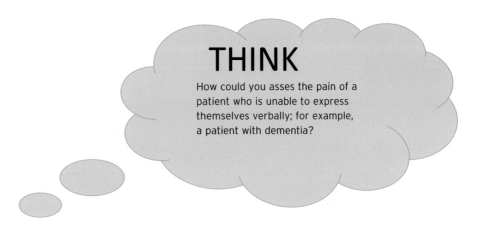

THINK

How could you asses the pain of a
patient who is unable to express
themselves verbally; for example,
a patient with dementia?

Assessing pain in cognitively impaired patients

Assessing pain in those with cognitive impairment may present particular difficulties and may lead to patient's being managed with sub-optimal analgesia. The degree of impairment will impact upon the ability of the patient to use the standard assessment tools so it will be useful for the paramedic to have alternative methods to supplement conventional tools. Several tools are available to measure pain in older adults with dementia but few have been comprehensively evaluated; each has strengths and limitations that need to be acknowledged.[28] The Pain Assessment in Advanced Dementia (PAINAD) has been shown to be a valid, and reliable instrument for measurement of pain in non-communicative patients[29] but may be a little over-complex for use in the prehospital environment. A simple checklist of non-verbal indicators was developed in 2000 (Table 15.2), which may be of some assistance in the acute setting. It should be noted that the low frequencies of observed behaviours at rest indicate that the tool is less useful during rest and may be more useful for observing activities such as transfers, standing, or ambulation.[30]

Recommendations[28]

Ask older adults with dementia about their pain. Even older adults with mild to moderate dementia can respond to simple questions about their pain.[31]

- Use a standardised tool to assess pain intensity, such as the numerical rating scale (NRS) (0–10) or a verbal descriptor scale (VDS). The VDS asks participants to select a word that best describes their present pain (e.g., no pain to worst pain imaginable) and may be more reliable than the NRS in older adults with dementia.
- Use an observational tool (e.g., Checklist of non-verbal indicators) to measure the presence of pain in older adults with dementia.
- Ask family or usual caregivers as to whether the patient's current behaviour (e.g., crying out, restlessness) is different from their customary behaviour. This change in behaviour may signal pain.

Table 15.2 Checklist of non-verbal indicators.[30]Reprinted from *Pain Management Nursing* 1(1), Karen S. Feldt, 'The checklist of nonverbal pain indicators (CNPI)', pp. 13-21, copyright 2000, with permission from Elsevier

	With movement	At rest
Vocal complaints - non-verbal expression of pain demonstrated by moans, groans, grunts, cries, gasps, sighs)		
Facial grimaces and winces - furrowed brow, narrowed eyes, tightened lips, dropped jaw, clenched teeth, distorted expression		
Bracing - clutching or holding onto side rails, bed, tray table, or affected area during movement		
Restlessness - constant or intermittent shifting of position, rocking, intermittent or constant hand motions, inability to keep still		
Rubbing - massaging affected area		
Vocal complaints - verbal expression of pain using words, e.g., 'ouch' or 'that hurts;' cursing during movement, or exclamations of protest, e.g., 'stop' or 'that's enough.'		
TOTAL SCORE		

Indications:
Behavioural Health adults who are unable to validate the presence of or quantify the severity of pain using either the Numerical Rating Scale or the Wong-Baker Faces Pain Rating Scale.
Instructions:
1. Write a 0 if the behaviour was not apparent
2. Write a 1 if the behaviour occurred even briefly during activity or rest
3. Results in a total score between 0 and 6.

This has not been validated for prehospital use, but may at least give the practitioner an indication of likely severity and appropriate interventions.

Overview of pain management techniques

Non-pharmacological Interventions

Non-pharmacological methods for managing pain include splinting (see Chapter 16), distraction, patient positioning, reassurance, elevation, dressings (e.g. burn dressings) and psychological approaches. Non-pharmacological methods should be used to complement pharmacological treatments as opposed to replacing them.

Distraction

Distraction techniques have particular relevance for children and have been shown to be an effective adjunct to analgesia for children with musculoskeletal pain in the emergency department.[32] Small-scale studies related to intravenous cannulation also suggest that parental positioning-distraction interventions have the potential to enhance positive clinical outcomes with a primary benefit of decreased fear.[33] It should be noted that distraction involves a variety of techniques, such as guided imagery, music therapy, reading or being read to, blowing bubbles, playing with toys, tapping a rhythm, and watching TV or videos.[34] Whilst some distraction techniques are not suitable for the prehospital environment or on the back of an ambulance, many simple techniques are. Paramedics could consider distraction through talking to children, reading to them, or letting them play with things on the ambulance that don't pose a health and safety hazard. It is also important to keep parents involved.

There is little literature available for distraction techniques in adults in the acute setting although distraction therapy is advocated in pain management for both chronic pain and post-surgery pain. It is likely that adults will also benefit from distraction in the acute setting, but be aware that patients distracted from their pain may not look like they are in pain, which could lead to an incorrect judgment. It is important to be aware that after the distraction is over, the pain may be increased and other pain relief measures may be needed.[35]

Patient positioning

Patient positioning may confer significant relief to patients and effort should be made to help the patient achieve a comfortable position. The paramedic should be guided by the patient's own preference but may be able to offer advice regarding movement of people with back pain for example. It is worth noting that ischaemic cardiac pain tends to be the same regardless of position, which may help with a provisional diagnosis.

Reassurance

Patients should be provided with ongoing reassurance, information and support from all involved in the prehospital care of a patient in pain. It has been known for over 30 years that information before surgery about procedures and expected discomforts help to minimise anxiety;[36] practitioners should provide information about what may happen to the patient in the next phase of care to help reduce anxieties. It has been suggested that is important that the patient chooses how much information they wish to have.[37]

Pharmacological Interventions

A number of drugs are available for paramedic administration and the decision as to the most appropriate medicine will be based upon guidelines and clinical judgement. Drugs available include opioid analgesics, non-steroidal anti-inflammatory drugs, paracetamol, and Entonox. The pharmacology behind the drugs is beyond the scope of this text; however, a discussion surrounding the principles guiding the appropriateness of analgesic drugs is warranted. The Joint Royal Colleges Ambulance Liaison Committee state that analgesia should normally be introduced in an incremental way, considering timeliness, effectiveness and potential adverse events.[38] This is very much in keeping with the 'Three Step Analgesic Ladder' espoused by the World Health Organization (WHO) in 1986.[39] The WHO philosophy was designed to improve pharmacological interventions in patients with cancer pain but has been adapted for use in cases of acute pain. The underlying objective is to provide adequate pain relief without necessarily exposing the patient to more potent analgesic agents. There are inherent problems with this in emergency care in the out-of-hospital environment, but the philosophy should help to guide initial thought processes when deciding upon analgesic medicines. Essentially, the paramedic should start at the most appropriate level for the patient's presenting pain and only step up to the next level if the pain is not controlled after a suitable trial period - i.e. the time in which the drug would be expected to have an effect. Orally administered paracetamol starts to have an analgesic effect at around 11 minutes but doesn't reach maximum effect until 37 minutes[40] so it could be argued that no step up should be taken until after that time. This may not be practical or desirable and the paramedic will need to make a clinical decision based upon the patient's needs.

The poor array of analgesics available to paramedics means that it is not really possible to create a three-step analgesic ladder in the manner proposed by WHO. Generally paracetamol and ibuprofen are indicated for mild to moderate pain and opiate-based analgesics are indicated for moderate to severe pain. Entonox (see Chapter 11) can feasibly be used for any severity of pain that warrants pharmacological intervention and is particularly useful as its short onset and duration of action mean that it can be used as a primary analgesic whilst other pain relief is administered. Entonox may also be used in conjunction with morphine during painful treatments such as splinting.[38]

Some patients with chronic pain may experience 'breakthrough' pain despite their usual regime of medicines. In situations like this it is likely that the patient will require large doses of analgesics in order to derive benefit; it is advisable to contact the patient's pain management team for advice and support.

Chapter Key Points

1. Pain is one of the most frequent symptoms presented by patients in the emergency care setting; it is a complex phenomenon that comprises both physical and emotional elements. Pain is a subjective experience and should rely heavily on the patient's self-report whenever possible.
2. Acute pain is a symptom with a discernible cause and usually subsides when injured tissues heal. Acute pain has a protective function.
3. Chronic pain is pain that has persisted beyond the time of healing; a classification based purely on causal agent is not achievable.
4. The history of the pain is very important when making a differential primary diagnosis.
5. Tools are available for the assessment of pain severity; the paramedic should be prepared to use more than one tool when required.
6. The use of non-verbal indicators may be helpful in those patients who have difficulty expressing themselves verbally.
7. Numerous non-pharmacological techniques can be used to alleviate pain; there is evidence to support their use.
8. Pharmacological interventions should be introduced in an incremental way bearing in mind the constraints of prehospital care and the needs of the patient.
9. The starting point for analgesia is a clinical decision.
10. Entonox is particularly useful as its short onset and duration of action mean that it can be used as a primary analgesic whilst other pain relief is administered.

References and Further reading

1 Cordell WH, Keene KK, Giles BK, Jones JB, Jones JH, Brizendine EJ. The high prevalence of pain in emergency medical care. *Am J Emerg Med* 2002;20(3):165-169.

2 Tuturro M. Pain, priorities and prehospital care. *Prehosp Emerg Care* 2002;6(4):486-488.

3 McLean SA, Maio RF, Domeier RM. The epidemiology of pain in the prehospital setting. *Prehosp Emerg Care* 2002;6(4):402-405.

4 Healthcare Commission. *Patient survey report 2004 - Emergency Department key findings.* London: Healthcare Commission, 2004.

5 Gray A, Johnson G, Goodacre S. Paramedic use of Nalbuphine in major injury. *Eur J Emerg Med* 1997;4:136-139.

6 LJ, Cooper JD, Chamber RM, Gradiesk RE. Prehospital use of analgesia for suspected extremity fractures. *Prehosp Emerg Care* 2000;4(3):205-208.

7 Vassiliadis J, Hitos K, Hill C. Factors influencing prehospital and emergency department analgesia administration to patients with femoral neck fractures. *Emerg Med* 2002;14:261-266.

8 McEachin CC, McDermott JT, Swor R. Few emergency medical services patients with lower-extremity fractures receive prehospital analgesia. *Prehosp Emerg Care* 2002;6(4):406-410.

9 Lord BA, Parsell B. Measurement of pain in the prehospital setting using a visual analogue scale. *Prehosp Disaster Med* 2003;18(4):353-358.

10 Kelly AM. Setting the benchmark for research in the management of acute pain in emergency departments. *Emerg Med* 2001;13(1):57-60.

11 Merskey H, Bogduk N (Eds) *International Association for the Study of Pain Task Force on Taxonomy, Classification of Chronic Pain*, 2nd edn. Seattle: IASP Press, 1994.

12 McCaffery M. *Nursing Practice Theories Related to Cognition, Bodily Pain and Non-Environmental Interactions.* Los Angeles: University of California, 1968.

13 Jones GE, Machen I. Pre-hospital pain management: the paramedics' perspective. *Accid Emerg Nurs* 2003;11:166-172.

14 Mann E, Carr E. *Pain Management.* Oxford: Blackwell Publishing, 2006.

15 Lamé IE, Peters ML, Vlaeyn JW, Kleef M, Patijn J. Quality of life in chronic pain is more associated with beliefs about pain, than with pain intensity. *Eur J Pain* 2005;9:15-24.

16 Newberry L, Barnett GK, Ballard N. A new mnemonic for chest pain assessment. *J Emerg Nurs* 2005;31:84-85.

17 Van Tubergen A, Debats I, Ryser L, Londono J, Burgos-Vargas R, Cardiel MH, Landewe R, Stucki G, Van Der HD. Use of a numerical rating scale as an answer modality in ankylosing spondylitis - specific questionnaires. *Arthrit Rheumat (Arthrit Care Res)* 2002;47:242-248.

18 Bijur PE, Latimer CT, Gallagher J. Validation of a verbally administered numerical rating scale of acute pain for use in the emergency department. *Acad Emerg Med* 2003;10(4):390.

19 Guyatt GH, Townsend M, Berman LB, Keller JL. A comparison of Likert and visual analogue scales for measuring change in function. *J Chron Dis* 1987;40:1129-1133.

20 Snow S, Kirwan JR. Visual analogue scales: a source of error. *Ann Rheumat Dis* 1988;47:526.

21 Williamson A, Hoggart B. Pain: a review of three commonly used pain rating scales. *J Clin Nurs* 2005;14:798-804.

22 Jensen MP, Turner JA, Romano JM. What is the maximum number of levels needed in pain intensity measurement? *Pain* 1994;58:387-392.

23 Jamison RN, Gracely RH, Raymond SA, Levine JG, Marino B, Herrmann TJ, Daly M, Fram D, Katz NP. Comparative study of electronic vs. paper VAS ratings: a randomized, crossover trial using healthy volunteers. *Pain* 2002;99:341-347.

24 Jensen MP, Karoly P, Braver S. The measurement of clinical pain intensity: a comparison of six methods. *Pain* 1986;27:117-126.

25 Carey SJ, Turpin C, Smith J, Whatley J, Haddox D. Improving pain management in an acute care setting: The Crawford Long Hospital of Emory University experience. *Orthopaed Nurs* 1997;16(4):29-36.

26 Krulewitch H, London MR, Skakel VJ, Lundstedt GJ, Thomason H, Brummel-Smith K. Assessment of pain in cognitively impaired older adults: A comparison of pain assessment tools and their use by nonprofessional caregivers. *J Am Geriat Soc* 2000;48:1607–1611.

27 Stuppy D. The Faces Pain Scale: reliability and validity with mature adults. *Appl Nurs Res* 1998;11(2);84–89.

28 Herr, K., Bjoro, K., & Decker, S. Tools for assessment of pain in nonverbal older adults with dementia: A state-of-the-science review. *J Pain Symptom Manage* 2006;31(2):170–192.

29 Warden Va, Hurley AC, Volicer L. Development and Psychometric Evaluation of the Pain Assessment in Advanced Dementia (PAINAD) Scale. *J Am Med Direct Ass* 2003;4(1):9–15.

30 Feldt KS. The Checklist of Nonverbal Pain Indicators (CNPI). *Pain Manage Nurs* 2000;1(1):13–21.

31 American Geriatrics Society Panel on Persistent Pain in Older Persons. Clinical practice guidelines: The management of persistent pain in older persons. *J Am Geriat Soc* 2002;50:S205–S224.

32 Tanabe P, Ferket K, Thomas R, Paice J, Marcantonio R. The effect of standard care, ibuprofen, and distraction on pain relief and patient satisfaction in children with musculoskeletal trauma. *J Emerg Nurs* 2002;28:118–125.

33 Cavender K, Goff MD; Hollon EC, Guzzetta CE. Parents' positioning and distracting children during venipuncture. Effects on children's pain, fear, and distress. *J Holist Nurs* 2004;22(1):32–56.

34 Joseph MH, Brill J, Zeltzer LK. Pediatric pain relief in trauma. *Pediatr Rev* 1999;20:75–83.

35 McCaffery M, Pasero C. *Pain: Clinical Manual for Nursing Practice*, 2nd edn. St. Louis: Mosby, 1999.

36 Hayward J. *Information, A Prescription Against Pain, The Study of Nursing Care*. Research project, series 2 (5). London: RCN, 1975.

37 Mitchell M. Patients' perceptions of pre-operative preparation for day surgery. *J Adv Nurs* 1997;26(2):356–363.

38 Joint Royal Colleges Ambulance Liaison Committee. *UK Ambulance Service Clinical Practice Guidelines version 4*. London: IHCD, 2006.

39 World Health Organization. *Cancer Pain Relief*. Geneva: WHO, 1986.

40 Moller PL, Sindet-Pedersen S, Petersen CT, Juhl GI, Dillenschneider A, Skoglund LA. Onset of acetaminophen analgesia: comparison of oral and intravenous routes after third molar surgery. *Br J Anaesth* 2005;94(5):642–648.

Chapter 16

Fracture and soft tissue injury management

Content

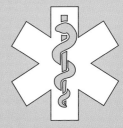

Despite the natural resilience of the human body extremes of force or weakening of structures can result in injury to bone, ligament and tendon. Whilst these conditions may vary markedly in their severity and aetiology, the similarity of the signs and symptoms of any injury to bone, ligament or tendon makes these conditions difficult to differentiate. As such a structured approach to the management of traumatic injury (and suspected non-traumatic injury such as pathological fractures) has core underlying principles that may be applied in any situation regardless of the eventual diagnosis. This chapter will set out generic guidance for the management of fractures, sprains, strains and dislocations in the acute emergency setting using current evidence where available.

Definitions: What are fractures, sprains, strains and dislocations?

A fracture is described as a break in the continuity of a bone; this can be the result of excessive force, repetitive load bearing activity (stress fracture) or abnormal bone structure (pathological fracture such as osteoporosis).[1] A sprain is defined as a stretching or tearing of a ligament, a ligament is a fibrous attachment that joins bone to bone and stabilises a joint.[2] A strain is a term used to describe the stretching and tearing of a muscle or tendon, a tendon being a fibrous continuation of the muscle that attaches muscle to bone and is essential for the leverage mechanisms of human movement.[2]

In a dislocation the bone is entirely displaced from the joint causing the articulating surfaces to no longer be intact. If the joint is only partially dislocated this is known as subluxation, this causes the articulating surfaces to only be in partial contact. In the event that the ligaments supporting a joint are disrupted causing an increased gap between the articulating surfaces, this is referred to as diastasis.[3] It is important to note that these conditions may not be present in isolation, the forces required to cause one type of injury may well cause a further injury.

General principles of musculoskeletal injury management

In the prehospital setting there are five key elements that underpin the management of musculoskeletal injury:

- Reduce pain
- Prevent further injury
- Ensure neurological and vascular supply distal to the injury
- Reduce the risk of fat embolism
- Promote recovery.

Pain control

Pain control in the acute management of musculoskeletal injury may take many forms ranging from simple reassurance, immobilisation of the limb (discussed later), pharmacological management (see Chapter 15, Pain Assessment and management) and the use of cold compresses. The use of reassurance as a method of pain relief is not based upon evidence; however reassuring patients is undoubtedly a major facet in the role of any prehospital and acute care practitioner.

The use of cold treatment for musculoskeletal injury has long been documented as a method of reducing pain and swelling at the site of an injury. There is little high level evidence to support this notion; however the application of a cold compress to an area will reduce the blood flow by vasoconstriction thus reducing inflammatory mediators and inflammation. The reduction in local body temperature will also slow nerve conduction, thus inhibiting pain sensation experienced. Care should be taken if using a cold compress as this may cause thermal burns to the site of application.

Immobilisation of the limb

The immobilisation of an injured limb is based upon the principles of general musculoskeletal injury management stated previously in this chapter. Through the application of splinting there are a number of benefits to the patient that are based upon sound pathophysiological reasoning. Splinting is applied as a method of reducing the movement of broken bone ends and to support the fracture site. Through the movement of broken bone ends pain is commonly experienced alongside an increased risk of damage to nerves, blood vessels, muscles and overlying skin. This can potentiate the injury increasing both mortality and morbidity; therefore the reduction in movement of the injured limb can reduce this risk. Immobilisation may reduce the occurrence of bleeding through allowing the formation of clots in damaged blood vessels and reduce the likelihood of potentially fatal fat emboli.

The placing of a limb in a splint of any form should reduce the pain for the patient and increase their comfort, thus subsequently reducing anxiety and the circulation of catecholamines which may cause peripheral vasoconstriction and reduced peripheral tissue oxygenation.[2,4]

Principles of splinting

The principles of splinting are a core element for any prehospital care provider ranging from the first aider to the advanced trauma specialist. The failure to effectively splint a musculoskeletal injury may result in increased pain and further injury, alongside the potential for increased damage to the injured area due to improper handling. The following principles of splinting should be considered whenever splinting is required (see Procedure below).

Procedure	Rationale
1. The injured area should be carefully visualised prior to splinting the limb.	It is imperative that the practitioner is aware of what potential injuries are present. Foreign bodies within the wound or severe bleeding from an open fracture should be considered prior to splint application as they are difficult to manage after a splint is applied.

Procedure	Rationale
2. Ensure that splinting is required.	Splinting as with all procedures is not without risk, the time taken to apply splinting may be detrimental in the multisystem trauma patient who requires rapid evacuation to an appropriate facility. The use of splints also limits the ability to visualise the patient, therefore the risks and benefits of splinting must be considered.
3. Prior to splinting assess the neurovascular status distal to the site of the injury and repeat after splinting.	A pre- and post-treatment assessment should always be considered to ensure that no harm is caused by your actions.
4. Manage wounds on the immobilised part prior to splinting.	Once the splint is applied it may be difficult to gain access to the wound to manage bleeding effectively.
5. The splint should immobilise the joint above and below the suspected injury site.	This will reduce the movement of the limb or injured part.
6. Pad the splint well.	This will reduce movement of the injured limb, increase comfort and reduce the likelihood of pressure injury.
7. Support the injured part proximally and distal to the injury whilst applying the splint.	This will provide manual stabilisation of the injured part whilst the splint is applied, this will reduce the pain experienced during the procedure.
8. If the injured limb is grossly deformed consider applying traction and straightening the limb.	This should only be considered if there is suspicion that the limb is being threatened by the injury. Signs include the loss of distal neurovascular supply and taut skin over the site of the suspected fracture (and suspicion that the bone fragment may pierce the skin).[5]
9. If it is not possible to straighten the limb to a near anatomical position, it should be splinted in the position of deformity.	Resistance or severe pain when attempting to re-align the limb should indicate that re-location is unlikely to be successful at that time therefore attempts should be ceased.
10. Splint firmly but not too tight.	Excessive tension may inhibit distal blood flow thus potentiating injury.
11. Try to avoid covering the finger or the toes of the patient when splinting (unless not feasible).	The fingers and toes are useful areas to check for distal neurovascular status following the application of a splint.

Types of splinting

Any device that is utilised to immobilise an injury can be considered a splint. There are a variety of widely used splinting devices within emergency care settings; this chapter will discuss the most commonly used; providing guidance on the benefits and limitations of each.

Slings and support bandages

A sling is commonly used for the splinting of a shoulder or arm injury, they may be used in isolation or as an adjunct to support additional devices such as a rigid splint (discussed later). A sling formed from a triangular bandage holds the injured limb to the body and takes some of the weight from the injured limb, potentially reducing pain caused by limb movement. Slings should be avoided in patients with a neck injury due to additional pressure being placed upon the neck. There are commonly two applications of a sling to the upper extremity, a broad arm sling and a high arm sling (or elevated sling). These differ in application however provide similar benefits to the patient. A broad arm sling is most commonly used for injuries at the elbow or below, whereas a high arm sling is used for injuries above the elbow; however there is little evidence to support either technique over the other therefore a sling should be applied to the comfort of the patient. A step-by-step guide to the application of a broad arm sling technique and high arm sling technique can be seen below.

The application of a broad arm sling

Procedure	Rationale
1. Gain informed consent and explain the procedure to the patient. Provide any required analgesia for the procedure to be undertaken.	A pain free and less anxious patient is easier to treat. Informed consent is essential in providing care for patients who are able to consent.
2. Ensure that the triangular bandage is clean and in good condition prior to use.	To reduce the risk of cross infection and ensure that the sling will not fail resulting in pain.
3. Lay the long side of the triangular bandage vertically down the uninjured side of the patient with the injured arm flexed at the elbow to 90° (if possible), the bandage should pass behind the injured arm (Figure 16.1).	A broad arm sling requires the injured arm to be flexed to approximately 90° for it to be effective, this will allow the arm to rest upon the sling. reducing pressure on the injury site.
4. Bring the bottom edge up and over the arm.	This will cradle the injured arm within the sling.
5. Tie the two ends together behind the patient's neck using a simple reef knot. Consider applying a pad beneath the knot (Figure 16.2). Pin or tie the point at the elbow to form a cradle.	A reef knot allows the knot to be easily undone, padding beneath the knot may reduce pain from friction or pressure from the knot upon the neck.

Procedure	Rationale
6. Re-check the distal neurovascular status of the limb.	This should be checked after any intervention to ensure that no harm is done.

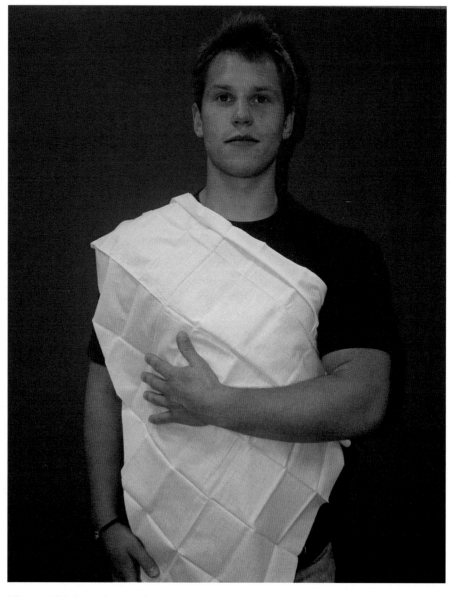

Figure 16.1 Broad arm sling step 1.

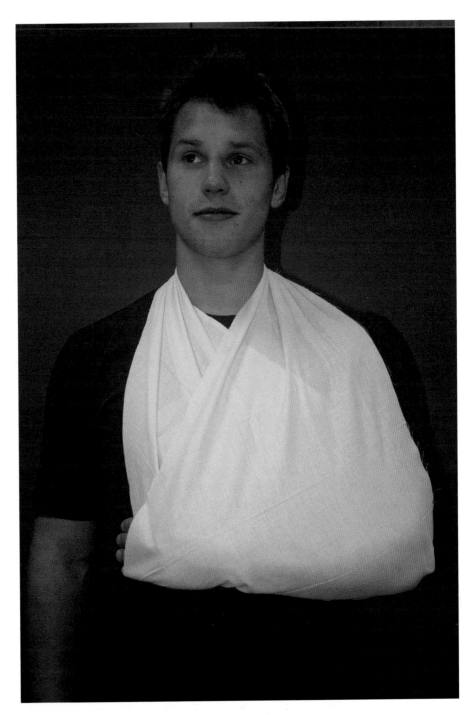

Figure 16.2 Broad arm sling step 2.

The application of a high arm sling

Procedure	Rationale
1. Gain informed consent and explain the procedure to the patient. Provide any required analgesia for the procedure to be undertaken. Ensure the triangular bandage is clean and undamaged.	A pain free and less anxious patient is easier to treat. Informed consent is essential in providing care for patients who are able to consent. All equipment should be checked to ensure it does not fail.
2. Place the sling over the injured arm with the arm elevated towards the opposing shoulder. The longest side of the triangular bandage should run from the shoulder of the uninjured arm towards the elbow of the injured arm.	The sling must be carefully applied to ensure it works as an effective cradle for the injured limb.
3. Pass the point of the longest side of the triangular bandage under the injured arm and behind the back of the patient. The end is then tied with the opposite end of the longest side behind the patient's neck using a reef knot (Figure 16.3). Consider padding beneath the knot.	A reef knot allows the knot to be easily undone, padding beneath the knot may reduce pain from friction or pressure from the knot upon the neck.
4. Ensure that the arm is comfortable and securely supported. Re-check the distal neurovascular status of the injured limb.	Always check that any interventions are effective, if not then re-consider your actions or remedy and problems.

With the application of a sling the support to the limb can be enhanced by the use of an additional support bandage around the torso. This will serve to further immobilise the limb and is particularly useful in shoulder dislocations and clavicle injuries.

Box splints

Box splints are a commonly carried by emergency care personnel, yet are often overlooked due to the simplicity of their use and due to the favourability of other devices. A box splint is most commonly used for lower leg injuries; however they may be used for knee and arm injuries also. These splints consist of three long padded sides and a foot piece (Figure 16.4) which is designed to place the foot at a 90° angle (anatomical position).

The splint forms a 'box' around the injured limb with one side exposed to allow for ease of application and review of the limb once it has been splinted. Box splints are effective in immobilising a straight limb, especially when combined with additional padding. However box splints are of limited use in a deformed limb due to their rigid structure which will not conform to the shape of the limb. A step by step guide to using a box splint is shown below.

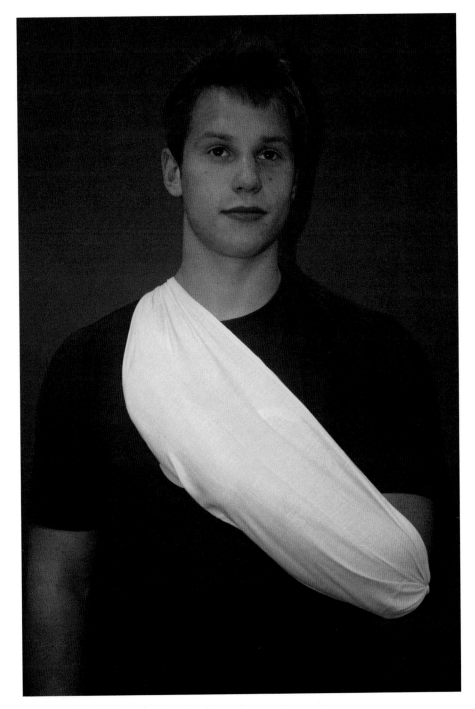

Figure 16.3 High arm sling step 2.

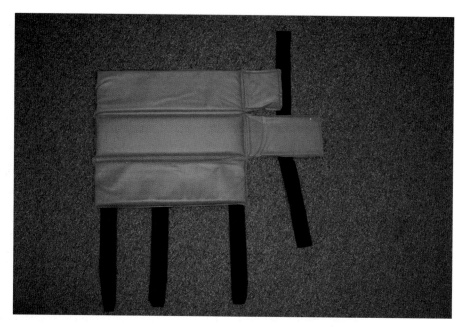

Figure 16.4 A box splint.

Application of a box splint

Procedure	Rationale
1. Gain informed consent and explain the procedure to the patient. Provide any required analgesia for the procedure to be undertaken. Ensure the equipment is clean and undamaged.	A pain free and less anxious patient is easier to treat. Informed consent is essential in providing care for patients who are able to consent. All equipment should be checked to ensure it does not fail or provide an infection risk.
2. The injured limb (leg) should be exposed and footwear removed if possible.	This is desirable for both examination and post immobilisation checks.
3. The leg should be supported manually and carefully raised, the splint should be passed under the leg.	Support is required to ensure that the injury is not worsened by the movement and also to reduce pain.
4. The two sides of the splint should be folded up against the leg to form a box around the limb, the foot piece should be placed against the sole of the foot at 90° or in a position that is comfortable.	This will box in the leg and provide stability, it may be necessary to add additional padding at this point to support the limb.

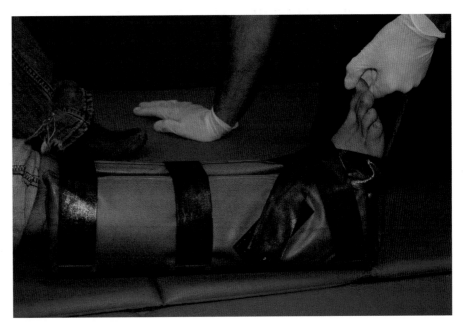

Figure 16.5 Application of a box splint.

Procedure	Rationale
5. The Velcro straps should be carefully placed over the leg avoiding the area of injury, the foot strap should be passed over the top of the foot (Figure 16.5).	This provides firm support for the limb, passing the straps tightly over the injured area may worsen the pain or injury and should be avoided.
6. Re-check the distal neurovascular status of the limb.	This should be checked after any intervention to ensure that no harm is done.

THINK

You are called to see a patient with an extremely deformed lower leg; will a box splint be appropriate? If not what can you do to immobilise the limb?

Vacuum splints

A vacuum splint consists of a sealed vinyl coated polyester mattress filled with polystyrene beads that is normally pliable; however when air is removed from within the mattress by a pump the splint becomes rigid and conforms to the set position. There are a variety of vacuum splint products used by emergency and voluntary services; therefore this section will discuss the general principles of use. Vacuum splints are particularly popular within the emergency services due to the versatility of the product and ability to conform to even the most deformed limb. The vacuum splint has the additional benefit of being suitable for spinal immobilisation on small children.

A step-by-step guide to the basic use of a vacuum splint upon an injured limb is given below.

Application of a vacuum splint

Procedure	Rationale
1. Gain informed consent and explain the procedure to the patient. Provide any required analgesia for the procedure to be undertaken. Ensure the equipment is clean, undamaged and in good working order.	A pain-free and less anxious patient is easier to treat. Informed consent is essential in providing care for patients who are able to consent. All equipment should be checked to ensure it does not fail or provide an infection risk.
2. Applying a vacuum splint requires a minimum of two operators.	This ensures that the injury site is stabilised during the splinting process.
3. Choose the correct splint size.	The splint should be large enough to extend beyond the joints above and below the injury, if the injury is a dislocation the splint should be large enough to extend beyond both sides of the dislocated joint.
4. One operator should stabilise the injury at all times, the other operator should lay the splint flat on the floor and smooth the splint to a uniform thickness.	The polystyrene balls are essential in making the splint rigid, therefore they are required to be uniformly spread; failure to do this may result in some areas of the splint remaining pliable.
5. Place the splint (pump valve on the outside) around the injury.	Access to the valve is essential or else the air cannot be removed.
6. Secure the splint in place using the Velcro straps (or equivalent) (Figure 16.6).	This supports the limb within the splint.
7. Connect the vacuum pump to the valve and gently withdraw the air, as this occurs the other operator should continue to support the injury and gently mould the splint if required.	Continual support is required until the splint application is fully completed.

Procedure	Rationale
8. Continue until the splint is as rigid as required, disconnect the pump and re-tighten the straps if necessary (Figure 16.7).	As the splint becomes more rigid the straps may become loose, therefore it may be necessary to re-apply the strapping.
9. Re-check the distal neurovascular status of the limb.	This should be checked after any intervention to ensure that no harm is done.

from Ferno-Washington 2000.[6]

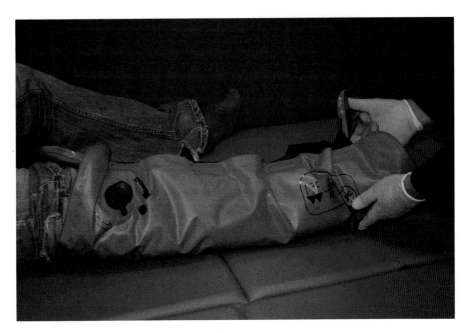

Figure 16.6 Vac splint wrap around leg.

Neighbour strapping

Neighbour strapping is a simple first aid principle that requires the strapping of an injured part to the neighbouring part, commonly used in finger or toe injuries the injured digit will be strapped to the one next to it to provide support. This concept may also be utilised in other injuries such as neck of femur fractures. These injuries are difficult to immobilise any other way in the prehospital setting therefore the strapping to another limb provides a quick and simple method of applying immobilisation principles. A number of methods of neighbour strapping can be used including the use of adhesive tape in finger or toe injury, however in the acute setting consideration must be given to the pain caused by the removal of adhesive tape. The more commonly used method of neighbour strapping is the use of either fracture straps (elasticated Velcro straps that stretch around the injured and non injured limb) or the use of broadly folded triangular bandages. These are commonly used in

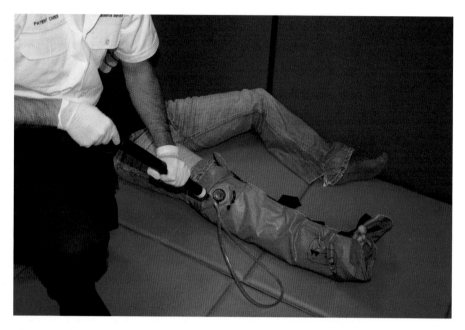

Figure 16.7 Vac splint around leg secure straps (completed).

the management of neck of femur fractures as other forms of splinting are not ideally suited to this injury. These straps can simply be placed around the injured limb securing it to the non-injured limb for support. Padding should be placed between the limbs to aid comfort and reduce pressure over bony processes. The straps should not be placed tightly over the injury site as this may cause increased pain and movement of bone ends.

Traction splints

Traction is a method commonly utilised in fracture management (especially that of femoral shaft fractures), through the application of distal traction to a deformed fractured limb there are a number of potential benefits. Firstly traction will act to reduce a deformed limb back towards its' anatomical shape, secondly applied traction will act to 'pull' apart the fractured bone ends to reduce the likelihood of neurovascular damage through impingement by bony fragments and reduce pain. A third benefit is the reduction of bleeding through re-shaping of the muscle mass surrounding the injury. In the event of shaft of femur fractures the strong muscles of the thigh will shorten the limb causing the bone ends to overlap causing an increased risk of neurovascular injury, pain and bleeding. When the normally cylindrical muscles of the thigh are shortened by a fracture they become more spherical in shape, this will increase the internal volume of the muscle and subsequently increase the potential space for accumulating blood. Through the application of traction bone ends are separated and the normal shape of the thigh muscles is restored thus reducing the likelihood of excessive bleeding.[4,7]

Traction may be applied using either manual means (by gentle pulling on the limb) or with the use of traction devices such as the Sager or Donway splint (which are used in mid-shaft of femur fractures only). Whichever means of traction is used careful consideration must be given as to the correct recognition of the need for traction and any detrimental effects that may be caused by such actions.

There are a number of potential contraindications to the application of traction splints; these can be seen below:

- Fractures around the knee
- Dislocation of the hip
- Fracture dislocation of the knee
- Ankle injuries
- Simple fractures of the lower third of the tibia and fibula
- Fractures of the pelvis
- Fractured neck of femur.

From Greaves et al. (2006)[4]; Lee & Porter (2005).[8]

These general principles of contraindications to traction are based upon the potential to potentiate injury to joints through applied force and therefore any potential joint injury should be considered prior to any traction. It is also essential to refer to manufacturer and local guidelines for contraindications for traction use as they may differ markedly.

Whilst traction splints are currently widely available in prehospital care there is little evidence to suggest that their use of benefit over traditional immobilisation methods, therefore the use must currently be based upon pathophysiological considerations.[9,10]

The Donway splint

The Donway splint is a device that cradles the injured limb with the ankle of the limb securely strapped by an ankle support and applied around the thigh to maintain stability. Using a pump, the upper and lower halves of the splint are pushed apart by increasing air pressure. Once the pressure reaches an effective level and the patient is comfortable securing screws are tightened to maintain the position of both ends of the splint and the pressure is released through a release valve.

A step-by-step guide to the application of the Donway splint can be seen below.

Application of the Donway splint

Procedure	Rationale
1. Gain informed consent and explain the procedure to the patient. Provide any required analgesia for the procedure to be undertaken. Ensure the equipment is clean, undamaged and in good working order.	A pain-free and less anxious patient is easier to treat. Informed consent is essential in providing care for patients who are able to consent. All equipment should be checked to ensure it does not fail or provide an infection risk.

Procedure	Rationale
2. Applying a splint requires a minimum of two operators, this allows for support of the limb and for manual traction to be applied if required.	This ensures that the injury site is stabilised during the splinting process.
3. Feed the ischial ring under the knee and adjusted around the thigh with the buckle fastened loosely.	The natural hollow of the knee provides a useful point of access around the leg with minimal movement.
4. Depress the air valve to ensure that there is no pressure retained within the system.	Excess pressure in the system can cause the equipment to be problematic to use and has a potential to cause injury.
5. Unlock the collets (securing screws), raise the footplate into the upright position and place the splint over the leg.	The foot must be securely strapped around the ankle to ensure adequate traction is applied.
6. Adjust the side arms to the desired length and attach to the ischial ring pegs (twist the side arms to lock in place).	If the side arms are to short there will be excessive movement of the splint when pressure is applied.
7. Open the ankle strap and carefully place the patient's heel in the padded portion of the strap with the heel against the footplate.	The placement of the ankle strap and footplate are of paramount importance as they are designed to ensure traction is along the axis of the limb and pressure is applied equally across the surface of the foot. Misplacement can cause maligned traction of the limb resulting I potentiating the injury.
8. Maintaining the foot against the footplate adjust the lower Velcro attachment to ensure that the padded support is positioned high on the ankle.	
9. Criss-cross the straps tightly over the instep starting with the longest strap. Tighten the straps around the footplate and secure with Velcro (Figure 16.8).	
10. Apply pneumatic pressure to the desired level using the pump, upon completion tighten the ischial strap to secure the ring in the ischial load position.	The recommended operating range of the splint is 10-40lbs of traction; excessive force will cause safety valves to release pressure. Pressure below this range will potentially be ineffective.
11. Align the leg supports with the calf and thigh and apply by passing the strap under the leg, passing back over the frame and back under the leg to form a cradle (Figure 16.9).	This will cradle the injured limb thus reducing movement.
12. Apply the knee strap by passing under the knee passing around the frame and fastening above the knee (Figure 16.9).	This will stop knee flexion and subsequent limb movement that may cause pain and mal-alignment of the limb.

Procedure	Rationale
13. The leg is now supported and in traction so the heel stand can be raised.	This will elevate the limb slightly to reduce pressure on the limb and reduce swelling.
14. Turn the securing screws (collets) until hand tight and apply a further quarter turn to secure the side arms, this will allow the pressure to be released from the system by pressing the release valve until the gauge shows zero pressure.	Releasing the pressure following locking the side arms will reduce the likelihood of further injury to the patient in the event of pressure loss within the system.
15. Re-check the distal neurovascular status of the limb.	This should be checked after any intervention to ensure that no harm is done.
16. The Donway splint should remain on the limb until definitive care is provided (usually surgical intervention).	The splint should only be removed if there are signs that the application is worsening the patient condition, premature release of the traction will result in pain and may potentiate injury.

From Thomas Biomedical.[11]

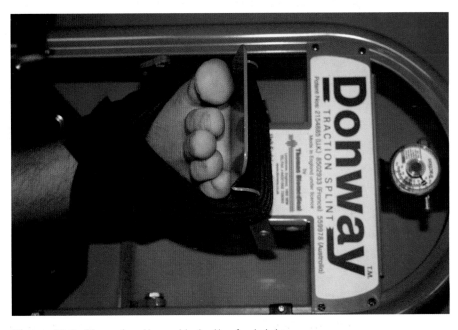

Figure 16.8 Strapping the ankle to the footplate.

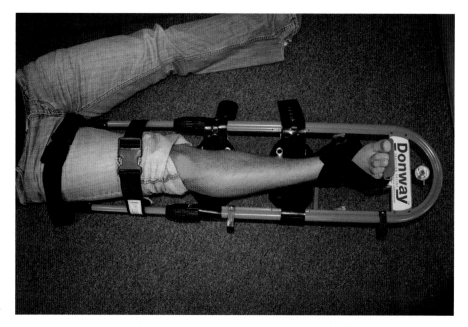

Figure 16.9 Completing the splinting process.

Whilst the Donway splint is carried by a number of prehospital care agencies, it is not without flaws and limitations. One major difficulty of the Donway splint is the size of the device that makes not only carriage of the device problematic but subsequent transfer of the patient difficult especially in small vehicles or air transport. Another reported issue with systems such as the Donway splint is that only one limb can be splinted using the device; devices such as the Sager splint (below) offer the ability to splint both legs (in the presence of bilateral femur fractures) and are smaller in size therefore easier to transport.

The Sager splint

The Sager splint is a traction splint that is lightweight and has the advantage of being smaller than other commercially available splint such as the Donway; this has the benefit of being easier for transport purposes and manual handling. An additional benefit of the Sager splint is the ability to splint and apply traction to either one or two legs using the same device. A step-by-step guide to the application of a Sager splint is provided below; as with all devices referral to manufacturer's guidelines is recommended:

The application of the Sager splint

Procedure	Rationale
1. Gain informed consent and explain the procedure to the patient. Provide any required analgesia for the procedure to be undertaken. Ensure the equipment is clean, undamaged and in good working order.	A pain-free and less anxious patient is easier to treat. Informed consent is essential in providing care for patients who are able to consent. All equipment should be checked to ensure it does not fail or provide an infection risk.
2. Applying a splint requires a minimum of two operators, this allows for support of the limb and for manual traction to be applied if required.	This ensures that the injury site is stabilised during the splinting process.
3. Position the splint between the patient's legs, resting the ischial/perineal cushion against the ischial tuberosity (midway between the femur and the symphysis pubis). Ensure that the scrotum is clear of the cushion. The shortest end of the ischial pad should be toward the ground.	The ischial tuberosity rests in the same plane as the femur, this will align the traction along the axis of the femur. Compression of the scrotum beneath the cushion will result in pain and injury.
4. Apply the securing bridle around the upper thigh of the injured limb.	This stabilises the splint around the limb, care is required if applying the bridle over the fracture site.
5. Lift the button latch and extend the inner shaft until the crossbar rests adjacent to the patient's heels.	Unnecessary extension of the inner shaft beyond the feet makes the device more difficult to use and transport.
6. Position and secure the ankle harnesses by passing beneath the heel and securing above the medial and lateral malleoli of the ankle, ensure that the harness is snugly fitted to the crossbar (Figure 16.10). This should be applied to both ankles.	Secure fitting of the harness to the ankle and the crossbar is essential to reduce the risk of slippage of the limbs and loss of traction.
7. Grasp the splint shaft with one hand and the traction bar with the other and gently extend the inner shaft until the desired amount of traction is reached (this is generally 10% of the patients body weight to a maximum of 15 lb).	It is important to stabilise the splint whilst applying traction so that control is maintained. Excessive pressure may cause further damage to the limb, therefore should be avoided.
8. Slide the elastic cravats beneath the hollow of the knee and firmly secure in position around both legs (large cravat to the thigh, smaller cravat around the calves). This can be seen in Figure 16.11.	This maintains limb stability and reduce movement.

Procedure	Rationale
9. Apply the figure of eight around the feet	This maintains foot stability and reduces movement.
10. Re-check the distal neurovascular status of the limb.	This should be checked after any intervention to ensure that no harm is done.
11. The Sager splint should remain on the limb until definitive care is provided (usually surgical intervention). If traction removal is required this can be achieved by lifting the pressure release spring (with support on the shaft to release pressure gently).	The splint should only be removed if there are signs that the application is worsening the patient condition, premature release of the traction will result in pain and may potentiate injury.

From Sager (2004).[12]

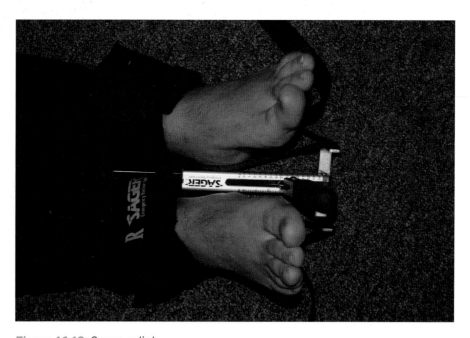

Figure 16.10 Sager splint.

SAM splints

SAM splints are formed from a thin layer of aluminium alloy sandwiched between two layers of closed cell foam. These splints are pliable and flexible when unrolled, however when bent into a curve become rigid and strong. The SAM splint has the benefit of exceptional diversity of usage and can potentially be used on any bone of the body (depending upon the size of the splint).[13] The Sam splint is designed for use as a rigid splint that can be conformed to any limb or bone, the splint can immobilise and provide compression of an injury site to potentially reduce haemorrhage.

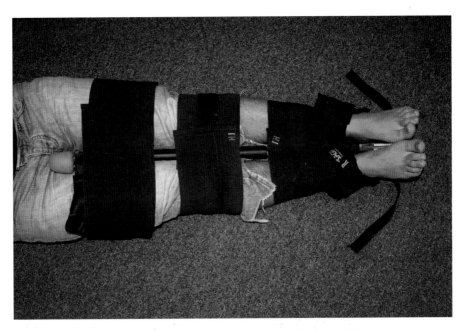

Figure 16.11 Sager splint.

Scenario

You are a spectator at a motorcross event that has no medical cover; a rider has come off of their bike and has a suspected fractured forearm and lower leg. You are called to assist but you have no equipment. What methods could you use to assist in immobilising the patient's injuries? What are the risks involved in this to both yourself and the patient?

Pelvic fractures

Despite being a relatively rare occurrence pelvic fractures are noteworthy due the specific needs for their management and the likelihood of severe haemodynamic instability from internal haemorrhage.[14] Pelvic fractures are estimated to occur in between 5 and 11.9% of patients with severe blunt trauma, with mortality rates ranging between 7.6 and 25%.[14-16] Pelvic stabilisation in the acute phases of management in pelvic fractures has been demonstrated as effective in reducing this severe haemorrhage.[17]

There are a number of methods that may be utilised for the reduction of pelvic fractures, including circumferential wrapping by a sheet, belt or pelvic circumferential compression device (PCCD), such as the SAM sling.[17,18] These methods seek to control haemorrhage by stabilising fracture sites to promote clot formation and through the reduction of potential pelvic volume for blood accumulation.[19] Whilst the use of sheets or belts are recommended by the American College of Surgeons Committee on Trauma[20] for advanced trauma life support, there is contention as to the efficacy of such methods with little research to support their use. Recent studies into the use of circumferential compression by the use of PCCD has demonstrated that the use of such devices is timely and may reduce pelvic width and subsequent potential for bleeding.[17,18,19,21]

The SAM sling

The SAM sling is a recent commercially available pelvic compression device that has been proven in a number of studies to provide stability and compression of pelvic fractures.[17,18,19,21] The SAM sling (from SAM Medical, 2007)[22] can be seen in Figure 16.12.

The SAM sling is scientifically and clinically proven to provide safe and effective force; stabilising pelvic fractures. The standard sling size fits 95% of population without cutting or trimming which facilitates ease of use in the prehospital setting. The sling has been designed to allow for application by a single user rapidly (usually less than one minute) and does not require fine touch to operate; it provides clear feedback by sound ('click') and feel to confirm correct application. The sling is also designed to comply with infection control procedures by cleansing with standard detergents or antimicrobial solutions.

The procedure for the application of a SAM sling can be seen below.

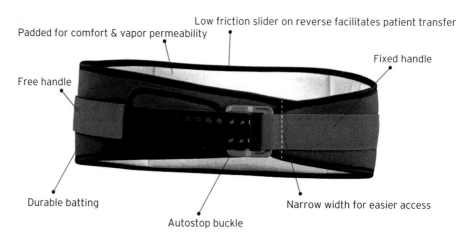

Figure 16.12 The SAM sling. Reproduced with permission of SAM Medical Products.

The application of the SAM sling

Procedure	Rationale
1. Unfold sling with the white surface facing up.	This allows for the easy to slide surface to be in contact with the ground thus facilitating sliding of the sling under the patient.
2. Place white side of Sling beneath patient at level of buttocks (greater trochanters/ symphysis pubis). This can be achieved by sliding under the natural hollow of the back or under the knees and sliding to the correct position.	This is the ideal area to provide compression of the pelvis.
3. Firmly close Sling by placing black Velcro® side of flap down on the black Velcro® strip. Fold back material as needed. Try to place buckle close to midline (Figure 16.13).	Central placement of the buckle aids the application of tension equally across the pelvis.
4. Grab orange free handle on outer surface of flap and release from flap by pulling upward. With or without assistance, firmly pull both orange handles in opposite directions to tighten sling.	The compression of the sling applies pressure to the pelvis thus stabilising potential pelvic fractures.
5. Keep pulling free handle until you feel or hear the buckle lock or click. As soon as the buckle clicks, maintain tension and firmly press orange handle onto the black Velcro® strip. Note: Do not be concerned if you hear a second 'click' after the sling is secured.	The sling is designed to apply a preset level of pressure across the pelvis excessive or inadequate force has the potential to be ineffective or potentiate injury.
6. To remove sling, lift orange free handle away from flap by pulling upward. Maintain tension and slowly allow sling to loosen.	The sling should ideally remain in place until definitive care is provided (i.e. surgery). Removal of the sling prematurely may cause subsequent bleeding.

From SAM Medical (2007).[22]

There are a number of alternative pelvic slings and compression devices, therefore please refer to individual policies and procedures for the devices available in your work area.

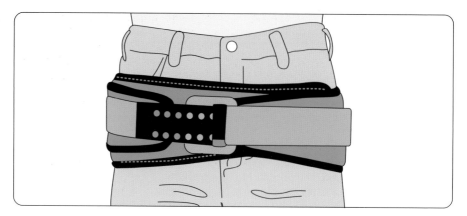

Figure 16.13 Application of the SAM sling. Reproduced with permission of SAM Medical Products.

Chapter Key Points

1. The management of sprains, strains, fractures and dislocations follows a number of core principles that should be followed to reduce pain and prevent further injury.
2. Any potential injury should be assessed before and after any intervention to ensure that no further damage is caused by healthcare staff.
3. Ensure that you are familiar with the immobilisation devices within your work area and that you are able to follow manufacturer's instructions.
4. Remember to consider appropriate analgesia prior to any immobilisation as the act itself may cause pain to the patient.

References and Further reading

1 Douglas G, Nicol F, Robertson C. *Macleod's Clinical Examination*, 11th edn. Edinburgh: Elsevier, 2005.
2 Marieb E, Hoehn K. *Human Anatomy and Physiology*, 7th edn. London: Pearson International, 2007.
3 Caroline N. *Emergency Care in the Streets*, 6th edn. London: Bartlett Publishers, 2008.
4 Greaves I, Porter K, Hodgetts T, Woollard M. *Emergency Care: A Textbook for Paramedics*. London: Elsevier, 2006.
5 Joint Royal Colleges Ambulance Liaison Committee. *UK Ambulance Service Clinical Practice Guidelines*. London: JRCALC, 2006.
6 Ferno-Washington. *Vacuum Splints Kit: User's Manual: 234-2124-00*. Ohio: Ferno-Washington Inc, 2000.
7 Borschneck A. Why traction? *JEMS*. 1985;44-45.
8 Lee C, Porter K. Prehospital management of lower limb fractures. *Emerg Med J* 2005;22: 660-663.

9 Wood S, Vrahas M, Wedel S. Femur fracture immobilization with traction splints in multisystem trauma patients. *Pre-Hosp Emerg Care* 2003;7(2):241-243.

10 Chu R, Browne G, Lam L. Traction splinting of femoral shaft fractures in a paediatric emergency department: Time is of the essence? *Emerg Med* 2003;15:447-452.

11 Thomas Biomedical. *Donway Traction Splint: Instructions for Use*. Herefordshire: Thomas Biomedical, 2000.

12 Sager. *Instructors' Manual: The Science of Traction Splinting*. Accessed on-line: www.sagersplints.com. [21/06/08]. California: Sager.

13 SAM Medical. *SAM Splint: The Pocket Cast*. Accessed on-line at: www.sammedical.com. [21/06/08]. Portland: SAMMEDICAL,

14 Lee C, Porter K. The prehospital management of pelvic fractures. *Emerg Med J* 2007;24: 130-133.

15 Poole G, Ward E. Causes of mortality in patients with pelvic fracture. *Orthopaedics* 1994;17:691-696.

16 Alonso J, Lee J, Burgess A, Browner B. The management of complicated orthopaedic injuries. *Surg Clin North Am* 1996;76:879-903.

17 Krieg J, Mohr M, Mirza A, Bottlang M. Pelvic circumferential compression in the presence of soft tissue injuries: A case report. *J Trauma* 2005;59:470-472.

18 Bottlang M *et al*. Noninvasive reduction of open-book pelvic fractures by circumferential compression. *J Orth Trauma* 2002;16(6):367-373.

19 Krieg J *et al*. Emergent stabilisation of pelvic ring injuries by controlled circumferential compression: A clinical trial. *Trauma* 2005;59:659-664.

20 American College of Surgeons. *Advanced Trauma Life Support for Doctors: Instructor Course Manual*. 1997;24:206-209.

21 Bottlang M. *et al*. Emergent management of pelvic ring fractures with the use of circumferential compression. *J Bone Joint Surg* 2002;84(suppl 2).

22 SAM Medical. *SAM Pelvic Sling: Powerpoint Presentation*. Portland: SAMMEDICAL, 2007.

Chapter 17

Spinal management

Content

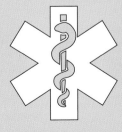

Spinal cord injury (SCI) most commonly affects young, fit people and generally leads to long-term disability that can seriously impact on a person's quality of life. In rare cases where the cord is damaged in the upper cervical regions, paralysis of the diaphragm and respiratory muscles can lead to immediate death. Increasingly, there are cases where the damage to the cord is only partial and considerable recovery is possible. Partial cord damage may affect individual sensory or motor nerve tracts, thereby producing varying long-term disability. Recovery is dependent upon recognition of the condition and application of the appropriate management.

Early data suggest that 3% to 25% of spinal cord injuries occur after the initial injury,[1] although the actual effect of spinal immobilisation on mortality, neurological injury, spinal stability and adverse effects in trauma patients remains uncertain. What is known and is of particular interest is that airway obstruction is a major cause of preventable death in trauma patients, and spinal immobilisation, particularly of the cervical spine, can contribute to airway compromise. This leads to the conclusion that immobilisation may potentially increase mortality and morbidity.[2]

Relevant gross anatomy

Please also refer to an appropriate anatomy textbook (see reference 3).

The spinal cord is approximately 42–45 cm in length and extends from the foramen magnum to the superior border of the second lumbar vertebra. Its diameter is approximately 2 cm at the mid-thoracic point, a little larger in both the inferior cervical and mid-lumbar enlargements, and narrowest at the inferior tip.[3] This means that there is more space for the cord in the superior cervical regions so that SCI may be ameliorated with adequate immobilisation. In the cervical and lumbar enlargements, the cord tends to be wide and the spinal canal relatively narrow and injury in these areas is likely to cause SCI.[4]

Evidence on how to immobilise the spine

The literature

There are no randomised controlled trials evaluating the various out-of-hospital spinal immobilisation techniques[2] so it is not possible to state categorically which method(s) should and shouldn't be used. However, certain known facts suggest that some methods may be better than others for immobilising the spine.

The UK ambulance services do not tend to use soft collars and with good reason. Soft collars do not limit movement[5,6] so are of no benefit where the risk of cervical spine injury is high. There are variances between different types of semi-rigid collars, but small studies have not demonstrated any clear reduction of movement,[7] suggesting that the application is more important than the actual device. What has been shown on healthy volunteers is that semi-rigid cervical collars when used alone only reduce movement by between 31% and 45%,[8] which clearly shows that a collar on its own is insufficient to protect the cervical spine. In the same study it was found that head blocks and straps produced a reduction of between 58-64% but when head blocks and straps were in place the addition of a collar was not beneficial. This is important when considering the impact of cervical collars on intracranial pressure (ICP), which is discussed later.

There has been a tendency for paramedics to routinely use long boards for the immobilisation of patients, but there may be alternatives to this approach. Long boards have been shown to be inferior to devices such as the vacuum mattress in terms of reduction of movement and patient comfort,[9,10] although the vacuum mattress is not suitable for extrication. Extrication devices such as the Kendrick extrication device (KED) have also proven to be better than long boards at reducing rotational movement and, where time is not critical, the use of such a device may be warranted.[11,12]

What is essential when using a rigid long board is to minimise the time a patient is on the board. It is suggested that a patient should be on an unpadded long board for no more than 45 minutes.[13,14] The problems related to pressure ulceration are discussed later in this chapter.

A further consideration is the method used to place the patient onto the immobilisation equipment and none are without their risks. There will inevitably be a small amount of spinal movement when transferring a patient to immobilisation equipment but there appears to be little consensus as to which method should be used.

Log rolling has been shown to cause significant motion of the head and thoracolumbar spine,[15,16] although it is not known if the range of movement would actually exacerbate the clinical condition. There is a suggestion that the variation in the amount of flexion and extension between different techniques is not clinically significant[17] although axial rotation appears to be more pronounced in the log-roll method than when using a 6-person lift or a lift-and-slide technique.[18] Log-rolling should not be used where there is suspicion of a pelvic fracture as it may disrupt clots and promote further blood loss.[19]

JRCALC[4] are suggesting that use of a scoop stretcher may be safer for lifting patients onto a long board. This is supported by research that has shown that the scoop stretcher causes significantly less movement on application compared with the long board.[20] It may be worth immobilising the patient on the scoop stretcher rather than transferring to a long board as this reduces the need for secondary transfers and a log-roll manoeuvre to remove the patient from the device. It has also been shown that immobilisation on the scoop provided increased comfort levels compared with the long spinal-board.[20]

The optimum positioning for cervical immobilisation cannot be achieved without some form of padding between the back of the head and the long board. In healthy adults, a slight degree of flexion equivalent to 2 cm of occiput elevation produces a favourable increase in spinal canal/spinal cord ratio at levels C5 and C6, a region of frequent unstable spine injuries.[21]

Hazards and complications associated with spinal immobilisation

There are numerous potential complications associated with spinal immobilisation, particularly cervical spine immobilisation using a semi-rigid collar. These include:

- Airway problems (including increased risk of aspiration)
- Increased intracranial pressure

- Restricted respiration
- Dysphagia
- Skin ulceration
- Pain.

THINK

Before reading the next section, make a list of how spinal immobilisation may cause airway problems and the strategies you have for managing them.

Airway problems

Airway management is made more difficult in patients with suspected spinal injury by the need to maintain in-line immobilisation of the patient's head and neck. This restricts access to the airway and also makes it more difficult to clear vomit or blood because the usual postural drainage manoeuvres may be contraindicated. Application of a semi-rigid cervical collar exacerbates the problem by significantly reducing mouth opening, which could hinder definitive airway placement.[22] Loosening the cervical collar or removing the anterior portion of the collar before attempts at tracheal intubation may improve the view that can be attained during laryngoscopy.[22] The flexible bougie is the preferred option for first-line use in all cases to maximise rates of intubation on first attempt.[23]

The risk of aspiration is increased for the supine trauma patient. Because trauma is unexpected, the patient is likely to have a full stomach and injury may reduce their ability to protect the airway.[24] In the supine position, passive regurgitation or vomiting may result in aspiration of gastric contents and impaired oxygenation.[24] There is debate about whether the long board helps to protect against aspiration, a belief borne out by the idea that it facilitates turning a vomiting patient onto their side. It has been suggested that rapid log-rolling is considered a more appropriate strategy to turn the trauma patient that is vomiting,[25] but this requires four people to carry out the manoeuvre and one person to suction the patient. One person holds the head and coordinates the roll, while three others roll the chest, pelvis, and limbs so that the head, neck, body and limbs move in an aligned manner. The fifth person carefully suctions the oral cavity and avoids inducing further gagging or vomiting.[26] Consideration may need to be given to administration of a suitable antiemetic and gastric decompression (where trained to do so).

The use of an extrication device such as the KED may help to alleviate some of these problems by allowing the patient to be managed in a position other than supine.

Increased intracranial pressure

Correctly fitted cervical collars cause an increase in intracranial pressure,[27-31] most likely because they reduce venous return from the head. Evidence suggests that in patients with head injury, loosening of the cervical collar once the patient is securely on the board may prevent compromise of venous return and exacerbation of raised intracranial pressure.[32]

Restricted respiration

Studies have shown clinically significant effects on respiration using both the long board and the vacuum mattress.[33] This is significant because restricted chest expansion can result in low tidal volumes and exacerbate the physiological effects of the supine position on respiratory function.[34] The supine position leads to a reduced functional residual capacity and means that fewer alveoli are available for external respiration. Given that trauma leads to an increased metabolic rate and oxygen demand, it is likely that high-concentration supplemental oxygen will be needed to help meet the patient's oxygen requirements. These physiological effects are of particular concern where patients have associated thoracic injuries that further compromise respiratory function; it is possible that these patients will require ventilator support.

Dysphagia

Dysphagia (difficulty swallowing) has been linked to the application of a semi-rigid cervical collar but this problem has been noted specifically in patients with unusual neck anatomy following neurosurgical procedures.[35] It is unclear whether this may also be a problem in prehospital emergency immobilisation but it is worth bearing in mind given the potential airway obstruction that may occur as a result of dysphagia.

Skin ulceration

Cutaneous pressure ulceration is of significant concern for the spinally injured patient and every effort should be made to minimise the amount of time a patient spends on high-pressure surfaces such as the long board and scoop. The duration of contact and high interface pressure are predictors of cutaneous pressure ulceration in the trauma patient.[36] Ischaemia occurs when the pressure between the immobilisation device and the skin exceeds or approaches capillary pressure. At 32 mmHg of pressure, capillary blood flow becomes compromised causing hypoxia, necrosis and ulceration.[37] The intensity of pressure is proportional to the time necessary to cause tissue damage so that the higher the pressure, the shorter the contact time required to cause irreversible tissue damage. It is suggested that a sustained interface pressure of 35 mmHg for 2 hours and 60 mmHg for 1 hour is sufficient to cause irreversible tissue damage.[37] Studies on healthy subjects have recorded interface pressures of 233.5 mmHg and 82.9 mmHg at the sacrum and thorax on a rigid spine board.[34,38]

Pain

Spinal immobilisation devices can induce pain, even in those with no injuries. Various studies have shown that healthy volunteers immobilised with rigid neck collars and long boards complain of pain and discomfort after approximately 30 minutes.[39,34,40] The pain is most often located at the heels, sacrum, thoracic spine, elbows, occipital region and chin where the interface pressures are at their highest.[2,34,40] It has been suggested that after 30 minutes it becomes difficult to differentiate the pain generated by the immobilisation devices from the pain caused by the initial trauma.[34,40] This will make it more difficult to assess the patient's condition and may also lead to unnecessary clinical imaging where physicians believe the pain is related to the initial trauma.[34,40]

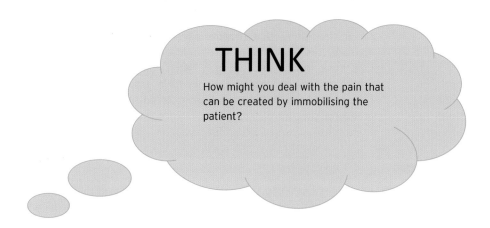

THINK

How might you deal with the pain that can be created by immobilising the patient?

Indications for spinal immobilisation

Penetrating trauma

Until recently there has been no discrimination between blunt and penetrating trauma when considering the need for spinal immobilisation. Most books and journals have recommended that all patients with such injuries should be immobilised, or merely state that such is the practice in their emergency department and pre-hospital trauma care.[41] However, a semi-rigid collar applied over a penetrating injury, such as high velocity bullets or projectiles, may conceal findings such as continuous oozing, subcutaneous emphysema and especially expanding haematoma.[41]

The recommendations from a study carried out in Israel suggest the following:[41]

- In penetrating injury to the neck without a clear neurological deficit, there is no place for using a collar or any other device for neck stabilisation.
- Neck stabilisation devices may be used when there is overt neurological deficit or the diagnosis cannot be made (i.e. unconscious victim). However, in this case it is obligatory to expose the neck by removing the anterior portion of the device every few minutes, at least in the initial phase of treatment.

- Neck stabilisation devices may be used for the unusual occurrence of a penetrating injury which is combined with blunt trauma. The stabilisation is then for the blunt mechanism only and not for the penetrating one.

JRCALC state that those with isolated penetrating injuries to limbs or the head do not require immobilisation. Those with truncal or neck trauma should be immobilised if the trajectory of the penetrating wound could pass near or through the spinal column.[4]

Blunt trauma

In blunt trauma, manual immobilisation should be commenced at the earliest time for any patient where the mechanism of injury suggests the possibility of SCI. The immobilisation can be released once the practitioner has ascertained that **ALL** of the following criteria are present:[4]

- No alteration in consciousness or mental state and patient is able to fully co-operate with examination
- No evidence of intoxication
- No complaint of spinal pain
- No vertebral tenderness
- No neurological deficit or complaint
- No significant distracting injury.

Note: Spinal pain does not include tenderness isolated to the muscles of the side of the neck.

THINK

How will you differentiate between a distracting injury and a non-distracting injury? This is important if you are to use the guidelines to good effect.

Equipment and procedures

- Cervical (semi-rigid) collars
- Extrication devices
- Long board and straps
- Vacuum mattress.

Cervical collars

There are numerous semi-rigid collars on the market and each has its own specific requirements. It is not possible to give guidance on all individual cervical collars so the practitioner should ensure that they are familiar with the techniques specific to the device being used.

A cervical spine collar needs to sit on the chest, posterior thoracic spine and clavicle, and trapezius muscle to be effective.[42] The head is immobilised by the collar beneath the mandible and at the occiput. The spine is not fully immobilised by a collar but its application aids in reducing head movement. The sizing of the collar is also of great importance; if the collar is too small it won't restrict the flexion motion of the neck, if too long it may cause hyperextension or allow for greater motion if the chin slips inside the front piece of the collar. In addition to sizing, it is also important to ensure that the collar is fastened correctly – too loose and it will not restrict motion of the head and neck, too tight and it may compromise the veins of the neck leading to a rise in ICP.

The collar should be applied only when the patient's head has been brought into neutral alignment. If the head cannot be brought into neutral alignment it will be very difficult and possibly dangerous to apply a semi-rigid collar. In those instances, improvisation with blankets or towels may be required.

Key Points

Cervical collars

1. Do not immobilise the head and neck on their own.
2. Must be sized correctly as per manufacturer guidelines.
3. Should be correctly fitted to ensure optimum support without obstructing venous return.
4. Should be applied only when the patient's head and neck have been brought into neutral alignment.
5. Should not hinder the ability of the patient to open their mouth or the practitioner to open the patient's mouth.
6. Should not hinder the patient's respiration.

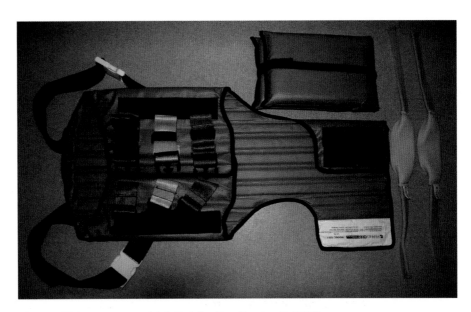

Figure 17.1 Ferno Kendrick Extrication Device® (KED).

Extrication devices

For the purposes of this section, the Ferno Kendrick Extrication Device® (KED) (Figure 17.1) will be discussed. Other extrication devices are available but tend to follow similar principles to the KED; the practitioner needs to be aware of any differences between the KED and the device that they use. The KED is used when spinal immobilisation is indicated for a sitting patient with non-time critical injuries.

The KED is constructed from vertically aligned slats which provide the rigidity required to help minimise the risk of further injury during extrication. It has wrap-around head and chest flaps to allow for immobilisation of the cervical, thoracic and part of the lumbar regions to help prevent rotation or angulation of the spine. The device is secured by means of a colour coded sequence of straps and the patient's head is held in place by adjustable head and chin straps. An adjustable neck pad is provided to help fill the gaps caused by the natural curvature of the spine. The chest flaps fold back to allow the KED to be used with heart monitoring equipment, pregnant patients and younger adolescents.

Procedure	Additional information/ rationale
1. Discuss the procedure and gain consent from the patient (where appropriate).	Consent is a legal requirement. Explanation of the procedure helps to gain cooperation from the patient.
2. Practitioner One should be positioned behind the patient to hold the head (where possible).	This stabilises the head and neck.

Procedure	Additional information/ rationale
3. Practitioner Two checks neurological and vascular response of all extremities and then measures and applies the cervical collar.	Assesses neurological status prior to movement and as a baseline for further observations. The collar helps to restrict movement of the head and neck.
4. The KED is slid into position behind the patient and wrapped around. The side flaps should be touching the patient's armpits.	

5. The torso straps should be positioned and fastened in the following order:
  (i) Middle chest strap
  (ii) Lower chest strap.	

6. The upper chest strap is optional at this time but should not be secured too tightly if used. It should be fastened just before the patient is moved.	If over-tightened, the top chest strap can impede respiration.
7. The groin straps should be positioned and fastened taking care not to trap the patient's genitalia. This can be achieved by working the strap in a backwards-and-forwards motion under the patient's thigh and buttock until it sits comfortably in the intergluteal fold. Once in place, the straps are tightened.	
8. It may be necessary to reappraise the torso straps and adjust as necessary.	
9. Use the padding behind the patient's head to maintain neutral alignment. Position the head flaps and, using the head straps, secure the patient's head.	Care needs to be taken when placing the head flaps as the practitioner holding the head will need to change their hand positions to facilitate this.
10. Recheck all straps before moving and ensure that the top chest strap has been connected.	Ensures security.
11. If possible, the ambulance cot should be placed close to the patient with either a long board or vacuum mattress placed upon it.	Minimises lifting and handling.
12. The best option is to place the long board beneath the patient's buttocks with the foot end securely placed on the patient's seat (i.e. car seat), and the head end on the ambulance cot. If this cannot be achieved, the patient may need to be lifted into position.	

Procedure	Additional information/ rationale
13. Rotate the patient so that their back is towards the long board. The legs will need to be lifted as the patient is extricated.	
14. Once square to the board, the patient can be lowered to the board whilst keeping the legs elevated. The two groin straps need to be released at this point and the patient's legs can be lowered.	
15. The patient should be positioned appropriately on the board and secured for transportation.	
16. The practitioner should consider releasing the top chest strap at this point.	To assist with respiration

Key Points

Extrication devices

1. Extrication devices are useful for immobilising a patient from a sitting position.
2. These devices do not fully immobilise the spine so full immobilisation using a long board or other suitable device is recommended.
3. They should NOT be used in time-critical patients.
4. Strapping should be attached and adjusted in the correct order according to the manufacturer.

Long board

The long board is made of either wood or plastic and is designed to be used to provide rigid support whilst moving a patient with suspected spinal, hip, pelvic or lower extremity injuries. Despite the limitations discussed earlier, long boards are useful for extrication from vehicles, full body immobilisation where SCI is a possibility or for victims of multiple trauma, an emergency stretcher during cardiopulmonary resuscitation or multiple casualty incidents, or for water rescue.

The board should be supplied with a complete head immobiliser and four body straps; it should never be used without the head immobiliser and at least three body straps.[43] Any void between the sides of the patient and the sides of the long board need to be filled with padding to help prevent lateral movement of the body on the board.[42] Securing of the patient can be accomplished in a number of different ways;

the techniques may need to be adapted depending on any other injuries that may have been sustained. The overriding aim is to prevent movement in any direction but care needs to be exercised to ensure that strapping does not impair the patient's ability to breathe. It will be necessary to immobilise both the upper torso (shoulders and chest) and lower torso (around the pelvis) to achieve effective immobilisation.

The Prehospital Trauma Life Support Manual suggests two alternatives for thoracic strapping.[42]

Either:

- Two straps (one going from each side of the board over the shoulder, then across the upper chest and through the opposite armpit to lock into place on the armpit side) produce an X, which stops lateral movement and upward movement of the torso.

Or:

- Fasten one strap to the board by the armpit, pass it under the armpit, over the upper chest and then under the opposite armpit, to fasten to the board on the second side of the board. A second strap is then attached to each side of the board and passed over the shoulders to fasten it to the armpit strap.

The lower torso should be secured by passing a single strap across the iliac crests and tightening them.[42]

If the patient needs to be upended it is useful to use a figure of 8 around the feet and ankles to prevent the patient from sliding down the board.

When strapping the patient, care needs to be taken not to exacerbate any other injuries such as pelvic or clavicular fractures.

If a patient is not trapped and is supine on the floor they should not be log-rolled onto the long board; instead they should be lifted using the orthopaedic scoop stretcher and either placed onto the long board or immobilised on the scoop stretcher. When using the long board as an extrication device it is important to slide the patient up the board rather than lifting them. This minimises the movement in all areas of the spinal column and reduces the risk of exacerbating an SCI.

Use of the long board for women in late pregnancy

The use of the supine position for a woman in the late stages of pregnancy can seriously compromise maternal cardiac output.[44] This is caused by the gravid uterus completely occluding the inferior vena cava[45] and laterally displacing the subrenal aorta.[46] It is necessary to either manually displace the uterus or to tilt the long board to the left. It is suggested that a 30° tilt is required to displace the uterus[4] although the full left lateral position has been shown to produce the best cardiac output in late pregnancy.[47] There are inherent difficulties in achieving this tilt in a spinally injured patient as there is a tendency for the patient to slip laterally on the board so causing spinal bending. This can best be managed by filling the voids between the sides of the patient and sides of the board but it is likely that some movement will still occur. It is unlikely that a 30° tilt will be accurately measured by the paramedic in the field, so constant observations of cardiac adequacy will be required and adjustments made as necessary. A better option may be to use a vacuum mattress loaded onto a long board and then tilted the requisite angle.

Procedure	Additional information/rationale
1. Explain procedure and gain consent from patient (where appropriate).	Consent is a legal requirement. Explanation of the procedure helps to gain cooperation from the patient.
2. Apply any appropriate cervical collar or extrication device.	Provides additional head and neck support until the patient is fully immobilised on long board.
3. Prepare the board. Head pad should be in place and straps connected to their respective clip pins but the buckles should be unfastened.	
4. Use appropriate technique to place patient on long board. The patient should be located centrally on the board with the head on the head pad to maintain neutral alignment.	Sliding techniques should be used rather than lifting when extricating a patient. If lifting an untrapped patient from supine, the orthopaedic scoop should be used.
5. Use blanket rolls to fill the voids between the sides of the patient and the sides of the board.	Reduces lateral movement of the patient's body on the board.
6. Apply body straps in the following order: (i) Chest (ii) Pelvis (iii) Thighs (iv) Ankles (v) Head immobiliser and straps.	Immobilises area of greatest mass first. Consider figure of 8 around the feet and ankles to prevent downward movement.
7. Lift patient onto a suitable ambulance cot using the side lifting handles of the long board.	An end-to-end lift should not be performed as the board may be flexible, which will cause curvature of the spine.
8. Loosen the cervical collar.	Helps to prevent compromise of venous circulation and reduces risk of increasing ICP.
9. Document the time the patient was placed on the board.	

Key Points

Long board

1. The long board is designed to be used to provide rigid support whilst moving a patient with suspected spinal, hip, pelvic or lower extremity injuries.
2. The board should be supplied with a complete head immobiliser and four body straps.
3. It should never be used without the head immobiliser and at least three body straps.
4. Log rolling should NOT be used for any patient who is untrapped and lying supine on the floor.
5. Log rolling should not be used for patients with possible pelvic fractures as it may dislodge clots and worsen bleeding.
6. Women in late pregnancy should not lie supine on the board in order to prevent aortocaval compression.
7. The time the patient is on the board should be kept to a minimum and application time should be recorded on the patient report form.

Vacuum mattress

The vacuum mattress is a lightweight but tough device used to provide rigid support whilst moving a patient with suspected spinal, hip, pelvic or lower extremity injuries. The device is filled with high density beads that conform to the patient when air is removed by means of a pump. This serves to cocoon the patient and reduce movement during transportation. It has advantages over the long board:

- Good insulation from the surroundings.
- It can be used in whatever position is appropriate for the patient, for example, it can be used for patients in a semi-reclined position.
- It provides comparable spinal immobilisation to the long board with increased comfort.[48]
- The patient is likely to be more secure if a lateral tilt is required.

The main disadvantages of the vacuum mattress are that it doesn't lend itself well to extrication and there is the risk of failure due to puncture and a leak of air back into the mattress once the patient has been secured. Typically, transferring a patient onto a vacuum mattress will require the use of an intermediate-stage immobilisation device such as a KED, and a device for lifting the patient.

The exact method required for immobilising a patient on a vacuum mattress will vary upon the device being used and the strapping system employed. The following guidelines are generic and the manufacturer's own instructions or employer guidelines should be followed where differences exist.

Procedure	Additional information/ rationale
1. Explain procedure and gain consent from patient (where appropriate).	Consent is a legal requirement. Explanation of the procedure helps to gain cooperation from the patient.
2. Apply any appropriate cervical collar or extrication device.	Provides additional head and neck support until the patient is fully immobilised on long board.
3. Prepare the mattress. Smooth out the beads in the mattress and undo the straps and lay by the side.	
4. Using appropriate technique, place the patient on the vacuum mattress (an orthopaedic scoop stretcher may be used to achieve this). There is often an appropriate point for location of the patient's shoulders on the mattress; the practitioner should ensure that the patient is correctly aligned with this point.	
5. Conform the vacuum mattress around the contour of the patient, starting at the head	
6. Apply body straps in the following order: (i) Chest (ii) Pelvis (iii) Thighs (iv) Ankles.	
7. Evacuate air from the vacuum mattress until it becomes rigid; ensure that the mattress remains rigid.	
8. Disconnect the vacuum pump and ensure that the valve is closed or secured.	
9. Reassess and adjusts the straps around the chest, hips, and legs.	
10. Stabilise the head in a neutral position and secure to the vacuum mattress LAST.	
11. Reassess patient's baseline observations.	Helps to prevent compromise of venous circulation and reduces risk of increasing ICP.
12. Lift patient onto a suitable ambulance cot using the side lifting handles of the vacuum mattress.	

Procedure	Additional information/ rationale
13. Loosen the cervical collar.	
14. Document the time the patient was placed on the device.	

Key Points

Vacuum mattress

1. The vacuum mattress provides comparable immobilisation to the long board but with greater comfort
It is not suitable to be used as an extrication device.
2. Although it is more comfortable than a rigid board, it still produces high interface pressures and the time the patient spends immobilised on the device should be kept to a minimum.

Summary

Spinal immobilisation is a necessary part of the management of many trauma patients but it is not without its complications. The practitioner needs to be aware of the problems associated with spinal immobilisation and ensure that only those patients with an indication for immobilisation are immobilised.

Each of the spinal immobilisation devices has advantages and disadvantages; the practitioner needs to be cognisant of this and use the most appropriate equipment available for the circumstances.

Chapter Key Points

There are numerous potential complications associated with spinal immobilization

Knowledge of the benefits and limitations of immobilisation equipment is essential

Manual immobilisation should be commenced at the earliest time for any patient where the mechanism of injury suggests the possibility of SCI

Immobilisation can only be released once the practitioner has ascertained that ALL criteria from the selective immobilisation algorithm have been satisfied

References and Further reading

1 Chi CH, Wu FG, Tsai SH, Wang CH, Stern SA. Effect of hair and clothing on neck immobilization using a cervical collar. *Am J Emerg Med* 2005;23(3):386-390.

2 Kwan I, Bunn F, Roberts I, on behalf of the WHO Pre-Hospital Trauma Care Steering Committee. *Spinal Immobilisation for Trauma Patients*. The Cochrane Database of Systematic Reviews, Date of Most Recent Substantive Amendment: 22 January 2001.

3 Tortora GJ, Derrikson B. *Principles of Anatomy and Physiology*, 11th edn. New Jersey: Wiley, 2006.

4 Joint Royal Colleges Ambulance Liaison Committee. *UK Ambulance Service Clinical Practice Guidelines* version 4. London: IHCD, 2006.

5 Podolsky S, Baraff LJ, Simon RR, Hoffman JR, Larmon B, Ablon W. Efficacy of cervical spine immobilization methods. *J Trauma* 1983;23(6):461-465.

6 Huerta C, Griffith R, Joyce SM. Cervical spine stabilization in pediatric patients: Evaluation of current techniques. *Ann Emerg Med* 1987;16(10):1121-1126.

7 Del Rossi G, Heffernan TP, Horodyski M, Rechtine GR, The effectiveness of extrication collars tested during the execution of spine-board transfer techniques. *Spine J* 2004;4:619-623.

8 Houghton L, Driscoll P. Cervical immobilization – are we achieving it? *Prehosp Immed Care* 1999;3:17-21.

9 Luscombe MD, Williams JL. Comparison of a long spinal board and vacuum mattress for spinal immobilisation. *Emerg Med J* 2003;20:476-478.

10 Hamilton RS, Pons PT. The efficacy and comfort of full-body vacuum splints for cervical-spine immobilization. *J Emerg Med* 1996;14(5):553-559.

11 Howell JM, Burrow R, Dumontier C, Hillyard A. A practical radiographic comparison of short board technique and Kendrick extrication device. *Ann Emerg Med* 1989;18(9):943-946.

12 Graziano AF, Scheidel EA, Cline JR, Baer LJ. A radiographic comparison of prehospital cervical immobilization methods. *Ann Emerg Med* 1987;16(10):1127-1131.

13 Cordell WH, Hollingsworth JC, Olinger ML, Stroman SJ, Nelson DR. Pain and tissue-interface pressures during spine-board immobilization. *Ann Emerg Med* 1995;26(1):31-36.

14 Chan D, Goldberg R, Tascone A, Harmon S, Chan L. The effect of spinal immobilization on healthy volunteers. *Ann Emerg Med* 1994;23(1):48-51.

15 McGuire RA, Neville S, Green BA, Watts C. Spinal instability and the log-rolling maneuver. *J Trauma* 1987;27(5):525-531.

16 Swartz EE, Nowak J, Shirley C, Decoster LC. A comparison of head movement during back boarding by motorized spine-board and log-roll techniques. *J Athlet Train* 2005;40(3): 162-168.

17 Del Rossi G, Horodyski M, Heffernan TP, Powers ME, Siders R, Brunt D, Rechtine GR. Spine-board transfer techniques and the unstable cervical spine. *Spine* 2004;29(7):E134-138.

18 Del Rossi G, Horodyski MH, Conrad BP, Di Paola CP, Di Paola MJ, Rechtine GR. The 6-plus-person lift transfer technique compared with other methods of spine boarding. *J Athlet Train* 2008;43(1):6-13.

19 Lee C, Porter K. The prehospital management of pelvic fractures. *Emerg Med J* 2007;24: 130-133.

20 Krell JM, McCoy MS, Sparto PJ, Gretchen L. Fisher, Stoy WA, Hostler DP. Comparison of the Ferno Scoop Stretcher with the Long Backboard for Spinal Immobilization. *Prehosp Emerg Care* 2006;10:46-51.

21 De Lorenzo RA, Olson JE, Boska M, Johnston R, Hamilton GC, Augustine J, Barton R: Optimal positioning for cervical immobilization. *Ann Emerg Med* 1996;28:301-308.

22 Goutcher CM, Lochhead V. Reduction in mouth opening with semi-rigid cervical collars. *Br J Anaesth* 2005;95(3):344-348.

23 Ollerton JE, Parr MJA, Harrison K, Hanrahan B, Sugrue M. Potential cervical spine injury and difficult airway management for emergency intubation of trauma adults in the emergency department – a systematic review. *Emerg Med J* 2006;23:3-11.

24 Braude D, Domeier R, Prehospital care for road traffic casualties: Spinal immobilisation should be done selectively. *Br Med J* 2002;325(7358):279.

25 Lerner B, Moscati R. Duration of patient immobilization in the ED. *Am J Emerg Med* 2000;18(1):28-30.

26 Emergency Nurses Association. Spinal Immobilisation, 5th edn. *Trauma nursing core course.* 2000;377:81.

27 Craig GR, Nielsen MS. Rigid cervical collars and intracranial pressure. *Int Care Med* 1991;17:504-505.

28 Raphael JH, Chotai R. Effects of the cervical collar on cerebrospinal fluid pressure. *Anaesthesia* 1994;49:437-439.

29 Davies G, Deakin C, Wilson A. The effect of a rigid collar on intracranial pressure. *Injury* 1996;27:647-649.

30 Kolb JC, Summers RL, Galli RL. Cervical collar induced changes in intracranial pressure. *Am J Emerg Med* 1999;17:135-137.

31 Ferguson J, Mardel SN, Beattie TF, Wytch R. Cervical collars - a potential risk to the head-injured patient. *Injury Internat J Care Injured* 1993;24(7):454-456.

32 Porter KP, Allison KM. The UK emergency department practice for spinal board unloading. Is there conformity? *Resuscitation* 2003;58(1):117-120.

33 Totten VY, Sugarman DB. Respiratory effects of spinal immobilization. *Prehosp Emerg Care* 1999;3(4):347-352.

34 Vickery D, The use of the spinal board after the pre-hospital phase of trauma management. *Emerg Med J* 2001;18:51-54.

35 Houghton DJ. Dysphagia caused by a hard cervical collar. *Br J Neurosurg* 1996;10(5): 501-502.

36 Brownlee AE. Managing spinal immobilisation devices in the emergency department. *Australas Emerg Nurs J* 2005;8(3):79-83.

37 Hampton S, Preventable pressure sores. *Care Crit Ill* 1997;(13):193-197.

38 Boitano M, Tait D, Petrovic R, Nicosia S. The spine board: peak pressure assessment design implications for wound prevention. *J Trauma Injury Infect Crit Care* 2004;57(2):460.

39 Chan D, Goldberg RM, Mason J, Chan L. Backboard versus mattress splint immobilization: a comparison of symptoms generated. *J Emerg Med* 1996;14(3):293-298.

40 Lerner B, Moscati R. Duration of patient immobilization in the ED. *Am J Emerg Med* 2000;18(1):28-30.

41 Barkana Y, Stein M, Scope A, Maor R, Abramovich Y, Friedman Z *et al.* Prehospital stabilization of the cervical spine for penetrating injuries of the neck - is it necessary? *Injury* 2000;31(5):305-309.

42 Association of Emergency Medical Technicians. *Prehospital Trauma Life Support*, 6th edn. Missouri: Elsevier, 2007.

43 Joint Royal Colleges Ambulance Liaison Committee. *UK Ambulance Service Clinical Practice Guidelines* version 3. London: IHCD, 2004.

44 Clark SL, Cotton DB, Pivarnik JM *et al.* Position change and central hemodynamic profile during normal third-trimester pregnancy and post-partum. *Am J Obstet Gynecol* 1991;164:883-887.

45 Kerr MG, Scott DB, Samuel E. Studies of the inferior vena cava in late pregnancy. *Br Med J* 1964;1:532-533.

46 Bieniarz J, Crottogini JJ, Curuchet E *et al.* Aortocaval compression by the uterus in late human pregnancy: an arteriographic study. *Am J Obstet Gynecol* 1968;100:203-217.

47 Bamber JH, Dresner M. Aortocaval compression in pregnancy: the effect of changing the degree and direction of lateral tilt on maternal cardiac output. *Anesth Analg* 2003;97: 256-258.

48 Ahmad M, Butler J. Spinal boards or vacuum mattresses for immobilisation. *Emerg Med J* 2001;18:379-380.

Chapter 18

Assessment and management of wounds and burns

Content

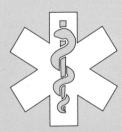

The assessment and management of wounds and burns is an important area of prehospital care and first aid. Many of the principles that underlie the techniques discussed are based upon many years of first aid intervention, as such little evidence surrounds the area. Where appropriate and available, evidence will be provided to support or dispute intervention or management options. Where no evidence is available guidance will provided based upon perceived best practice.

The circulatory system is a closed network of vessels including arteries, veins and capillaries that carry blood to all parts of the body.[1] If this network suffers any damage or break in its' continuity then haemorrhage occurs, this can be either internal (occult) or external bleeding. If this bleeding is not controlled either by the body's own physiological processes or by external influence (i.e. first aid measures or surgery) then hypovolaemic shock and ultimately death can occur.

Definitions

A wound is defined as a break in an organ or tissue caused by an external agent; this can be divided into seven broad categories[2] that will be discussed later.

Sources of bleeding

Internal bleeding

Normally concealed within the body, internal bleeding can be difficult to detect and may only be suspected due to mechanism of injury and the presence of signs of shock in the absence of external haemorrhage. There are no first aid or wound management techniques that can be used to control such bleeding; therefore definitive care is required at a suitable receiving hospital.

External bleeding

External bleeding is bleeding that is exhibited on the outside of the body and should be rapidly detected during the primary or secondary surveys. The seriousness and severity of an injury is dependent upon the source of the haemorrhage (arterial, venous, capillary), the degree of vascular disruption and the amount of bleeding that the patient can compensate for. In most cases of bleeding the practitioner should be able to stem the flow of blood loss.

Arterial bleeding

Arteries are the thick walled blood vessels that carry blood away from the heart. This blood is typically oxygen rich (aside from the pulmonary arteries).[1] Blood within these vessels is under the highest pressure of the vascular circuit and therefore damage to arteries results in potential high volumes of blood loss. Arterial bleeding is characterised by bright red spurting of blood with each heart beat (oxygenated blood is brighter than deoxygenated blood). Due to the high pressure blood volume losses can be great unless controlled urgently.

Venous bleeding

Veins are blood vessels that carry blood back to the heart; typically this is deoxygenated blood (aside from the pulmonary veins). The blood within the veins is described as dark red/blue in colour as oxygen has been removed. The venous system is a lower pressure circuit than that of the arterial. There is a loss of pulsatile movement of blood, with blood flowing more freely. This causes venous bleeding to typically be free flowing rather than spurting, however blood loss from venous injury can be severe, especially in the leg and the neck where large wide veins are present.

Capillary bleeding

Capillaries are the smallest blood vessels in the body and are found throughout the body as they provide a rich circulation supply to most of the tissues of the body.[1] Capillaries generally have exceedingly thin walls which may pass very near to the surface of the skin and are easily damaged. As blood volumes are small in individual capillaries and under low pressure blood will typically ooze from the wound. Capillary blood may be a mix of oxygenated or deoxygenated blood therefore the colour may vary.

Classification of wounds

Wounds are classified by mechanism and physiological disturbance. Whilst differing classifications are used they commonly fit into seven broad categories (excluding burns – discussed later in this chapter). It is important that the practitioner can describe a wound for documentation and referral purposes, especially in today's increasingly litigious society.

Incised wound

An injury to the skin that may be superficial or deep. Incisions are caused by sharp objects such as a knife or broken glass. Incisions are typically clean wounds (unless the object is dirty), with neat edges.

Lacerations

Lacerations are a tearing or splitting of the skin caused by blunt trauma. Commonly lacerations are caused by either direct or indirect blow to the skin by a heavy or fixed object such as furniture or the floor.

Puncture/penetrating wounds

These wounds have a small opening where the object has penetrated the skin causing potential underlying damage. It can be very difficult to assess these wounds as the damage may not be indicated by the entry wound. Careful assessment of the wound is required in a controlled environment by a competent and experienced practitioner; this is usually undertaken in an operating theatre or Emergency Department. The investigation of depth and underlying damage is not recommended in the prehospital environment. A concise history is paramount in providing a level of suspicion of underlying injury. Common causes of these wounds range from stab wounds to standing on a nail.

Abrasion

An abrasion (often referred to as a graze) is a superficial removal of the skin by rubbing or friction. This can be painful due to the exposed nerve endings and may have embedded dirt in the skin. These wounds may range from carpet burns from a fall to severe 'gravel rash' following a fall from a moving motorcycle.

Crush Injury

These are caused by severe crushing pressures causing the skin to split. Crush wounds are often associated with underlying injury to bone or organs due to the forces involved.

Bite wounds

These wounds are naturally caused by the teeth which may be human or animal. Bite wounds are often ragged edged and involve bruising from the crushing forces involved. Bite wounds are associated with a high risk of infection due to the natural bacteria in the mouth of the human or animal.

Contusions

Also referred to as bruising, a contusion is bleeding from damaged blood vessels beneath the skin that result in a bluish/purple discoloration beneath the skin. These are typically caused by blunt trauma, although contusions may form around the site of other wounds.

Other wounds

These include amputation which is the complete detachment of a part of the body that may be cut or torn away. This may result in significant bleeding due to the damage to arteries, veins and bone. If tissue still connects the amputated body part then it is termed as partial amputation. Avulsion injuries are a flap of skin and underlying tissue that is partially torn or cut away, one such injury is the tearing away of the scalp in blunt head trauma.

Wound healing

Wound healing is a dynamic process involving physiological processes in a series of stages whereby damaged or destroyed tissues are restored to normal function.[3]

Phases of wound healing

Wound healing is a complex process that occur s in a predictable order. The processes of wound healing are generally described in four stages[4]:

- Haemostasis
- Inflammatory stage
- Proliferation or reconstructive stage
- Maturation or re-modelling stage.

Whilst these stages are not distinct and may overlap, for simplicity they will be discussed individually, due to the complex nature of wound healing only brief discussion will be provided, further reading suggestions are provided at the end of this chapter that will provide more information.

Haemostasis

This occurs within seconds and minutes of injury. Blood vessels constrict to reduce blood loss. When platelets come into contact with collagen from damaged blood vessels chemical mediators are released that promote coagulation.[4] Platelets adhere to vessel walls and damaged edges where they are stabilised by fibrin threads to form a clot.

Inflammatory stage

Neutrophils, monocytes and keratinocytes (white blood cells) migrate to the damaged area over the first 2-3 days following injury. Histamine release causes vasodilatation and increased permeability of capillary walls to cause leucocytes, antibodies, proteins and electrolytes to exude into the surrounding tissues. This causes the wound to be red, swollen and hot.[4] White blood cells (neutrophils and macrophages) begin the process of repair by destroying and ingesting bacteria and devitalised tissue. This increases the oxygen demand in the tissues through the increase in cellular activity; therefore hypoxic wounds are more susceptible to infection and poor healing.

Proliferation or reconstructive stage

This stage lasts from about 3-24 days. As macrophages accumulate at the site of injury chemical mediators are released that attract fibroblasts to the site. Fibroblasts produce proteins such as collagen and elastin that leads to the formation of new connective tissue that increases the strength of the wound.[5] New blood vessel formation is also stimulated and will begin to grow in the matrix of connective tissue. The new tissue at the site of injury is referred to as granulation tissue; this is generally pink/red in appearance and is very fragile. Wound contraction also occurs, with specialised fibroblasts pulling the wound edges together to reduce the surface area of the wound. During this time re-epithelialisation occurs as epithelial tissue migrates across the surface of the wound to eventually cover the wound.

Maturation or re-modelling stage

This stage commences at about 21 days after the injury and may continue for over a year. There is a gradual reduction in the vascularity of the wound and collagen fibres are re-modelled to a more organised structure that strengthens the wound. During this time stronger avascular tissue may replace the highly vascular granulation tissue, this may lead to scarring.[4]

Complications in wound healing

There are a variety of complications that can affect wound healing; this section will briefly discuss some of the key issues that may affect wound healing.

Factors that affect wound healing

Table 18.1 Factors that affect wound healing. From Timmons (2003)[6] and Dougherty and Lister (2006)[4]

Factor	Complication(s)
Nutrition	There is a clear correlation between sub clinical nutrition and poor wound healing. The process of wound healing requires a number of nutritional factors to be present to meet demand. For example fats and proteins are required and cannot always be synthesised by the body.
Diabetes	Diabetes mellitus is linked to a number of issues that can influence wound healing, for example reduction in vascular supply to wound sites and a pre-disposition to infection in raised blood glucose levels. These can lead to poor or delayed wound healing.
Renal disease	Renal disease comprises of a variety of key pathophysiological changes that may affect wound healing. For example fluid and electrolyte imbalance may result in reduced cellular efficiency and subsequent healing processes. Also the presence of anaemia due to decreased erythropoietin production may lead to reduced oxygen supply to the wound site.
Steroid use and other medications	Steroids have been linked to poor wound healing by inhibition of collagen synthesis and a reduction in the tensile strength of collagen. Other drugs noted to delay wound healing include alcohol, penicillin, nicotine and non-steroidal anti-inflammatory drugs.
Other factors	Complications include; foreign body in the wound, infection, obesity, stress, location of the wound (e.g. highly mobile areas).
Age	The aging process presents a number of factors that may influence wound healing. These include reduced cardiovascular functioning resulting in poor tissue perfusion; poor nutritional status; reduced glucose tolerance and potential decrease in hygiene standards and self-care.

Principles of wound management

Whilst wounds may present in a variety of forms as previously discussed the principles of wound management can be generalised to deal with each situation with little adaptation.

Control of bleeding (no foreign body)

Procedure	Rationale
1. Ensure the area is safe.	This is a key objective in any primary survey.
2. Protect yourself and the patient with appropriate infection control measures such as gloves, eye wear and apron.	To reduce the risk of cross infection and blood borne virus exposure.
3. Reassure the patient.	An anxious patient is more difficult to manage and anxiety will increase cardiac output and potentially bleeding.
4. Elevate and support the wounded part above the height of the heart.	This will allow for postural reduction in blood flow to the injured part, thus reducing potential blood loss.
5. Expose the wound to identify the wound type and site.	This will aid describing of the wound and identification of any debris in the wound. If there is a foreign body within the wound – refer to later in this chapter.
6. Apply direct pressure to the wound.	Direct pressure to a wound site will reduce blood flow/loss and encourage coagulation.
7. Apply a sterile or clean dressing pad and bandage over the wound; this should be tight enough to stem the flow of the bleeding but not tight enough to restrict circulation distal to the injury.	If circulation is disrupted beyond the site of bandaging there is a risk of tissue necrosis.
8. Check the distal circulation (pulses or capillary refill time).	To ensure distal blood flow.
9. If the bleeding is not controlled by the first dressing apply a further dressing over the top.	This will add further pressure to the wound.
10. If the initial dressings do not stem the bleeding: • Maintain elevation and pressure upon the wound and remove the dressings • Re-position the dressings to apply the best pressure possible • Re-check distal circulation.	The re-positioning of the dressings may apply pressure more directly over the wound. After any intervention the effect of the treatment should be checked to ensure efficacy and detriment to the patient.
11. If the bleeding is severe and not controlled by these initial methods then consider indirect pressure.	See later in chapter.

Control of bleeding (foreign body present)

In the presence of a retained foreign body in a wound, it is important that the object is not removed from the wound as this may cause further tissue damage, dislodge blood clots or unseal blood vessels causing an increase of bleeding. The following principles apply to the management of bleeding with a retained foreign body:

- Do not remove the object, unless small and sitting on top of the wound as opposed as embedded in the wound. If debris is sitting upon the wound it may be brushed away gently using a sterile pad.
- Do not apply pressure upon the object as this may cause further damage.
- Pressure should be applied to the sides of the wound, holding the wound together.
- Pad around the object to apply pressure to the sides of the wound and to ensure the object is not dislodged. When padded a bandage can be applied over the top to secure the padding.
- Consider primary principles of wound management, such as elevation.
- In the event of failure to stem bleeding then indirect pressure may be required.

THINK

You are called to a patient who is impaled on a fence post. How will you deal with a wound and such a large embedded object? How will this change your management and transportation?

Indirect pressure

If bleeding is not controlled by initial first aid measures then application of indirect pressure should be considered. This requires pressure to be placed upon the artery that supplies the area of bleeding. Applying pressure will reduce blood flow to the area and subsequent blood loss during which time more substantial or definitive bandaging can be applied.

Common sites for indirect pressure include:

- The brachial artery for arm wounds
- The femoral artery for leg wounds
- The temporal artery for scalp wounds.

The carotid artery should not be compressed when dealing with head or scalp wounds.

The use of tourniquets and haemostatic dressings

In the presence of severe haemorrhage that is uncontrolled by direct and indirect pressure (for example amputation) there are few options available for wound control; in such occasions it is suggested that a tourniquet could be used. The tourniquet was initially used by battlefield surgeons in ancient Rome to control bleeding during amputations; subsequently the use of the tourniquet has undergone fluctuations in popularity with a recent resurgence in military settings.[7] Arterial tourniquets work by compressing muscle and other tissues surrounding extremity arteries, therefore compressing the lumen of the artery and reducing distal blood flow.[7] The tension required to achieve this is dependent upon the size of the extremity[8] and the width of the tourniquet.[9] Wider tourniquets are more effective at stopping arterial flow at a given tension than a narrow tourniquet due to an increased area of vasculature being compressed.[9]

Complications of tourniquet use

There are a variety of potential complications associated with the application of a tourniquet. The time a tourniquet is applied for has often been a concern over its' use, even application for a matter of minutes leads to changes in muscle and nerve physiology. In an early study by Heppenstall *et al.* (1979)[10] found that after 1 hour there was no evidence of muscle damage, however at 2 hours of ischaemia elevated levels of lactic acid and creatinine phosphokinase were found (these are linked to skeletal muscle damage or injury). Surgical guidelines and studies support no more than 60-90 minutes of use, with a suggested upper limit of 2 hours.[11] However these studies are not prehospital based, so there is little guidance upon a safe duration of application.

There has been documented evidence of post-tourniquet complications known as post-tourniquet syndrome (weakness/parasthesia/pallor/stiffness) in the distal limb. This has been related to the damage caused to muscle, nerves and blood vessels during tourniquet use of over 1.5 hours in surgical intervention. This syndrome appears common but the effects are limited to approximately 3 weeks.[12] There are further concerns over issues such as worsened venous bleeding with an incorrectly applied tourniquet that allows for arterial flow to continue but venous return to be stemmed.[7] Compartment syndrome is a further complication that may occur with prolonged use, however little evidence surrounds this area and it is suggested the it may be the injury itself, not the tourniquet, which causes the presence of compartment syndrome.[13] Whilst there are numerous concerns and potential complications of tourniquet use the evidence surrounding these issues is unclear.[14,15]

Can they be used safely?

Recent military experience supports the safety of short-term tourniquet use in prehospital care[16,17,18] with a small-scale study finding limb salvage with arterial injury in 11 of 14 patients despite tourniquet times averaging 2 hours.[19]

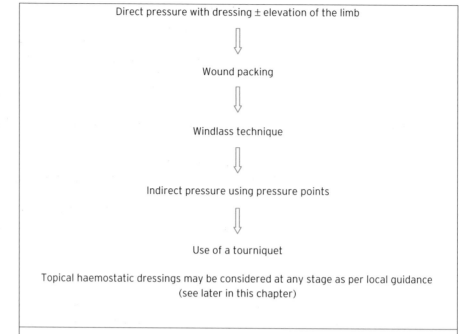

Figure 18.1 A stepwise approach to haemorrhage control.[20]

Indications for use

Whilst little evidence surrounds the use of tourniquets in the civilian setting, systematic reviews of haemorrhage control suggest that there may well be a role in a stepwise approach[7,20] as shown below. Whilst it is recognised that there limitations and complications associated with the use of a tourniquet, the ability to stem severe bleeding in the event of all other methods failing or in the presence of multiple casualties with other priorities of care, evidence suggests that tourniquet use may be appropriate (Figure 18.1).[7,20]

Doyle *et al.* (2008)[7] and Lee *et al.* (2007)[20] propose indications for tourniquet use in the prehospital care setting that allows for the technique to be used when the benefits will outweigh the complications, these can be seen below:

- Failure to stop bleeding using pressure dressings.
- Injury does not allow for the use of pressure dressings.
- Significant extremity bleeding in the face of any of the following:
- Need for airway management
- Need for breathing support
- Circulatory shock
- Need for other emergency interventions or assessment

- Bleeding from multiple sites.
- Impaled foreign body with ongoing extremity bleeding.
- Benefits of preventing death from hypovolaemic shock by cessation of ongoing external haemorrhage are greater than the risk of limb damage or loss from ischaemia caused by tourniquet use.
- Dangerous situations for the caregiver or adverse environmental factors (i.e. darkness).
- Mass casualty events whereby priorities of care are inhibited by the number and/ or severity of injuries.

Whilst the use of tourniquet application looks set to return it is important that any practitioners that use such techniques are adequately prepared and understand the underlying concepts of such an intervention. If applied it is imperative that the tourniquet is not covered as it may remain unseen for a long period of time and it is essential that the time of application is recorded to ensure that prolonged usage is avoided.

Haemostatic dressings

Haemostatic dressings are topical agents that use a variety of physiological mechanisms to stem bleeding. The method of action is determined by the nature of each product, current haemostatic dressings include:

- Fibrin glues and sealants
- Microporous Polysaccharide Hemosphere® (MPH)
- Mineral zeolite
- Poly-N-acetylglucosamine.

Fibrin glues and sealants

These contain high concentrations of fibrinogen and thrombin (and sometimes other clotting factors) that work by mimicking the latter stages of the clotting process. This will produce more rapid clot formation.[21] Multiple animal studies have proven that these bandages decrease blood loss and maintain blood pressure significantly better than a standard dressing and direct pressure.[22,23]

Microporous Polysaccharide Hemosphere® (MPH)

This is a powder that is poured into open wounds and absorbs water and low molecular weight products from blood thus allowing clotting factors and platelets to become more concentrated (therefore active).[24] Studies suggest that this powder is effective in accelerating haemostasis time in human and animal subjects.[25] However further studies have questioned the efficacy in severe haemorrhage with no improvements in mortality in animal subjects.[26]

Mineral zeolite

These products work by adsorbing water and concentrating clotting factors. This encourages and enhances the natural clotting process. In an animal study by Alam et al.[26] this substance was found to significantly reduce mortality in comparison to no interventions and the use of absorbent pad and elastic bandage, and also had the lowest blood loss volume (not statistically significant). There are concerns that the temperature rise that occurs from this exothermic reaction may result in burns; however this risk appears minimal in terms of potential benefit from the haemorrhage control.[27]

Poly-N-acetylglucosamine

These dressings are fabricated from chitosan, a naturally occurring polysaccharide. This has a positive electrical charge and attracts negatively charged red blood cells that become woven into the bandage to form a seal. In addition this dressing forms an antibacterial barrier. Positive results have been found with these products in simulated combat wounds and animal studies, with reduced blood loss and improved mortality rates.[28]

Scenario

You are called to a patient as a solo responder.
The patient is unresponsive and has a noisy airway that requires intervention. The patient also has a significant arterial bleed from the femoral artery and has lost a large amount of his blood volume. What are your priorities for this patient? What actions would you take?

Burns assessment

In the UK burns patients account for approximately 175,000 emergency department attendances and 15,000 hospital admissions each year.[29] As such the care and assessment of this large group of patients is of great importance. The following guidance for the assessment and management of the burns injured patient is taken from current international literature and meta-analytical reviews including The National Burn Care Review (2000);[29] Management of Burns and Scalds In Primary Care - New Zealand Guideline Group (2007)[30] and further research as indicated.

This guidance will look at burns specific management and will not therefore look at the full assessment and management of a patient.

Definition

A burn is defined as tissue damage caused by such agents as heat, chemicals, electricity, sunlight or nuclear radiation.[2]

Assessment of burns

There are three key areas for the assessment of a burn, these are the type of burn; the size of the burn and burn depth. Whilst the majority of evidence supporting burns assessment is based upon a consensus of expert opinion there are an increasing number (often small) of studies into this area.[30]

Type of burn

Burn type is the defined by the source of the energy that causes the tissue damage, this includes:

- Thermal burn – this is caused by exposure to extreme heat and may include wet (scalds) or dry (i.e. flame) sources. These are direct burns that are directly related to the level of heat and duration of contact with the heat source.
- Chemical burn – These are caused by the chemical properties of acids and alkalis. The severity is dependent upon the time of contact and the concentration of the substance.
- Electrical burn – Electrical burns are caused by contact with electrical sources such as exposed cables; these injuries commonly produce an entry and exit burn as the charge passes through the body. There may well be underlying damage on the path between the entry and exit points.
- Radiation burns – Radiation burns are most commonly caused by radiation from the sun (sunburn); however they may be caused by exposure to other radioactive isotopes.
- Friction burns – This is the result of friction between the body and another object resulting in heat production. This mechanism may also result in abrasion injuries.
- Cold burns – This is caused by contact with extremely cold objects/gases/liquids. The extreme temperature causes damage to the tissues.

Assessment of burn area

There are a variety of methods for the estimation of total burn surface area (TBSA) currently in use, these commonly include:

- Palmar surface method
- The rule of nines
- Lund and Browder charts
- Serial halving.

Palmar surface method

This method is based upon the supposition that the palmar surface of the patient's hand (including the fingers) represents approximately 1% of the total body surface area and can therefore be used as a guide for estimating burn size. However this technique is poorly validated[31] and should be used with caution especially in children and obese patients, as the method does not allow for age changes and variations in individual body weight.[30] Recent studies suggest that a value of approximately 0.8% should be used as it may provide a more accurate assessment.[30,32] The palmar surface method is more commonly used in small or irregular burns (<15%) or relatively large burns (>85% where the unburnt tissue can be estimated).[33]

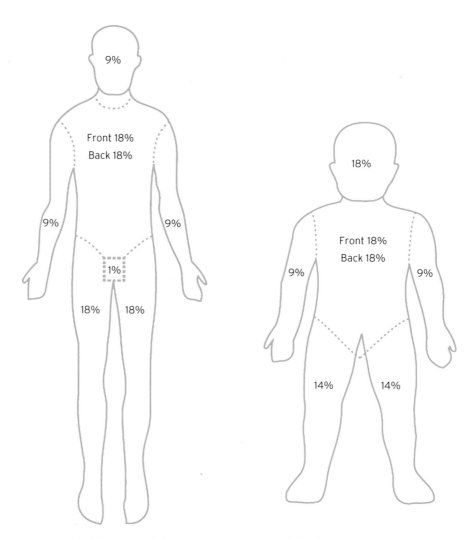

Figure 18.2 The rule of nines burns assessment chart.

The rule of nines

This estimation method (Figure 18.2) is based upon the principle that the adult body can be split into areas that equate to 9% and subsequently calculated. The rule of nines has been demonstrated to be swift method of burn surface area estimation however there are suggestions that it may overestimate burn surface area[34] and can potentially be inaccurate in children despite an adapted child model.[30] However it is accepted that the rule of nines method can provide a reasonable estimate of burn area.

Lund and Browder charts

The Lund and Browder chart is a burn area assessment chart that has been derived from a set of norm data for the body surface areas in children and adults. The

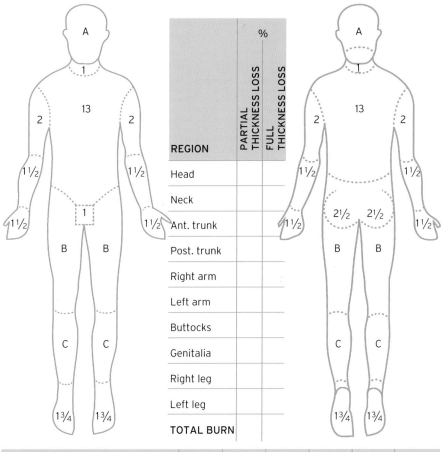

REGION	PARTIAL THICKNESS LOSS	FULL THICKNESS LOSS
Head		
Neck		
Ant. trunk		
Post. trunk		
Right arm		
Left arm		
Buttocks		
Genitalia		
Right leg		
Left leg		
TOTAL BURN		

AREA	AGE 0	1	5	10	15	ADULT
A = ½ of head	9½	8½	6½	5½	4½	3½
B = ½ of one thigh	2¾	3¼	4	4½	4½	3¾
C = ½ of one lower leg	2½	2½	2¾	3	3¼	3½

Figure 18.3 The Lund and Browder chart.

model (Figure 18.3) is suggested to be more accurate than the rule of nines but however takes longer to use than other methods.[30] As the model provides differing age ranges it can compensate for variations in body size with age for a more accurate measurement.

Differing models have been proposed for large breasted women as this can lead to underestimation of burn size by up to 5%[35] and for use in obese patients.[30] However these models are not essential and commonplace as the focus is often upon other clinical priorities.

Serial halving

This is a relatively new method of burns area assessment proposed by the Royal College of Surgeons Edinburgh - Faculty of Prehospital Care[36] that aims to provide a swift 'ball park' estimate. There has been little research undertaken to validate the use of such a model but has an appeal as a swift approach to estimation. This approach is split into three stages:

- Does the burn cover more than half of the body? For example if the back of the patient is completely without burns then it must be less than or equal to 50% of the body. This will distinguish between greater or less than 50% total burn surface area. If the answer is no then stage two is undertaken.
- Does the burn cover more than half of the remaining half of the body? If it does then the burn size is greater than 25% of total body surface area. If the answer is no then the burn must cover less than 25% of the body and stage three is undertaken.
- Does the burn cover more than or is equal to half of the remaining body surface area? If the answer is yes the then burn surface area is greater than 12.5% of the body surface area, if the answer is no then the burn must be less than 12.5%.

As can be seen this is a rough estimation tool but can be undertaken quickly with a brief visual inspection. In a small scale study serial halving has been found to be as reliable as the rule of nines in burn size estimation and much simpler to follow.[37]

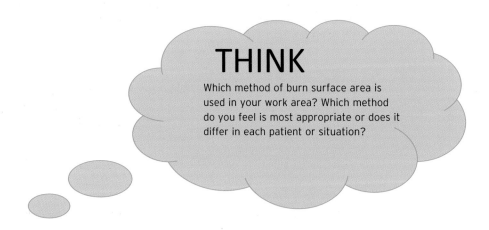

THINK

Which method of burn surface area is used in your work area? Which method do you feel is most appropriate or does it differ in each patient or situation?

Assessment of Burn Depth

There is no agreed methods for the assessment of burn depth with suggested techniques including capillary refill time (as dermal circulation will be lost in deeper burns) and the use of pin prick testing.[30] However these tests are not reliable within the first 24 to 48 hours following an injury due to oedema and inflammatory response.[30] Burn depth is generally assessed in the prehospital or emergency environment by appearance and the presence of pain. The classification of burn depth can be seen in Table 18.2.

Table 18.2 Burn depth assessment From New Zealand Guideline Group (2007)[30]

Classification	Superficial (epidermal)
Example	UV light (sun burn), very brief flash burns
Appearance	Dry and red, will blanch with pressure, no blistering present
Sensation	May be painful
Healing time	7 days
Scarring	No scarring
Classification	Superficial dermal (superficial partial thickness)
Example	Scalds, short flash burns
Appearance	Pale pink, with fine blistering, blanches to pressure
Sensation	Usually extremely painful
Healing time	Up to 14 days
Scarring	May be some colour mismatch in healed tissue
Classification	Mid-dermal (partial thickness)
Example	Scald, flame, oil or grease burns
Appearance	Dark pink with large blisters, capillary refill time may be prolonged
Sensation	May be painful
Healing time	Up to 21 days
Scarring	Scarring may be present (moderate risk)
Classification	Deep dermal (deep partial thickness)
Example	Scalds, flame burns
Appearance	Blotchy red, may blister, no capillary refill due to damaged capillaries
Sensation	No sensation present due to damaged nerves
Healing time	Over 21 days
Scarring	Scarring is likely
Classification	Full thickness
Example	Scald (prolonged exposure), high voltage electricity, chemical
Appearance	White, waxy or charred, no capillary refill due to vessel damage, no blistering. It may be lobster red and mottled in children
Sensation	No sensation due to nerve damage
Healing time	Will not heal without grafting
Scarring	Definite scarring

It is important to note that burn depth will vary in each patient and a burn may consist of a variety of depths.

Burn management principles

There is limited research into the initial management of burn injuries therefore many principles of management are based upon a consensus of opinion and common sense approaches. The management of a burn has three general stages:

- Remove the source of the burn
- Cool the burn
- Dress/cover the burn.

One area that may differ in terms of first aid measures in the management of chemical burns, as such this will be discussed separately.

Remove the source of the burn

The evidence for stopping the burning process is derived from expert opinion and common sense. As burn depth and size often relates to the length of exposure to the source of the burn removal of the source can undoubtedly reduce the severity of burn injury. Common steps include:

- Douse any flames using an appropriate medium (i.e. water).
- If electrical ensure the power source is turned off.
- Consider the use of a fire blanket or techniques such as stop, drop and roll.
- Remove any burnt clothing (unless adhering to the wounds) as this may retain heat.
- In tar burns do not remove the tar as this may seriously damage the underlying tissue. The burn should be cooled instead.

Cool the burn

There is good evidence that suggests the immediate cooling of a burn can reduce the severity of tissue damage.[30] In a series of studies into the use of cool water to cool a burn site it was found that such first aid measures significantly reduced the depth of the burn and reduced subsequent need for skin grafting and hospital admission times.[38-40] The use of ice or iced water is not recommended as it may lead to intense vasoconstriction and subsequent burn progression.[41] In a small animal study it was found that the application of ice for 10 minutes following a burn injury that burn depth was increased in comparison to a wound that had no treatment at all.

The presence of large burn surface area and subsequent cooling of the skin as a first aid measure may lead to hypothermia; this is especially evident in children and may be exacerbated by the use of ice or iced water.[42] It is therefore recommended that when cooling a burn that consideration is given to keeping the patient warm. Whilst there is limited evidence to provide an ideal temperature for water in cooling a burn, 15°C is suggested as ideal as it provides adequate cooling and reduction in tissue damage without the associated risks of cooling at lower temperatures.[30] There is little evidence to support a specific or minimum duration of cooling for a burn; however a single animal study sought to investigate this, proposing that 30 minutes of cooling provided the most effective treatment.[43] Due to the lack of data it is suggested that cooling be continued for approximately 30 minutes, although the patient condition (i.e. pain level) may dictate that this is prolonged or reduced. Cooling should be commenced as soon as is practically possible following injury as early cooling of a burn is significantly linked with improved wound healing.[44]

Whilst water is considered the medium of choice for burns cooling it is recognised that this may not always be available and expert opinion suggests that in the absence of running or clean water, other liquids such as milk or soft drinks may be used.[30] Over recent years products known as hydrogels have been introduced into UK ambulance services and first aid equipment. These products are a gel-like material that due to its chemical properties is able to hold large quantities of water (up to 90%). These products have the benefit of being portable and simple to use and act as both a cooling agent and a protective barrier from infection/debris. However there is still limited evidence comparing the use of such products versus running water.[30] When compared to air cooling or no treatment, small-scale studies have found these products to significantly reduce cooling times[45] and have a reduced risk of inducing hypothermia.[46]

Whilst there is little evidence to support such products at present, the availability and simplicity of the product is likely to make them a mainstay of treatment in prehospital care, especially in the absence of running water.

Covering the burn

There are a variety of materials that may be used to cover burns; however these generally have the following qualities:

- Clean (preferably sterile) material
- Non-adhesive
- Pliable.

Current practice for burn covering includes the use of clear plastic bags for hand burns (this allows for movement of the limb), hydrogel dressings, non-adherent dressings and polyvinyl chloride film (cling film). There has been little research into what constitutes an optimal burns dressing and current practice is limited by availability of products for use. The general principles of burn covering are to reduce the risk of infection, reduce pain (by covering exposed nerve endings) and to continue the cooling process.

When applying a burn dressing it is important that the dressing is not 'wrapped' around the limb as this may lead to a tourniquet effect in the presence of swelling and oedema[47], instead the dressing should be layered upon the burn to allow for expansion of damaged tissues. The use of cling film for a burn dressing is common in first aid practice as it is cheap, easily available and may provide a transparent covering to allow for inspection, whilst also reducing pain.[30] In addition PVC film has the benefit of being essentially sterile after the first few centimetres upon the roll. There is little evidence to support or dispute the use of this technique, however a dated microbiology study[48] suggests that PVC film is effective in reducing bacterial infection in wounds. In the absence of any of these dressings or coverings it is suggested that a clean, dry cotton sheet may be used.[30] Overall there is little consensus on a 'gold standard' burn dressing, with considered opinion suggesting that any one of a variety of products may be used in the initial setting. Within the secondary stages of care there are a large number of coverings that may be used; however the expense and nature of these products makes their use limited in first aid or emergency care.

Chemical burns

Burn injury due to chemicals usually occurs in the workplace, although they may occur in the domestic environment. There are currently over 25,000 products capable of causing chemical injury, therefore the potential for injury is high.[49] Chemical burns differ from thermal burns as they do not actually burn but cause tissues to liquefy or coagulate due to damage to proteins. Chemical injuries are often classified as either acid or alkali burns; however there are a wider range of classifications that include:

- Acid burns
- Alkali burns
- Organic hydrocarbon burns
- Miscellaneous burns (i.e. phosphorous)
- Extravasation injury
- Chemical warfare agents

From Seth, Chester and Moiemen (2007).[49]

This classification demonstrates that chemical injury can be caused by a broader range of substance than just acids or alkali, as some agents do not fit well into broad categories.

Management of chemical burns

The general management of any chemical burn has three steps:

- Remove the source of the burn - remove contaminated clothing.
- Irrigate the area thoroughly using running water.
- Provide supportive measures (i.e. analgesia).

The majority of chemicals are treated with copious irrigation with water as opposed to the neutralisation of the chemical with a specific agent. This is due to two factors; the availability of neutralising agents and the potential for exothermic (heat producing) reactions when the agent is neutralised which can result in increased tissue damage.[30,49] It is recommended that chemical burns are irrigated for a minimum of one hour;[30,49] however alkali burns may require as long as 8-24 hours of irrigation.[50] The use of copious irrigation without delay after initial injury has been demonstrated to significantly reduce the severity of a burn and the length of hospital admission.[30,51,52] However not all chemicals can be treated simply using this generic principle, as shown below.

Specific chemical burns

Lime (cement)

Cement or lime burns can be irrigated; however it is recommended that any dry cement is brushed off prior to irrigation as combining calcium oxide (lime) and water may cause an exothermic reaction and subsequently worsen a burn injury.

Phenol

Phenol is a carbolic acid that is commonly used in industry. It is recommended that the affected area is wiped prior to irrigation with water, as this may will lead to dilution and allow more rapid penetration into the skin.[49]

Elemental sodium/potassium and lithium burns

These agents are rare, however they are used in industry today. Burns from these materials *should not* be treated with irrigation with water as this may cause the compounds to spontaneously ignite,[53] as the metals react with water to form a very strong alkali.

Phosphorous

This is found in many products and may also be seen in military situations as phosphorous is a component of many hand grenades, mortar rounds and artillery rounds. Phosphorous spontaneously ignites upon contact with air, therefore management should be aimed at removing the source (brushing off the agent and removal of contaminated clothes) and at reducing air contact with the chemical. Recommended management for phosphorous burns is immersion in water or continuous irrigation with water or saline, in the absence of such irrigation fluid saline or water soaked dressings should be applied.[30,49]

THINK

What actions can you take to determine the likely source of a burn? What actions would you take if confronted with a chemical burn from an unknown source? Think about both patient safety and your own.

Chapter Key Points

1. The assessment and management of wounds and burns follows a set of core principles that can generally be followed to provide safe and effective patient care.
2. However there are chemical burns that require specific management strategies; it is therefore of great importance to identify the agent that has caused the injury so that damage is not potentiated.
3. Patients with lime, phenol, elemental sodium/potassium and lithium burns should not have their burns treated with water as this may worsen the injury.
4. Whilst tourniquets have been out of favour in previous years, current evidence suggests that they may have a role in the management of severe uncontrolled haemorrhage.

References and Further reading

1   Marieb E, Hoehn K. *Human Anatomy and Physiology*, 7th edn. San Francisco: Pearson Education, 2007.

2   Martin A. (Ed) *Oxford Concise Medical Dictionary*. Oxford: Oxford University Press, 2003.

3   Morison M, Ovington L, Wilkie K. *Chronic Wound Care: A Problem Based Learning Approach*. Edinburgh: Mosby, 2004.

4   Dougherty L, Lister S. (Eds) *The Royal Marsden Hospital Manual of Clinical Nursing Procedures*, 6th edn. Oxford: Blackwell Publishing, 2006.

5   Johnstone C, Farley A, Hendry C. The physiological basis of wound healing. *Nurs Stand* 2005;19(43):59-65.

6   Timmons J. Factors that compromise wound healing. *Primary Health Care* 2003;13(5):43-49.

7   Doyle G, Taillac P. Tourniquets: A review of current use with proposals for expanded prehospital use. *Prehosp Emerg Care* 2008;12(2):241-256.

8   Shaw JA, Murray DG. The relationship between tourniquet pressure and underlying soft-tissue pressure in the thigh. *J Bone Joint Surg Am* 1982;64(8):1148-1152.

9   Crenshaw AG, Hargens AR, Gershuni DH, Rydevik B. Wide tourniquet cuffs more effective at lower inflation pressures. *Acta Orhtop Scand* 1988;59(4):447-451.

10 Heppenstall RB, Balderston R, Goodwin C. Pathophysiologic effects distal to a tourniquet in the dog. *J Trauma* 1979;19(4):234-238.

11 Wakai A, Winter DC, Street JT, Redmond PH. Pneumatic tourniquets in extremity surgery. *J Am Acad Orthop Surg* 2001;9(5):345-351.

12 Kam PC, Kavanagh R, Yoong FF. The arterial tourniquet: pathophysiological consequences and anaesthetic implications. *Anaesthesia* 2001;56(6):534-545.

13 Angus PD, Nakielny R, Goodrum DT. The pneumatic tourniquet and deep venous thrombosis. *J Bone Joint Surg Br* 1983;65(3):336-339.

14 Townsend HS, Goodman SB, Schurman DJ, Hackel A, Brock-Utne JG. Tourniquet release: systemic and metabolic effects. *Acta Anaesthesiol Scand* 1996;40(10):1234-1237.

15 Naimer SA, Chemla F. Elastic adhesive dressing treatment of bleeding wounds in trauma victims. *Am J Emerg Med* 2000;18(7):816-819.

16 Lakstein D, Blumenfeld A, Sokolov T, Lin G, Bssorai R, Lynn M, Abraham R. Tourniquets for hemorrhage control on the battlefield: a 4-year accumulated experience. *J Trauma* 2003;54(5-Suppl):S221-S225.

17 Beekley A, Sebesta J, Blackbourne L, Holcomb J. *Prehospital Tourniquet Use in Operation Iraqi Freedom: Effect on Hemorrhage Control and Outcomes*. Paper no. 27. Presented at Western Trauma Association Annual Meeting, Big Sky, MT, March 2, 2006.

18 Chambers LW, Green DJ, Sample K, Gillingham BL, Rhee P, Brown C, Narine N, Uecker JM, Bohman HR. Tactical surgical intervention with temporary shunting of peripheral vascular trauma sustained during Operation Iraqi Freedom: one unit's experience. *J Trauma* 2006;61(4):824-830.

19 Walker A, Kershaw C, Nicholas S. *Home Office Statistical Bulletin*. Crime in England and Wales 2005/06. London: Home Office, 2006.

20 Lee C, Porter K, Hodgetts T. Tourniquet use in the civilian prehospital setting. *Emerg Med J* 2007;24:584-587.

21 Sierra D. Fibrin sealant adhesive systems: a review of their chemistry, material properties and clinical applications. *J Biomat Appl* 1993;7:309-352.

22 Jackson Mr, Gillespie DL, Longnecker EG, Goff JM, Fiala LA, O'Donnell SD, Gomperts ED, Navalta LA, Hestlow T, Alving BM. Hemostatic efficacy of fibrin sealant (human) on expanded poly-tetrafluoroethylene carotid patch angioplasty: a randomized clinical trial. *J Vasc Surg* 1999;30(3):461-466.

23 Larsen MJ, Bowersox JC, Lim RC. Efficacy of a fibrin hemostatic bandage in controlling hemorrhage from experimental injuries. *Arch Surg* 1995;130:420-422.

24 Gilbert DJ. New bandage stops hemorrhaging. *Journal American Forces Press Service. NNMC The Journal* January 22 1999. *Available at* www.dcmilitary.com/navy/journal/archives/jan22/j_c12299.html

25 Medafor Hemostatic Polymer Technologies homepage, MPH research. Available at http://medafor.com//research.html. Accessed 12/04/2008.

26 Alam HB, Uy GB, Miller D, Koustova E *et al*. Comparative analysis of hemostatic agents in a swine model of lethal groin injury. *J Trauma* 2003;54:1077-1082.

27 Rhee P, Brown C, Martin M, Salim A, Plurad D, Green D, Chambers L, Demetriades D, Velmahos G, Alam H. QuikClot use in trauma for hemorrhage control: case series of 103 documented uses. *J Trauma* 2008;64(4):1093-1099.

28 Pusateri AE, McCarthy SJ, Gregory KW *et al*. Effect of chitosan based hemostatic dressing on blood loss and survival in a model of severe venous haemorrhage and hepatic injury in swine. *J Trauma* 2003;54:177-182.

29 National Burn Care Review. National Burn Care Review, 2000. Http://www.baps.co.uk/documents/ncbr.pdf.

30 New Zealand Guideline Group. *Management of Burns and Scalds in Primary Care*. New Zealand: Accident Compensation Corporation, 2007.

31 Amirsheybani HR, Creccelius GM, Timothy NH *et al*. The natural history of the growth of the hand: 1. Hand area as a percentage of body surface area. *Plat Reconstr Surg* 2001;107(3):726-733.

32 Blackhurst H. Estimation of burn surface area using the hand. *Bestbets: Best Evidence Topics*. [On-line] www.bestbets.org/cgi-bin/bets.pl?record-01516.

33 Hettiaratchy S, Papini R. Initial management of a major burn: II – Assessment and resuscitation. *Emerg Med*. 2004;329:101-103.

34 Wachtel, TL. Berry, CC, Frank, HA. The inter-rater reliability of estimating the size of burns from various burn area chart drawings. *Burns* 2000;26:156-170.

35 Hidvegi N, Nduka C, Myers C *et al*. Estimation of breast burn size. *Plast Reconstr Surg* 2004;113(6); 1591-1597.

36 Allison K, Porter K. Consensus on the prehospital approach to burns patient management. *Emerg Med J* 21; 112-114.

37 Smith JJ, Malyon AD, Scerri GV, Burge TS. A comparison of serial halving and the rule of nines as a prehospital assessment tool in burns. *Br J Plast Surg* 2005;58:957-967.

38 New Zealand Guideline Group. *Management of Burns and Scalds in Primary Care*. New Zealand: Accident Compensation Corporation, 2007.

39 Nguyen NL, Gun RT, Sparnon AL *et al*. The importance of initial management: A case series of childhood burns in Vietnam. *Burns* 2002;28(2):167-172.

40 Tung K, Chen M, Wang H *et al*. A seven-year epidemiology study of 12,381 admitted burn patients in Taiwan – using the internet system of the childhood burn foundation. *Burns* 2005;31S:S12-S17.

41 British Burn Association. *Prehospital Approach to Burns Patient Management*. Manchester: British Burn Association, 2002. http://www.britishburnassociation.org/Downloads/prehosp.pdf [accessed August 2006].

42 Australian and New Zealand Burn Association. *Emergency Management of Severe Burns: Course Manual*, 8th edn. Australian and New Zealand Burn Association Limited, 2004.

43 Blomgren I, Eriksson E, Bagge U. Effect of cold water immersion on oedema formation in the scalded mouse ear. *Burns* 1982;9(1):17-20.

44 Raine TJ, Heggers JP, Robson MC *et al*. Cooling the burn wound to maintain microcirculation. *J Trauma* 1981;21(5):394-397.

45 Mertz PM, Davis SC, Cazzaniga AL *et al*. *To assess second-degree burn wound treatment with water-jel*. Carlstadt NJ: Trilling Medical Technologies Inc, 1990.

46 Castner T, Harz C, Schlor J. *Cooling out of the bag. Water-jel burn dressings*. Markdorf, Germany: Institute for Emergency Medicine, 2000.

47 PRODIGY Knowledge. *Burns and Scalds*. Revised November 2004. Sowerby Centre for Health Informatics at Newcastle Limited. (SCHIN), 1998. http://www.prodigy.nhs.uk/burns_and_scalds [accessed August 2005].

48 Milner RH, Hudson SJ, Reid CA. Plasticized polyvinyl chloride film as a primary burns dressing: A microbiological study. *Burns Incl Therm Inj* 1988;14(1):62-65.

49 Seth, R. Chester, D, Moiemen, N. A review of chemical burns. *Trauma* 2008;9:81-94.

50 Yano K, Hata Y, Matsuka O *et al.* Experimental study on alkaline skin injuries – periodic changes in subcutaneous tissue. *Burns* 1993;4:320-323.

51 Singer A, Sagi A, Ben Meir P *et al.* Chemical burns: Our 10-year experience. *Burns* 1992;18(3):250-252.

52 Sykes RA, Mani MM, Hiebert JM. Chemical burns: Retrospective review. *J Burn Care Rehabil* 1986;7(4):343-347.

53 Clare RA, Krenzelok EP. Clinical burns secondary to elemental metal exposure; 2 case reports. *Ann Emerg Med* 1988;6:355-357.

Chapter 19

Moving and handling procedures

Content

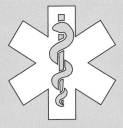

The moving and handling of patients is an area of great risk to both staff and patients within the prehospital and in hospital environment, as such this chapter will provide a theoretical underpinning of the legal, ethical and technical aspects of patient moving and handling. This chapter is not intended to provide information on how to use all manual handling aids in current use within the health service at this time, but to provide an overview for all healthcare professionals to ensure appropriate risk management and health and safety legislation is complied with. There is little evidence to support many principles of manual handling, therefore a consensus opinion is provided in many cases. Prehospital and emergency care staff are often exposed to patients who are in positions where patient handling or movement are restricted by a number of factors such as the number of personnel, the space available and underlying medical conditions. All of these may hamper manual handling processes; therefore the adherence to core principles are key in minimising injury and maximising efficacy of movement.

Definitions

The risks associated with manual handling have been recognised by the Ambulance Service Association and the Health and Safety Executive who state:

> *'Any work activity that involves lifting, pushing, pulling, carrying or moving can be considered as a moving and handling risk. Also, any work activity that could lead to musculoskeletal strain or injury needs to be considered, for example activities that include potentially long periods of static position, regular stooping or bending. Often musculoskeletal disorders are the result of a cumulative effect and therefore may not be easily attributable to one particular incident or accident'.*

Ambulance Service Association and Health and Safety Executive (2003).[1]

Why is moving and handling important?

More than one-third of all injuries lasting over three days reported to the Health and Safety Executive (HSE) and Local Health Authorities are a result of manual handling.[2] In a survey in 2001/2002 it was found that over 1.1 million staff suffered musculoskeletal injury or disorder as a result of their work or previous work duties.[2] Epidemiological studies into ambulance staff and healthcare workers suggest that these groups represent a high risk area of musculoskeletal injury.[3,4] A recent survey of accident and incident data collated from six UK ambulance Trusts showed that between 30 and 51% of all recorded incidents resulting in injury were a result of the moving and handling of loads; the mean incidence rate was 178 per 1000 staff members.[5] Where data were available it was noted the Emergency Medical Services had an increased prevalence of manual handling related incidents compared with patient transport services, with 90% of the cases from EMS personnel. Analysis of the incidents found three root causes: the use of the carry chair; the use of stretchers; and patient transfers (from bed to chair, floor to bed). These accident statistics represent a worrying picture for ambulance staff and highlight the need to introduce appropriate measures to reduce manual handling injury.

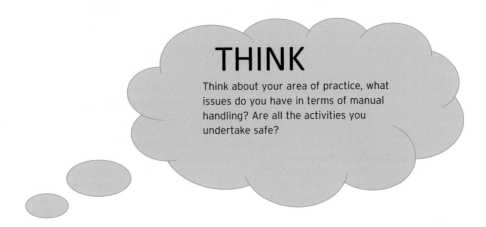

THINK

Think about your area of practice, what issues do you have in terms of manual handling? Are all the activities you undertake safe?

Key legislation

There are numerous pieces of key legislation that relate to manual handling policy and procedure. These are explained briefly below:

Health and Safety at Work etc Act [HSAWA] (1974)[6]

The overall objective of this act was to:

'make further provision for securing the health, safety and welfare of persons at work, for protecting others against risks to health or safety in connection with the activities of persons at work.'

The act established two bodies: The Health and Safety Commission and the HSE, to promote the objectives of the act and ensure the implementation of its provisions. This act set out a series of duties for employers, employees and designers, manufacturers and suppliers of equipment. HSAWA set out that the employer has an overall objective and responsibility to employees to:

'ensure, so far is reasonably practicable, the health, safety and welfare at work of all of their employees.'

These responsibilities include:

- Provision and maintenance of plant and safe systems of work.
- Safety in the collection, use, storage and transport of loads and substances.
- Provision of information, instruction, training and supervision of employees.
- Maintaining a safe workplace, access and egress.
- Maintaining a safe and healthy working environment including providing adequate welfare facilities.

The HASAWA, whilst implementing duties for the employer also set out a series of duties for the employee which requires any employee to take reasonable care for their own and others health and safety in the workplace. This includes taking positive steps to ensure that hazards in the workplace are understood and to comply with policy and guidance. Any failure to comply with these duties can make the employer of the employee liable for prosecution.

Manual Handling Operations Regulations [MHOR] (1992 – amended 2002)[7]

These regulations resulted from the 1990 'Manual Handling of Loads – European Directive[8] which legally obliged each member of the European Community to introduce legislation which would harmonise standards. These regulations placed a duty upon employers to:

- So far as is reasonably practicable to avoid the need for employees to undertake any manual handling operations at work which involve a risk of their being injured.
- Assess any hazardous manual handling operations that cannot be avoided.
- Reduce the risk of injury from manual handling operations so far as is reasonably practicable.
- To regularly review any assessment if there is reason to believe the previous assessment is no longer valid or there has been a significant change in the operations to which it relates.

From HSE (1992) MHOR – Regulation 4.[3]

In addition the MHOR placed a duty upon the employee to ensure that they make full and proper use of any system of work provided for his/her use by his employer in compliance with regulation 4.

Management of Health and Safety at Work Regulations [MHSAW] (1999)

These regulations set out a range of responsibilities for the employer with a primary focus upon risk assessment in the workplace. MHSAW set out regulations that ensured that each employer must undertake a risk assessment of any activity or environment that an employee or non-employee may experience. In the occurrence of any risks being identified, these must be reduced and those affected informed of their presence. Reduction of risk may be through the avoidance of such tasks if practicable to do so, through the provision of equipment (i.e. hoists) or training to those undertaking the activity. Again the individual is also given a duty to ensure the health and safety of themselves and others in the workplace.

Lifting Operations and Lifting Equipment Regulations [LOLER] (1998)[9]

These regulations apply to the use of lifting equipment in all industries and work activities. The regulations aim to reduce risks to people's health and safety from lifting equipment provided for use at work. In addition to the requirements of LOLER, lifting equipment is also subject to the requirements of the Provision and Use of Work Equipment Regulations 1998 (PUWER); see below. The regulations apply to any piece of equipment that is designed to lift or lower any load. LOLER requires that any equipment meets the following standards:

- Strong and stable enough for the particular use and marked to indicate safe working loads.
- Positioned and installed to minimise any risks.
- Used safely, i.e. the work is planned, organised and performed by competent people.
- Subject to ongoing thorough examination and, where appropriate, inspection by competent people.

Whilst these regulations do not directly apply to employees, all staff have a responsibility to ensure equipment meets the required standard under previous regulations such as HSAWA.[2]

Provision and Use of Work Equipment Regulations [PUWER] (1998)[10]

These regulations cover all equipment used at work including manual handling equipment. The act places a responsibility upon the employer to ensure that the correct equipment is available, is well maintained and used in situations where it is suitable. The regulations also state that the employer has a duty to ensure that staff are adequately trained in the use of any such equipment.

Manual handling and no lift policies

This is always a contentious area for prehospital care staff with many calls to areas in which a 'no lift' policy appears to exist. A duty of care exists under professional registration[11] and under the Human Rights Act[12] that contradicts the guidance of the earlier regulations and policy that suggest that manual handling tasks should only be undertaken if the risk is deemed low. The Human Rights Act[8] states that no one should be subjected to inhuman or degrading treatment and has the right to liberty and security of person. This means that the patient has the right to refuse to be handled in a certain way and the practitioner has the right to refuse to endanger themselves with a manual handling procedure.

In a high profile legal case surrounding no lift policies the High Court Judge ruled that a blanket no lift policy may be unlawful.[13] This case went on to highlight that under the Human Rights Act the refusal to undertake manual handling (in the event that mechanical aids cause great distress) could be considered an unlawful breach. This is an area in which there is no specific guidance other than to undertake a risk assessment and act accordingly in each individual case.

Risk assessment and manual handling

Risk assessment is the first step in the manual handling and risk management process. Assessment involves five steps as shown below:

- Identify the hazards.
- Identify who may be harmed and how.
- Evaluate the risks and decide upon precautions.
- Record the findings and implement them.
- Review the assessment and update accordingly.

From The HSE (2006) *Five Steps to Risk Assessment*.[14]

Table 19.1 A systematic method of risk assessment[7]

Environment	Are there: Constraints on posture? Poor flooring? Variation in floor level? Hot/cold/wet environment? Poor lighting conditions? Noise?
Load	Is the load: Heavy? Difficult to grasp? Unstable? Unpredictable? Harmful (i.e. hot)? Are there handles?
Individual capability	Does the lift require: Special training or information? Present a hazard? Are you capable of performing the lift?
Task	Does the lift involve: Holding the load away from the body? Covering large distances? Strenuous effort? Twisting? Insufficient rest? A new or unusual task? Large amounts of movement?
Equipment/other factors	Is the equipment: Available? Maintained? Suitable? Clean? Are you competent to use the equipment?

These steps provide a basis for employers to review any manual handling tasks that may be undertaken in the course of work duties. However they do not provide an active risk assessment for the practitioner at the time of the manual handling process, for this element the Manual Handling Operations Regulations (1992)[7] recommend the use of a systematic approach as shown in Table 19.1.

This list is not exhaustive; however each element should be considered prior to undertaking any manual handling task.

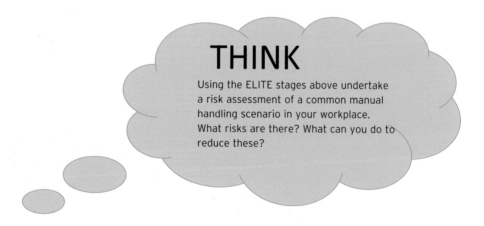

THINK

Using the ELITE stages above undertake a risk assessment of a common manual handling scenario in your workplace. What risks are there? What can you do to reduce these?

Biomechanical principles

Biomechanics are the study of mechanical laws relating to the movement or structure of the body (or living organisms).[15] When a person stands erect gravity applies forces to the spine from the head and the trunk, these forces are applied directly down the spine (compressive forces) using very little muscle activity to maintain the stable upright position.[16] However if the trunk is moved forwards or laterally the forces acting upon the spine change according to the lever principle, therefore the further away from the upright position a person is the greater the shearing forces that are exerted upon the spine. The change from compressive forces to shearing, twisting or torsional can be damaging upon the spine and intervertebral discs.[16]

There are three key biomechanical principles that underlie manual handling procedures: centre of gravity; a stable base; and external levers. The will be discussed briefly below.

Principle 1: Using the centre of gravity

Everything has a centre of gravity; this is the point where total body mass is concentrated. With uniform objects such as boxes and cylinders the centre of gravity will always be in the middle.[15] Humans however are not uniform as the body shape and dimensions can change rapidly; this can cause the centre of gravity to move even to points outside of the body.

In the upright standing position the centre of gravity commonly lies within the pelvis. This makes the pelvic control paramount in manual handling procedures both for the handler and the patient.

Principle 2: A Stable base

A base is the area of contact with a supporting surface (i.e. the floor),[15] therefore in the common manual handling position it is the feet of the handler and the area in between. If the line of gravity (a vertical line running from the centre of gravity to the supporting surface) falls within the area of the base then the object (person) is considered stable. However if the line of gravity falls outside of the base the object is unstable and therefore likely to fall or require additional forces to maintain stability. Using this principle a wider base is more likely to be stable than a small base. Typically in a human being the most stable base is with the feet apart (shoulder width or slightly wider) with one foot in front of the other.[17]

Principle 3: External levers

A lever is a solid object that is used to transfer force over its distance. If the external levers (i.e. the arms) are long (outstretched) then the centre and line of gravity are shifted to give an unstable base and apply greater pressure upon the muscles and ligaments of the spine and limbs to maintain balance. However if the levers are short, then the line and centre of gravity are within the area of the base thus reducing forces upon the spine. In addition this will allow power to be provided by the major muscle groups.

Principles of manual handling

1. Stop and think (plan the lift)
2. Place the feet
   - Have the feet apart, giving a balanced and stable base for lifting.
   - Have the leading leg as far forward as is comfortable.

3. Adopt a good posture
   * Bend the knees so that the hands when grasping the load are as nearly level with the waist as possible; but do not kneel or over-flex the knees.
   * Keep the back straight, maintaining its natural curves (tucking in the chin while gripping the load helps).
   * Lean forward a little over the load if necessary to get a good grip.
   * Keep the shoulders level and facing in the same direction as the hips.
4. Get a firm and secure grip
   * Try to keep the arms within the boundary formed by the legs.
   * The optimum grip may vary, but it should be secure.
   * If you vary the grip while lifting, do this as smoothly as possible.
5. Don't jerk
   * Carry out the lifting movement smoothly, raising the chin as the lift begins, keeping control of the load.
6. Move the feet
   * Don't twist the trunk when turning to the side.
7. Keep close to the load
   * Keep the load close to the trunk for as long as possible.
   * Keep the heaviest side of the load next to the trunk.
   * Slide the load towards you before attempting to lift it.
8. Put the load down, then adjust its position.

When handling at or near floor level, preferably use handling techniques which make use of the relatively strong leg muscles rather than those of the back, provided the load is small enough to be held close to the trunk. Bear in mind however that such techniques impose heavy forces on the knees and hip joints which must carry the weight of the load and the weight of the rest of the body.

1. Place feet beneath or adjacent to the load.
2. Move close to the load before beginning the manual handling operation.
3. Hold the load (as) close to the body (as possible) during the manual handling operation.
4. Address the load squarely before beginning the manual handling operation.
5. Preferably face the intended direction of movement before beginning the manual handling operation.
6. If possible, avoid lifting loads from the floor when seated.
7. If possible, avoid twisting, stooping or stretching when handling.
8. Where a load is bulky rather than heavy it may be easier to carry it at the side of the body if it has suitable handholds, or if slings or other devices can be provided.

From HSE (2003) *The Principles of Good Manual Handling: Achieving a Consensus.*[17]
  There is no such thing as a completely safe lift; therefore general principles should be adhered to, to reduce the potential for injury. Figure 19.1 suggests the safe recommended limits for weight in manual handling operations. It can be seen that the weight significantly reduces at extremes of height and distance from the body as this is when injuries are most likely to occur.

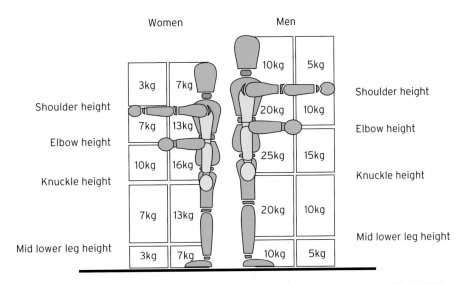

Figure 19.1 Guideline weights for safe lifting and handling. From HSE (2007) *Getting to Grips with Manual Handling: A Short Guide.*[17]

Additional principles

There are certain situations in which the basic principles cannot and do not apply, for example one-handed lifting; lifting large bulky loads and lifting in confined spaces. Under these circumstances the risks involved and the principles required may alter, therefore these are discussed individually below.

One-handed lifting

Early studies suggest that the biomechanical requirements and demands of one-handed lifting can significantly increase the likelihood of injuries such as intervertebral disc prolapse.[18] In a study of data upon one-handed lifting techniques the HSE (2003)[17] recommend that if the load is in front of the body and it is practicable to do so, that two hands should be used. However if the load is to the side of the body a one-handed lift should be used to reduce the lateral twisting of the spine. If possible support should be provided by the free hand as this can reduce the forces involved.

Lifting large bulky loads

In lifting large, bulky loads from lower heights, the bulk of the load prevents it from being brought between the knees. Even with a 'correct' foot posture, the centre of gravity of the load is beyond the knees and therefore at or around arm's length away from the body, this will increase the forces acting upon the spine and increase the risk of injury. The HSE[17] state in their analysis of data from numerous studies that there appears little evidence to support a specific technique in the lifting of large loads; however it is suggested that the key factor is to keep the load as close to the body as possible.

Lifting in confined spaces

The difficulty in lifting in confined spaces, for example in limited headroom, is often the need to move with the load during the lift. Lifting in limited headroom does place additional stress upon the operator with maximum safe weight limits being reduced by up to 60% in a reduction of headroom of only 10%.[17] There is very limited research into this area with studies reporting conflicting evidence over the use of kneeling or stooping as the preferred method in compensating for a lack of headroom. The HSE suggest that a stooping posture may be utilised as it allows for the load to be moved, whereas kneeling does not allow for any movement; however there is a caveat that the other principles of safe manual handling should be observed.[17]

Lifting aids

MHOR[7], LOLER[9] and PUWER[10] set out regulations that require employers to provide aids to manual handling to reduce risk and reduce the requirements for manual handling. Since these regulations a variety of aids to manual handling have been introduced into the health and social care arena. These include:

* Patient handling slings: These are available in a variety of forms and sizes. They are commonly used to assist the patient in sitting forward, slide up a bed or lifting, they are used in combination with other manual handling equipment.
* Handling belts: These are used to aid the handler in assisting the patient to stand and to aid the patient in walking. They are designed to allow the handler to maintain good posture whilst assisting.
* Slide sheets: These are made of a slippery material that allows a patient to be 'slid' removing the need to manually lift a patient.
* Transfer boards/banana boards: These are hard plastic boards that allow for a patient to be slid from one point to another; this is commonly chair to chair or chair to bed.
* Turntables: These are discs that are placed under the feet that are used to pivot or swivel patients.
* Hoists: These can be mobile or static devices that are used in combination with a sling to lift and move patients. They can be electric or hydraulic.

For more information upon these aids see Further reading or refer to manufacturer guidelines.

Scenario

You are called to a patient who is unconscious and unrousable; the patient is in an upstairs bathroom and is profoundly hypotensive. There is poor access to the property and the stairs are narrow with a number of turns involved. What methods would you use to get the patient out of the property? What risks are there both to you and the patient? Does the patient's condition affect the methods that you would use?

Chapter Key Points

1.   Moving and handling operations are not without risk. It is essential that a thorough risk assessment is carried out and key principles adhered to reduce the likelihood of injury or incident.
2.   It is recognised that moving and handling in emergency situations may not always be ideal and suited to all principles; however risk must be kept as low as is practically possible and lifting aids considered in each individual occasion.
3.   Keep external levers short and maintain a stable base.

References and Further reading

1   Ambulance Service Association and Health and Safety Executive. *National Policy and Strategy Framework for NHS Ambulance Services – Safer Handling*. London: ASA, 2003.
2   Health and Safety Executive. *Getting to Grips with Manual Handling*. London: HSE, 2003.
3   Health and Safety Executive. *Musculoskeletal Disorders in Health and Social Care*. London: HSE, 2007. Accessed on-line@ http://www.hse.gov.uk/healthservices/msd/index.htm [accessed 25/3/08].
4   Rodgers LM. A five-year study comparing early retirements on medical grounds in ambulance personnel with those in other groups of health staff. Part II: Causes of retirement. *Occupat Med* 1998;48:119-132.
5   Health and Safety Executive. *Evaluation of Manual Handling Tasks Involving the Use of Carry Chairs by UK Ambulance Personnel*. London: HSE, 2005.
6   United Kingdom Government. *The Health and Safety at Work etc Act*. London: HMSO, 1974.
7   Health and Safety Executive. *Manual Handling Operations Regulations*. London: HSE, 1992.
8   The Council of the European Communities. *Council Directive 90/269/EEC of 29 May 1990 on the minimum health and safety requirements for the manual handling of loads where there is a risk particularly of back injury to workers*. Office for Official Publications of the European Communities, 1990.
9   Health and Safety Executive. *Lifting Operations and Lifting Equipment Regulations*. London: HSE, 1998.
10   Health and Safety Executive. *Provision and Use of Work Equipment Regulations*. London: HSE, 1998.
11   Health Professions Council. *Code of Conduct, performance and ethics*. London: HPC, 2007.
12   United Kingdom Government. *The Human Rights Act*. London: OPSI, 1998.
13   R (on the application of A & others) v East Sussex County Council and Another. EWHC 167 (Admin) CO/4843/2001, 2003.
14   Health and Safety Executive. *Five Steps to Risk Assessment*. London: HSE, 2006.
15   Smith J. (Ed) *The Guide to the Handling of People*. Middlesex: Backcare, 2005.
16   Dougherty L, Lister S. *The Royal Marsden Hospital Manual of Clinical Nursing Procedures*, 6th edn. London: Blackwell Publishing, 2006.
17   Health and Safety Executive. *The Principles of Good Manual Handling: Achieving a Consensus*. London: HSE, 2003.
18   Allread W, Marras W, Parnianpour M. Trunk kinematics of one handed lifting and the effects of asymmetry and load weight. *Ergonomics* 1996;39:322-334.

Index